T0329676

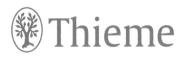

Navigation and Robotics in Spine Surgery

Alexander R. Vaccaro, MD, PhD, MBA
Richard H. Rothman Professor and Chairman
Department of Orthopaedic Surgery
Professor of Neurosurgery
Thomas Jefferson University and Hospitals
President
The Rothman Institute
Philadelphia, Pennsylvania, USA

Jaykar R. Panchmatia, MA, MPH, MB BChir, FRCS
Consultant Spine Surgeon
Guy's and St. Thomas' Hospitals
London, United Kingdom

I. David Kaye, MD
Assistant Professor of Orthopaedic Surgery
Thomas Jefferson University and Hospitals
Spine Surgeon
The Rothman Institute
Philadelphia, Pennsylvania, USA

Srinivas K. Prasad, MD, MS
Associate Professor of Neurological Surgery
Director, Neurosurgical Spine Fellowship
Thomas Jefferson University and Hospitals
Philadelphia, Pennsylvania, USA

125 illustrations

Thieme
New York • Stuttgart • Delhi • Rio de Janeiro

Library of Congress Cataloging-in-Publication Data

Names: Vaccaro, Alexander R., editor. | Panchmatia, Jaykar R., editor.
 | Kaye, I. David, editor. | Prasad, Srinivas K., editor.
Title: Navigation and robotics in spine surgery / [edited by] Alexander R. Vaccaro,
 Jaykar R. Panchmatia, I. David Kaye, Srinivas K. Prasad.
Description: New York : Thieme, [2020] | Includes bibliographical references and
 index. | Summary: "The past decade has seen major advances in image-guided
 spine surgery techniques, with robotically assisted approaches emerging in the
 last five years. While early adopters of this technology paved the way for more
 widespread use of navigated and robotic systems, barriers still exist. Navigation
 and Robotics in Spine Surgery by master spine surgeon Alexander Vaccaro and
 esteemed co-editors Jaykar Panchmatia, David Kaye, and Srinivas Prasad
 addresses existing issues such as the perception of increased upfront costs,
 intrusion on current workflow, and a lack of understanding about the potential
 ways these technologies can enhance the surgical experience and improve
 patient outcomes. Organized into six sections, the book starts with evidence-
 based fundamentals of navigated spine surgery and robotics including discussion of instrumentation and mechanics. Sections 2-5 serve as a surgical
 handbook for spine surgeons who wish to introduce these technologies into
 practice or augment their current repertoire with more complex techniques.
 Topics range from more routine procedures such as navigated and robotic
 minimally invasive TLIF to complex approaches like intraoperative ultrasound
 guided intradural spinal tumor resection. The final section looks at future
 directions and potential new applications for these technologies. Key High-
 lights An impressive group of international spine surgeons who pioneered
 navigation and robotic surgery techniques share invaluable tricks of the trade
 Discussion of fluoroscopy- and intraoperative CT-based platforms, applications
 for intraoperative sonography, and radiation exposure and minimization strategies Special topics include OR set-up and workflow, surmounting the learning
 curve, artificial intelligence, and lessons learned from other industries"– Provided by publisher.
Identifiers: LCCN 2019033234 | ISBN 9781684200313 (hardback)
 | ISBN 9781684200320 (eISBN)
Subjects: MESH: Spine–surgery | Spinal Diseases–surgery | Spinal
 Injuries–surgery | Robotic Surgical Procedures–methods
Classification: LCC RD768 | NLM WE 727 | DDC 617.5/6059–dc23
LC record available at https://lccn.loc.gov/2019033234

Copyright © 2020 by Thieme Medical Publishers, Inc.

Thieme Publishers New York
333 Seventh Avenue, New York, NY 10001 USA
+1 800 782 3488, customerservice@thieme.com

Thieme Publishers Stuttgart
Rüdigerstrasse 14, 70469 Stuttgart, Germany
+49 [0]711 8931 421, customerservice@thieme.de

Thieme Publishers Delhi
A-12, Second Floor, Sector-2, Noida-201301
Uttar Pradesh, India
+91 120 45 566 00, customerservice@thieme.in

Thieme Revinter Publicações Ltda.
Rua do Matoso, 170 – Tijuca
Rio de Janeiro RJ 20270-135 - Brasil
+55 21 2563-9702
www.thiemerevinter.com.br

Cover design: Thieme Publishing Group
Typesetting by Thomson Digital, India

Printed in the United States of America by
King Printing Co., Inc.   5 4 3 2 1

ISBN 978-1-68420-031-3

Also available as an e-book:
eISBN 978-1-68420-032-0

Important note: Medicine is an ever-changing science undergoing continual
development. Research and clinical experience are continually expanding our
knowledge, in particular our knowledge of proper treatment and drug therapy.
Insofar as this book mentions any dosage or application, readers may rest
assured that the authors, editors, and publishers have made every effort to
ensure that such references are in accordance with **the state of knowledge at
the time of production of the book.**

Nevertheless, this does not involve, imply, or express any guarantee or
responsibility on the part of the publishers in respect to any dosage instructions
and forms of applications stated in the book. **Every user is requested to examine
carefully** the manufacturers' leaflets accompanying each drug and to check, if
necessary in consultation with a physician or specialist, whether the dosage
schedules mentioned therein or the contraindications stated by the manufacturers differ from the statements made in the present book. Such examination is
particularly important with drugs that are either rarely used or have been newly
released on the market. Every dosage schedule or every form of application used is
entirely at the user's own risk and responsibility. The authors and publishers
request every user to report to the publishers any discrepancies or inaccuracies
noticed. If errors in this work are found after publication, errata will be posted at
www.thieme.com on the product description page.

Some of the product names, patents, and registered designs referred to in this
book are in fact registered trademarks or proprietary names even though specific
reference to this fact is not always made in the text. Therefore, the appearance of a
name without designation as proprietary is not to be construed as a representation by the publisher that it is in the public domain.

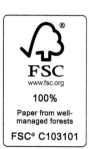

I would like to dedicate this book to the figures in my life who served as mentors, innovators, and most importantly as true friends in guiding my life's journey: Jerry Cotler, Steven Garfin, and Richard Rothman.

—Alexander R. Vaccaro

I dedicate this book to my parents, for providing me with a strong foundation for life; to my wife, for inspiring me to build on that foundation; and to my sons, for making it all worthwhile.

—Jaykar R. Panchmatia

This book is dedicated to my loving wife Talya, who has been there with and for me from the start, and our children Olivia, Jordyn, and Mattie, who pushed for a chapter about Transformers but settled for a book about spine surgery.

—I. David Kaye

To my parents, Rathna and Maheswara Prasad, for their decades of tireless love, support, and sacrifice. To my wife, Gita, and my kids, Krishna and Leela, who give my life meaning and define my every day.

—Srinivas K. Prasad

Contents

Contents

Foreword

Localizing functions of the body is a pursuit that has occupied physicians since the beginning of recorded history. Imhotep, a counselor to the Egyptian pharaoh Djoser, is credited with the first description of the term "brain," found in the Edwin Smith papyrus (ca. 2655-2600 BC). The ancient Egyptians believed that the heart was the seat of the soul, but the Greeks mostly leaned toward a cephalocentric doctrine. Centuries later, the cardiocentric/cephalocentric debate was still hotly contested. Utilizing anatomical studies, Galen postulated that the brain was the body's command center. It wasn't until the 1800s that John Hughlings-Jackson, David Ferrier, and others began to anatomically localize specific brain pathologies. Sir Victor Horsely took these experiments to a higher level by performing detailed anatomical studies of the brain. In 1908, Horsely developed the first stereotactic device to accurately lesion the brain in animals. Since then, the field of stereotaxy has evolved rapidly.

Advances in imaging have been critical in our understanding of the human body. Roentgen's X-ray ushered in a new method of visualizing anatomy that had never before been possible. This was soon followed by Walter Dandy's introduction of pneumoencephalography and Egaz Moniz's cerebral angiography. The Nobel Prize-winning developments of computed tomography and magnetic resonance imaging gave us unprecedented access to the internal anatomy and functions of the human body.

It was not until stereotactic principles were combined with precise imaging that we truly entered the era of computer-assisted surgery. Three-dimensional localization in real time has transformed the field of intracranial surgery, making the removal of brain neoplasms less invasive and safer. Although these same disciplines were combined for use in the spine, adoption stalled for many years as early registration paradigms were cumbersome and negatively impacted workflow. As technology has improved, there has been a resurgence in the use of image guidance in spinal surgery. Advantages include improved accuracy and decreased radiation exposure for the surgeon and the operative team.

In his 1920 science fiction play *R.U.R.*, Czech writer Karel Čapek introduced the word "robot" to the English language. The play tells the story of a factory that produces roboti, living creatures that resemble humans and have the capacity for individual thought. While at first the roboti seem content to work for their human masters, they later rebel, ultimately leading to the extinction of the human race. This play and similar depictions of robots in literature and film are probably responsible for the slightly negative reputation of robots in general. Only recently has this perception changed, thanks to the advent of robots that can vacuum our houses and perform other mundane chores. Raymond Goertz, while working for the US Atomic Energy Commission, is credited with the development of the first robotic arm in 1951. The first working definition of the word "robot" was published, fittingly, by the Robotics Institute of America in 1980: "...a reprogrammable, multifunctional manipulator designed to move materials, parts, tools, or specialized devices through various programmed motions for the performance of a variety of tasks."

In 1985, the six-degrees-of-freedom flexible arm PUMA 560 was used to guide a needle under CT guidance into the brain. The United States military, having a vested interest in telepresence surgery, helped fund the development of the da Vinci Surgical System, which was approved for use by the FDA in 2000 and designed to facilitate complex, minimally invasive intracavitary surgeries. In 2004, the FDA cleared the first commercially available positioning device for the placement of spinal instrumentation. New robots used for the first time and existing robots used for novel applications graphically demonstrate how the field of spinal surgery field is evolving. The days of fearing robots are behind us, as members of our specialty begin to embrace the concept of automation. Thankfully, unlike Čapek's rogue roboti, the likelihood of surgical robots rising up against us and causing world destruction is low!

This book is based upon the extensive experience of experts in the fields of image guidance and robotics and gives the reader an in-depth understanding of the practical aspects of bringing these technologies into the operating room. Although the field of spinal surgery is ever-changing, the adoption of advanced technologies finally seems to be gaining traction, and this book serves as the most up-to-date guide on the state of the art of these technologies, offering us a glimpse of what the future may hold.

Nicholas Theodore, MD, FACS, FAANS
Donlin M. Long Professor
Professor of Neurosurgery, Orthopaedics & Biomedical
Engineering
Department of Neurosurgery
Johns Hopkins University
Baltimore, Maryland

Preface

The past decade has seen an increasing performance of navigated techniques in spine surgery and, over the past five years in particular, an emergence of robotically assisted spine surgeries. In 2016, the robotics industry market was worth $4 billion and is expected to grow by 75% to almost $7 billion by 2026. The robotics market in spine surgery is expected to grow in turn, expanding from the current market capitalization of approximately $75 million to $320 million by 2026.

As these technologies become more mainstream, early adopters are paving the way for more widespread adoption and navigated and robotic systems are now routinely found in community medical centers. However, several barriers to broader acceptance exist. Among these are the perception of increased upfront costs, an intrusion on the current workflow, and a general lack of understanding of precisely how these technologies can enhance the surgical experience and potentially improve patient outcomes.

Navigation and Robotics in Spine Surgery aims to precisely address some of those concerns and make these emerging technologies more approachable for novices, or those looking to incorporate navigation and robotics into their practice. Simultaneously, the book provides expert techniques for those already comfortable with more routine procedures and looking to expand the scope of their navigated/robotic practice.

While there are, as of this writing, 290 publications in the PubMed database dealing with robotics in spine surgery and approximately 1,000 publications mentioning navigation in spine surgery, there is a relative dearth of techniques-based literature. The goal of this book is to fill this void and serve as a de facto manual, written by experts, early adopters, and frequent users of this technology. The editors of this book are all themselves proponents of this technology and have sought out surgeons who are experts in particular techniques and bring their own experience and "tricks of the trade."

This textbook has been divided into several sections. The first section is designed as an introduction to navigation and robotics in spine surgery. We present an evidence-based approach to the current use of navigation and robotics with specific chapters dedicated to the description of contemporary robotic and navigation systems and an overview of outcomes.

The second through fourth sections of the textbook serve as a handbook for those looking to introduce these technologies to their practice or augment their current armamentarium with more complex techniques. Topics range from more commonly performed procedures, with a navigation/robotic flair, such as "Navigated minimally invasive TLIF," to more complex ones such as "En bloc resection of spinal tumors using navigation," where navigation and robotics have made these procedures safer and more effective.

Equally as important as the description of techniques is a description of setting up an OR and operative workflow. Among the barriers to more widespread adoption of these technologies has been the intrusion on surgeons' current operative flow and the potential for increased operative times. The fifth section of the textbook can serve as a template for beginners with navigation and robotics until they have developed their own optimization.

The last section deals with avenues for the future. Currently, spine robots primarily are used for pedicle screw placement and although they provide consistent accuracy (albeit with a learning curve), its utility is limited. But with a little imagination, the potential for robotics in spine surgery is much more expansive. With increasingly sensitive imaging modalities, a robotically assisted spinal decompression may be on the horizon. The last section specifically deals with directions for future research and incorporating technology from other fields such as autonomous vehicles. There is even a chapter on artificial intelligence, a field that may inform the development of next generation spinal robotics and contribute to the evolution of this technology.

Finally, a video section is available on MedOne illustrating the concepts and procedures covered in this book.

Despite the proliferation of computer-assisted navigation and robotics in spinal surgery, in the current healthcare climate, stakeholders will demand improved outcomes in order to justify their costs. These technologies, which aim to supplant either fluoroscopically based or freehand procedures, must on balance produce improvements that are at least as valuable as those technologies they seek to supplant. Advantages of navigation and robotics include improved accuracy and consistency and decreased radiation exposure. Both can translate into cost savings; direct savings in terms of potentially reduced revision rates as a result of improved screw accuracy, and potentially invaluable cost savings to the surgical team with potential decreased carcinogenesis.

Additionally, some have suggested that as these technologies become more sophisticated, they have the potential to render even the most challenging surgical cases more approachable in more varied hospital settings, similar to the urologists' experience with increased performance of minimally invasive prostatectomy. In that setting, even traditionalists who almost exclusively were performing open procedures became minimally invasive surgeons after introduction of the da Vinci robotic system, which itself became an enabling technology. Similarly, navigation and robotics in spine surgery can help surgeons mount the learning curve for alternative techniques such as minimally invasive spine surgeries, and in that sense, provide even more cost savings; MIS surgeries have demonstrated decreased length of stay and infection, translating into reduced hospital costs and lower rates of revision.

As familiarity with technologies improves, these efficiencies will likely improve in tandem. We hope that this textbook allows surgeons to become more familiar with emerging technologies and enables incorporation into their daily practice.

Alexander R. Vaccaro, MD, PhD, MBA
Jaykar R. Panchmatia, MA, MPH, MB BChir, FRCS
I. David Kaye, MD
Srinivas K. Prasad, MD, MS

Contributors

A. Karim Ahmed, BS
MD Candidate
Department of Neurosurgery
Johns Hopkins School of Medicine
Baltimore, Maryland, USA

Ori Barzilai, MD
Assistant Attending
Department of Neurosurgery
Memorial Sloan Kettering Cancer Center
New York, New York, USA

Mark H. Bilsky, MD
Attending Neurosurgeon
Department of Neurosurgery
Memorial Sloan Kettering Cancer Center
New York, New York, USA

Christopher M. Bono, MD
Professor of Orthopaedic Surgery
Executive Vice Chair, Orthopaedic Surgery
Department of Orthopaedic Surgery
Harvard Medical School, Massachusetts General Hospital
Boston, Massachusetts, USA

Barrett S. Boody, MD
Assistant Professor of Clinical Orthopedic Surgery, Indiana University
Orthopedic Spine Surgeon, Indiana Spine Group
Carmel, Indiana, USA

Stefano Boriani, MD
Spine Tumor Surgeon at GS4
Istituto Ortopedico Galeazzi
Milano, Italia

Wesley H. Bronson, MD, MSB
Assistant Professor
Department of Orthopedic Surgery
Mount Sinai Health System
New York, New York, USA

John A. Buza III, MD, MS
Chief Resident
NYU Langone Orthopedic Hospital
NYU Medical Center
New York, New York, USA

Ali Bydon, MD
Professor
Department of Neurosurgery
Johns Hopkins University
Baltimore, Maryland, USA

Donald F. Colantonio III, MD
Captain, U.S. Army Medical Corps
Department of Orthopaedic Surgery
Walter Reed National Military Medical Center
Bethesda, Maryland, USA

Michael R. Conti Mica, MD
Orthopaedic Spine Surgeon
Division of Spine Surgery
DuPage Medical Group
Chicago, Illinois, USA

Erika A. Dillard, MD, PhD
Resident
Department of Neurosurgery
Thomas Jefferson University Hospital
Philadelphia, Pennsylvania, USA

Jian Dong, MD, PhD
Department of Orthopaedic Surgery
Zhongshan Hospital
Fudan University
Shanghai, China

James Dowdell, MD
Orthopedic Resident
Orthopedic Surgery
Mount Sinai Hospital
New York, New York, USA

Thomas J. Errico, MD
Pediatric Orthopedic Spine Surgeon
Nicklaus Children's Hospital
Miami, Florida, USA
Adjunct Professor of Orthopedic and Neurologic Surgery
NYU School of Medicine
New York, New York, USA

Darian R. Esfahani, MD, MPH
Chief Resident
Department of Neurosurgery
University of Illinois at Chicago
Chicago, Illinois, USA

James J. Evans, MD, FACS, FAANS
Professor
Department of Neurological Surgery
Thomas Jefferson University
Philadelphia, Pennsylvania, USA

Mingxing Fan, MD, PhD
Spine Department
Beijing Jishuitan Hospital
Beijing, China

Taolin Fang, MD, PhD
Research Fellow
Department of Orthopaedic Surgery
Rothman Institute, Thomas Jefferson University
Philadelphia, Pennsylvania, USA

Elvis L. Francois, MD
Orthopedic Surgeon
Department of Orthopedic Surgery
Mayo Clinic
Rochester, Minnesota, USA

Tristan Blase Fried, MD
Resident
Department of Orthopaedics
Thomas Jefferson University
Philadelphia, Pennsylvania, USA

Haruki Funao, MD, PhD
Associate Professor
Department of Orthopaedic Surgery
School of Medicine, International University of Health and
  Welfare
Minato-ku, Tokyo, Japan

Raj J. Gala, MD
Spine Surgery Fellow
Department of Orthopaedics
Emory University
Atlanta, Georgia, USA

Howard J. Ginsberg, MD, PhD
Neurosurgeon, St Michael's Hospital
Assistant Professor of Neurosurgery and Biomedical
  Engineering
University of Toronto
Toronto, Ontario, Canada

Christine L. Hammer, MD
Department of Neurosurgery
Thomas Jefferson University Hospitals
Philadelphia, Pennsylvania, USA

James S. Harrop, MD, FACS
Professor, Depts of Neurological and Orthopedic Surgery
Director, Division of Spine and Peripheral Nerve Surgery
Neurosurgery Director of Delaware Valley SCI Center
Thomas Jefferson University
Philadelphia, Pennsylvania, USA

Andrew C. Hecht, MD
Chief Spine Surgery
Associate Professor of Orthopaedic and Neurosurgery
Icahn School of Medicine
Mount Sinai Hospital and Health System
New York, New York, USA

Joshua E. Heller, MD, MBA
Associate Professor of Neurological and Orthopaedic
  Surgery
Department of Neurological Surgery
Thomas Jefferson University
Philadelphia, Pennsylvania, USA

Langston T. Holly, MD
Professor of Neurosurgery, Vice Chair of Clinical Affairs
Department of Neurosurgery
David Geffen UCLA School of Medicine
Los Angeles, California, USA

Kimberly Hu, BS
MD/MPH Candidate
Department of Neurosurgery
University of Illinois at Chicago College of Medicine
Chicago, Illinois, USA

Jeff Jacobson, MD
Professor of Neurosurgery
Medstar Georgetown University Hospital
Washington, DC, USA

Alex A. Johnson, MD
Orthopaedic Surgery Sports Medicine Fellow
American Sports Medicine Institute
Birmingham, Alabama, USA

Bradley C. Johnson, MD
SpineCare Medical Group
Daly City, California, USA

James D. Kang, MD
Chairman, Department of Orthopaedic Surgery
Brigham and Women's Hospital
Thornhill Family Professor of Orthopaedic Surgery
Harvard Medical School
Boston, Massachusetts, USA

I. David Kaye, MD
Assistant Professor of Orthopaedic Surgery
Thomas Jefferson University and Hospitals
Spine Surgeon
The Rothman Institute
Philadelphia, Pennsylvania, USA

Khaled M. Kebaish, MD
Professor of Orthopaedic and Neurosurgery
Department of Orthopaedic surgery
Johns Hopkins University
Baltimore, Maryland, USA

A. Jay Khanna, MD, MBA
Vice Chair and Professor of Orthopaedic Surgery, Neuro-
    surgery and Biomedical Engineering
Johns Hopkins University
Bethesda, Maryland, USA

Nikola Kocovic, MD
Resident Physician
Department of Internal Medicine
Icahn School is Medicine at Mount Sinai
New York, New York, USA

Prateek Kumar, MD
Resident
Department of Neurology
University of Illinois at Chicago
Chicago, Illinois, USA

Eric B. Laxer, MD
Associate Professor of Orthopaedic Surgery
Spine Section Chief, Director of Spine Residency Education,
Carolinas Medical Center Orthopaedic Surgery Residency
    Program
Vice Chair, Division of Spine Surgery, Atrium Musculoskel-
    etal Institute
OrthoCarolina Spine Center
Charlotte, North Carolina, USA

Ilya Laufer, MD
Associate Professor
Department of Neurosurgery
Memorial Sloan Kettering Cancer Center
New York, New York, USA

Nathan H. Lebwohl, MD
Chief of Spinal Deformity Surgery
Department of Orthopaedics
University of Miami Miller School of Medicine
Miami, Florida, USA

Yajun Liu, MD, PhD, FRCS
Spine Department
Beijing Jishuitan Hospital
Beijing, China

Richard M. McEntee, BS
Sidney Kimmel Medical College
Thomas Jefferson University
Philadelphia, Pennsylvania, USA

Ankit I. Mehta, MD, FAANS
Assistant Professor
Department of Neurosurgery
University of Illinois at Chicago
Chicago, Illinois, USA

Marco C. Mendoza, MD
Spine Surgeon
Tahoe Fracture Orthopedic & Spine
Carson City, Nevada, USA

Christopher M. Mikhail, MD
Resident Physician
Orthopaedic Surgery
Mount Sinai Hospital
New York, New York, USA

R. Alden Milam IV, MD
Assistant Professor
OrthoCarolina Spine Center
Atrium Health Department of Orthopedic Surgery
Charlotte, North Carolina, USA

Andrew H. Milby, MD
Assistant Professor
Department of Orthopaedic Surgery
University of Pennsylvania
Philadelphia, Pennsylvania, USA

Camilo A. Molina, MD
Spine Fellow
Department of Neurosurgery
Johns Hopkins Hospital
Baltimore, Maryland, USA

Kyle W. Mombell, MD
Resident Physician
Department of Orthopaedic Surgery
Naval Medical Center San Diego
San Diego, California, USA

Patrick B. Morrissey, MD
Assistant Professor
Department of Orthopaedic Surgery
Naval Medical Center San Diego
San Diego, California, USA

Yusef I. Mosley, MD
Marion Bloch Neuroscience Institute
Saint Lukes Hospital
Kansas City, Missouri, USA

Jay K. Nathan, MD
Chief Resident
Department of Neurosurgery
University of Michigan
Ann Arbor, Michigan, USA

Brandon L. Neisewander, BA
MD Candidate
Department of Neurosurgery
University of Illinois at Chicago College of Medicine
Chicago, Illinois, USA

Brian J. Neuman, MD
Assistant Professor
Department of Orthopaedics
Johns Hopkins University
Baltimore, Maryland, USA

Mark E. Oppenlander, MD, FAANS
Assistant Professor
Department of Neurosurgery
University of Michigan
Ann Arbor, Michigan, USA

Sohrab Pahlavan, MD
Spine Surgeon
Ventura Orthopedics
Ventura, California, USA

Trishan Panch, MD, MPH
Chief Medical Officer
Wellframe Inc.
Boston, Massachusetts, USA

Jaykar R. Panchmatia, MA, MPH, MB BChir, FRCS
Consultant Spine Surgeon
Guy's and St. Thomas' Hospitals
London, United Kingdom

Peter G. Passias, MD, MS
Associate Professor
Departments of Orthopaedic and Neurological Surgery
NYU School of Medicine
New York, New York, USA

Justin C. Paul, MD, PhD
Spine Surgeon
Department of Spine Surgery
OrthoConnecticut
Danbury, Connecticut, USA

Zach Pennington, BS
Medical Student
Department of Neurosurgery
Johns Hopkins University School of Medicine
Baltimore, Maryland, USA

Alfred J. Pisano, MD
Chief Resident
Department of Orthopaedic Surgery
Walter Reed National Military Medical Center
Bethesda, Maryland, USA

Srinivas K. Prasad, MD, MS
Associate Professor of Neurological Surgery
Director, Neurosurgical Spine Fellowship
Thomas Jefferson University and Hospitals
Philadelphia, Pennsylvania, USA

Glenn S. Russo, MD, MS
Connecticut Orthopaedics
Clinical Assistant Professor
Department of Surgery
Frank H. Netter School of Medicine at Quinnipiac University
Hamden, Connecticut, USA

Yamaan S. Saadeh, MD
Neurosurgery House Officer
Department of Neurosurgery
University of Michigan
Ann Arbor, Michigan, United States

Ralph T. Schär, MD
Neurosurgeon and Fellow in Complex Spine Surgery
Division of Neurosurgery, St. Michael's Hospital
University of Toronto
Toronto, Ontario, Canada

Adam M. Schmitt, MD
Assistant Attending
Department of Radiation Oncology
Memorial Sloan Kettering Cancer Center
New York, New York, USA

James M. Schuster, MD, PhD
Associate Professor of Neurosurgery
Director of Neuro-Trauma
Chief of Neurosurgery, Penn Presbyterian Medical Center
University of Pennsylvania
Philadelphia Pennsylvania, USA

Daniel M. Sciubba, MD
Professor
Department of Neurosurgery
Johns Hopkins University
Baltimore, Maryland, USA

Jonathan G. Seavey, MD, MS
Staff Surgeon
Department of Orthopedics
Naval Health Clinic Oak Harbor
Oak Harbor, Washington, USA

Arjun S. Sebastian, MD, MSc
Assistant Professor
Department of Orthopedic Surgery
Department of Neurosurgery
Rochester, Minnesota, USA

Kartik Shenoy, MD
Orthopaedic Spine Fellow
Department of Orthopaedic Surgery
Rothman Orthopaedic Institute
Philadelphia, Pennsylvania, USA

Michael P. Silverstein, MD
Orthopaedic Spine Surgeon
Jewett Orthopaedic Clinic
Orlando, Florida, USA

Brian T. Sullivan, MD
Orthopaedic Surgery Resident
Department of Orthopaedic Surgery
Johns Hopkins Hospital
Baltimore, Maryland, USA

Patricia Zadnik Sullivan, MD
Resident
Department of Neurosurgery
University of Pennsylvania
Philadelphia, Pennsylvania, USA

Zachary Tan, BS
Research Assistant
Department of Neurosurgery
University of Illinois at Chicago
Chicago, Illinois, USA

Nicholas Theodore, MD, FACS, FAANS
Donlin M. Long Professor
Professor of Neurosurgery, Orthopaedics & Biomedical
    Engineering
Department of Neurosurgery
Johns Hopkins University
Baltimore, Maryland, USA

Wei Tian, MD, PhD, FRCS
Professor
Spine Department
Beijing Jishuitan Hospital
Beijing, China

Alexander R. Vaccaro, MD, PhD, MBA
Richard H. Rothman Professor and Chairman
Department of Orthopaedic Surgery
Professor of Neurosurgery
Thomas Jefferson University and Hospitals
President
The Rothman Institute
Philadelphia, Pennsylvania, USA

Arya Varthi, MD
Assistant Professor
Department of Orthopedic Surgery
Yale University
New Haven, Connecticut, USA

Kaitlyn Votta, BS
Sidney Kimmel Medical College
Thomas Jefferson University
Philadelphia, Pennsylvania, USA

Scott C. Wagner, MD
Assistant Professor of Surgery
Department of Orthopaedics
Walter Reed National Military Medical Center
Uniformed Services University of the Health Sciences
Bethesda, Maryland, USA

William C. Welch, MD
Vice Chair Department of Neurosurgery
University of Pennsylvania
Professor of Neurosurgery and Orthopaedic Surgery
Philadelphia, Pennsylvania, USA

Jefferson R. Wilson, MD, PhD, FRCSC
Neurosurgeon, St. Michael's Hospital
Assistant Professor, University of Toronto
Toronto, Ontario, Canada

Jingwei Zhao, MD, PhD
Spine Department
Beijing Jishuitan Hospital
Beijing, China

John E. Ziewacz, MD, MPH
Neurosurgeon
Carolina Neurosurgery and Spine Associates
Charlotte, North Carolina, USA

Part I
Introduction to Navigation and Robotics

I

1 Principles of Navigated Pedicle Screw Placement

Yusef I. Mosley and Srinivas K. Prasad

Abstract

Treatment of spinal pathology often necessitates spinal instrumentation. The methods used for spinal instrumentation have changed significantly of the past decade. Most of the recent advancements in spinal instrumentation involve technology that allows the surgeon to place pedicle screws with minimal risk of complications. This chapter is a review of the steps a surgeon should take in order to reduce the risk of complication and to establish an efficient workflow in the operating room.

Keywords: intraoperative navigation, spine surgery, pedicle screw placement

1.1 Introduction

The evolution of spinal instrumentation has improved significantly over the last few decades with transpedicular instrumentation becoming the favored tool of the spine surgeon for a wide variety of spinal stabilization procedures. However, new techniques in any surgical specialty also come with new complications. The rate of misplaced pedicle screws ranges from 14 to 55% with standard nonnavigated insertion techniques. Approximately 7% of these misplaced screws result in neurological injury.[1,2,3]

Introduction of navigation techniques for spinal instrumentation came about around 1995 with the goal of improving instrumentation placement accuracy and reduced injury to neurovascular structures.[4] The advantages of spinal navigation for pedicle screw placement have been reported in multiple studies.[5,6] The use of image guidance systems has proven to reduce the number of pedicle breaches to less than 5%.[7,8]

The purpose of this chapter is to discuss operative planning for cases that utilize navigation for posterior spinal instrumentation and discuss various types of image-guided systems available on the market.

1.2 Consideration for Operative Planning

1.2.1 Operating Room Setup

When utilizing intraoperative navigation systems there are a number of factors that should be considered prior to bringing the patient to the operating room. First is the region of the spine that is being instrumented (i.e., cervical, thoracic, thoracolumbar, lumbar, or lumbosacral). Each region requires a different positioning technique and different strategies for placement of registration trackers to minimize registration error.

The patient's body habitus is another factor that should be considered prior to the operative intervention. Obese patients have increased soft tissue, which can create difficulties in positioning, beam penetration, exposure of the operative site,

line-of-sight requirements for navigation systems, and the limited ability to maneuver the registering devices for accurate navigation.[8]

Selection of the appropriate operative table is of utmost importance. Some of the most common operative tables include radiolucent Wilson frame and Jackson OSI table. There should be consideration for any special attachments for cervical cases in which the head should be fixated to the table to ensure accurate registration.

1.3 Types of Image-Guided Navigation

1.3.1 2D Navigation

This method utilizes fluoroscopic anteroposterior and lateral images that are acquired during surgery with a tracker affixed to the patient. The navigation system tracks the relative position of known instruments with respect to the patient and generates a synthetic view of these instruments in the fluoroscopic images. The advantages of this system are its speed, decreased radiation exposure, and ease of use. However, the next-generation three-dimensional (3D)-guided navigation systems have been shown to have better accuracy.

1.3.2 3D Navigation

This form of navigation once again requires a registration tracker on the patient's body that is paired to a CT-based form of imaging. The registration process involves identification of landmarks that are identifiable both within the CT scan and on the patient's anatomy. Using these common points, a transformation matrix is calculated to generate and complete the registration process. Cameras are used to optically track reflected infrared light from spheres or light-emitting diodes that are attached to surgical instruments. This technology enables the surgeon to navigate the patient's spine anatomy using a visual image that shows the position of tracked instruments in the CT scan. The surgeon can view projections in the axial, coronal, and sagittal planes via a monitor in the operating room (OR).

Advantages with the use of this technology include the ability to image multiple levels in a single sequence, imaging accuracy in patients who had undergone prior spine surgeries at the same levels, decreased radiation exposure to the OR staff, improved accuracy because the patient's anatomy is registered in the surgical position, and portability of the system so it can be easily transported between ORs.

Cone-Beam CT Scan

Cone-beam CT produces multiple fluoroscopic images acquired by an imaging device that rotates isocentrically around the patient. This technology brought about a significant change by enabling intraoperative registration of the surgical space to take place following surgical exposure and delineation of bone anatomy and eliminating the need for identification of common landmarks—the CT volume is registered in aggregate to the tracker placed on the patient.

A reference arc is secured at some anatomical location (e.g., spinous process, posterior superior iliac spine) or previous hardware and tracked.

Types of Cone Beam CT Scanners

- Arcadis Orbic 3D isocentric C-arm (Siemens AG; ▶ Fig. 1.1).
- Ziehm Vision RFD 3D (Ziehm Imaging; ▶ Fig. 1.2).
- O-arm (Medtronic; ▶ Fig. 1.3).

The biggest weakness of these systems is that there is greater intraoperative radiation to the patient and potentially staff in the OR at the time of the intraoperative image acquisition. Additionally, there are limits to how many levels can be imaged within the same volume, sometimes requiring numerous scans and/or numerous tracker placements to image the whole region of interest. Additionally, image quality can be somewhat limited because of patient factors, the presence of instrumentation, and technical factors with the intraoperative scanners.

CT Scan

This type includes intraoperative CT scan platforms that can be integrated with navigation systems.

Types of CT Scanners

- Airo (Brainlab; ▶ Fig. 1.4).
- BodyTom (NeuroLogica Corp.; ▶ Fig. 1.5).

1.3.3 Registration Modes

Material Fiducials

One of the pitfalls of material fiducials is the requirement of attaching the fiducials prior to surgery. This can increase the inaccuracy when used with spinal navigation and is not currently used.

Anatomical Fiducials

Anatomical fiducials are placed on accessible intraoperative targets to be identified by the surgeon. These targets are then registered to a CT-based image. This process is known as paired-point matching.

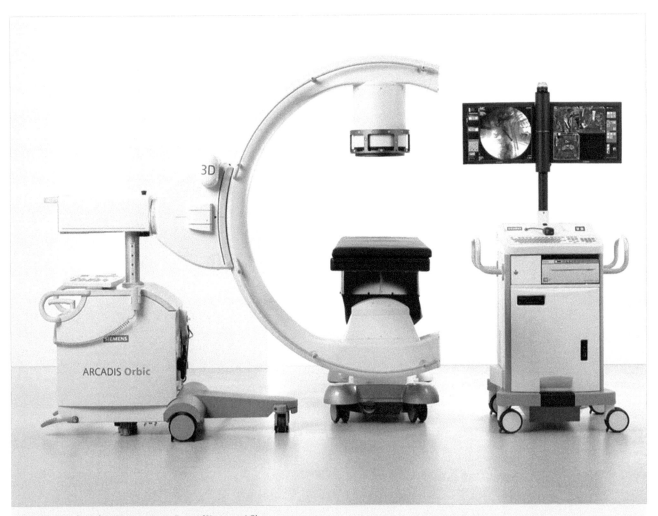

Fig. 1.1 Arcadis Orbic 3D isocentric C-arm (Siemens AG).

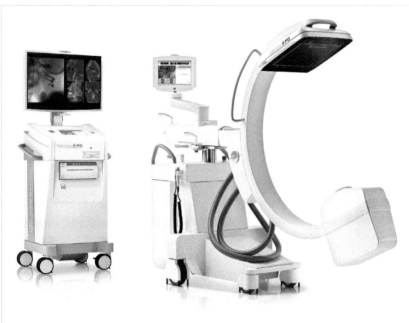

Fig. 1.2 Ziehm Vision RFD 3D.

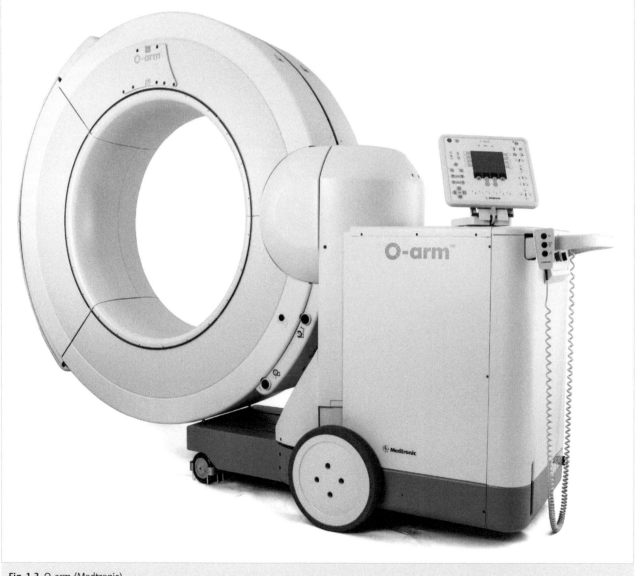

Fig. 1.3 O-arm (Medtronic).

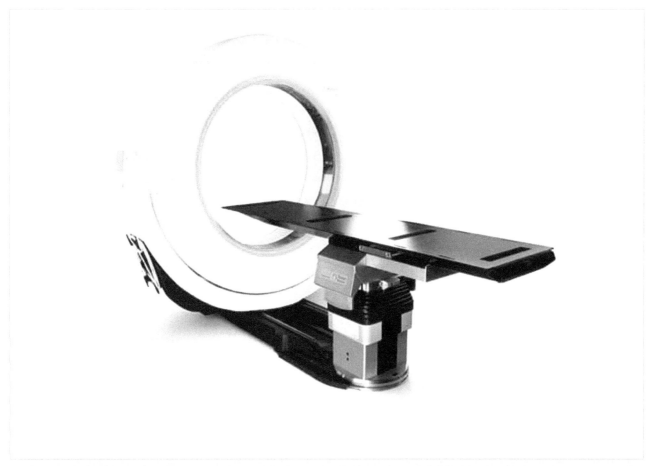

Fig. 1.4 Airo (Brainlab).

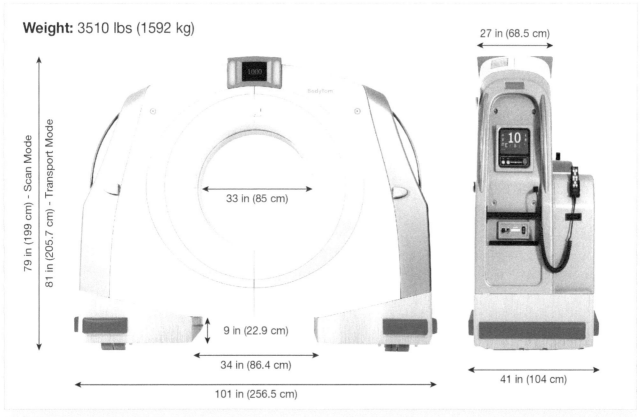

Weight: 3510 lbs (1592 kg)

27 in (68.5 cm)

79 in (199 cm) - Scan Mode

81 in (205.7 cm) - Transport Mode

33 in (85 cm)

9 in (22.9 cm)

34 in (86.4 cm)

101 in (256.5 cm)

41 in (104 cm)

Fig. 1.5 BodyTom (NeuroLogica).

The surgeon must identify the exact target/anatomical location, which can present many challenges. There is a variant of anatomical registration that includes the surface-based point-pairing techniques.

Automated Registration

This registration method is currently the most popular method employed in spine surgery today and involves acquisition of a CT scan intraoperatively with the patient positioned. Since it registers the full CT volume to the patient-based tracker, it does not require point matching of any sort.

1.4 Conclusion

The usage of navigation systems as an adjunct for spinal arthrodesis has made significant changes to the safety and accuracy of spinal surgery. Spine surgeons who decide to utilize these technologies should be updated on the current products available and the OR set up in order to ensure a safe surgical environment for the patient. Moreover, consistent use will help surgeons understand the relative strengths and weaknesses of these technologies and help surgeons handle accuracy issues that may arise in more complex cases.

References

[1] Amiot LP, Lang K, Putzier M, Zippel H, Labelle H. Comparative results between conventional and computer-assisted pedicle screw installation in the thoracic, lumbar, and sacral spine. Spine. 2000; 25(5):606–614

[2] Laine T, Lund T, Ylikoski M, Lohikoski J, Schlenzka D. Accuracy of pedicle screw insertion with and without computer assistance: a randomised controlled clinical study in 100 consecutive patients. Eur Spine J. 2000; 9(3): 235–240

[3] Laine T, Schlenzka D, Mäkitalo K, Tallroth K, Nolte LP, Visarius H. Improved accuracy of pedicle screw insertion with computer-assisted surgery. A prospective clinical trial of 30 patients. Spine. 1997; 22(11): 1254–1258

[4] Nolte L, Zamorano L, Arm E, et al. Image-guided computer-assisted spine surgery: a pilot study on pedicle screw fixation. Stereotact Funct Neurosurg. 1996; 66(1–3):108–117

[5] Ebmeier K, Giest K, Kalff R. Intraoperative computerized tomography for improved accuracy of spinal navigation in pedicle screw placement of the thoracic spine. Acta Neurochir Suppl (Wien). 2003; 85:105–113

[6] Girardi FP, Cammisa FP, Jr, Sandhu HS, Alvarez L. The placement of lumbar pedicle screws using computerised stereotactic guidance. J Bone Joint Surg Br. 1999; 81(5):825–829

[7] Tormenti MJ, Kostov DB, Gardner PA, Kanter AS, Spiro RM, Okonkwo DO. Intraoperative computed tomography image-guided navigation for posterior thoracolumbar spinal instrumentation in spinal deformity surgery. Neurosurg Focus. 2010; 28(3):E11

[8] Vaidya R, Carp J, Bartol S, Ouellette N, Lee S, Sethi A. Lumbar spine fusion in obese and morbidly obese patients. Spine. 2009; 34(5):495–500

2 Three-Dimensional Computer-Assisted Navigation Platforms

Barrett S. Boody

Abstract:

Intraoperative navigation technology for spine utilizes existing neurosurgical core concepts utilized with brain surgery. Over the past 50 years, advancements in imaging and computing have facilitated integration of real-time three-dimensional imaging to core neurosurgical principles of stereotaxy which utilizes external frames to provide references for difficult to visualize anatomy and pathology. With the recent advances of intraoperative fluoroscopic and CT scanning techniques along with intraoperative navigation platforms allowing instrument referencing and tracking, current spine navigated techniques for spinal surgery allow safe, effective, and accurate identification of complex spinal anatomy and assists with accurate spinal instrumentation placement. The core principles of intraoperative navigation involve successful performance and integration of imaging, tracking, registration, and image synthesis/visualization. Acquisition of intraoperative CT scans or fluoroscopy and subsequent integration with navigation platforms allows for three-dimensional recreation of the patient s anatomy. While a variety of tracking platforms are available, optical systems using a camera emitting infrared light and passive optical arrays in the surgical field are the most commonly utilized techniques. In order to register and associate the patient s imaging to the navigation platform, a rigid registration array is secured to the patient and mobile arrays are fixed to the navigated instruments. Last, image synthesis and visualization is performed, where the navigation platform integrates the patient s anatomy to the reference arrays within the surgical field, providing real-time visualization and integration of surgical instruments with patient anatomy. Intraoperative spine navigation has been shown to have accurate identification of intraoperative anatomy and improved accuracy with pedicle screw placement over conventional open and fluoroscopic techniques.

Keywords: computer-assisted navigation, intraoperative navigation, intraoperative CT scan, history of intraoperative navigation, navigated pedicle screws, spine navigation outcomes

2.1 Introduction

As surgical techniques have improved so have intraoperative technologies. Computer-assisted navigation platforms, a newer class of assistive modalities, have been developed with these techniques in mind, aiming to complement and enable the performance of increasingly complex cases. Prior to intraoperative navigation, surgeons would have to synthesize a great deal of information in their minds' eye; the preoperative advanced imaging would be correlated with intraoperative topography and anatomy to allow successful performance of a given procedure. With the advent of intraoperative navigation, real-time three-dimensional (3D) localization and orientation of instrumentation and pathology has been enabled. This has afforded an improved understanding of the pathology and has

potentially provided risk mitigation for more high-risk surgical procedures and possibly for even more routine techniques such as pedicle screw placement.

Recent publications suggest that intraoperative navigation can improve the accuracy and safety of instrumentation placement, can be time efficient, can be low risk, and can be cost-effective especially in complex spinal procedures. Despite the potential benefits of intraoperative navigation, widespread adoption has been lacking. Choo and colleagues reported that 63.4% of members in the Spine Arthroplasty Society and Society for Minimally Invasive Spine Surgery have minimal experience with navigated techniques.[1] Despite the available evidence, Härtl et al reported that only approximately 11% of north American and European surgeons routinely use navigation.[2] Adopters of the technology cite the increased accuracy, facilitation of complex surgery, and reduction in radiation as advantages, while nonusers note a lack of equipment or training and high overhead costs as obstacles to adoption of navigation techniques.[2]

2.2 Evolution of Intraoperative Navigation

Navigated spine surgical techniques were conceptually designed using neurosurgical principles of stereotaxy. Due to the complex cerebral anatomy encountered, Drs. Horsley and Clarke proposed the initial use of static frames to hold the skull motionless, providing a fixed external reference for the surgeon while accessing known landmarks to improve accessing obscure areas of the brain.[3] Spiegel and colleagues built off the concepts of Drs. Horsley and Clark to create the first frame-based intraoperative referencing for use in humans, noting the advantages of limited access minimize the morbidity of the craniotomy.[3,4]

In the 1970s and 1980s, advancements in imaging and computing allowed for the development of individualized intraoperative referencing.[5] Improved imaging techniques allowing 3D re-creations of anatomy, such as CT and MRI, and the integration of referencing computer guidance systems have facilitated development of frameless navigation techniques. In 1979, the Brown-Roberts-Wells stereotactic system allowed pairing of stereotactic instruments with CT data.[6] Roberts and colleagues in 1986 published a frameless stereotaxy technique utilizing emitted acoustic clicks from an operating microscope and detected by an array of microphones within the operating room (OR), allowing triangulation and reference of the discrete point in space. These intraoperative referenced points could be correlated with the preoperative CT scan and assist with positioning of the microscope.[7]

Barnett et al described an armless and frameless stereotactic instrument in 1993 consisting of a mobile ultrasonic probe localized by microphone arrays placed in the OR, allowing for less cumbersome intraoperative triangulation of neurosurgical anatomy.[8] A subsequent technique for intraoperative navigation utilized an articulated arm, whose arm lengths and joint positions could be computed and visualized on a monitor. The position of the articulated arm could then be coregistered by referencing arm locations to known points on preoperative imaging prior to the operation.[9,10]

Current intraoperative systems utilize optical camera arrays to detect either light-emitting diodes or reflective spheres placed statically on the patient. These "anchor" referencing points can be compared in real time to the position of reflective spheres or LEDs on surgical instruments and correlated to preoperative imaging. The superimposed position of the surgical instruments and preoperative imaging is then displayed on a monitor. Although these systems are reliant on continuous "line-of-sight" monitoring between the reference probes and tracked surgical instrument and the camera array, they continue to be a widely utilized technique for intraoperative navigation. Unlike cranial surgery, spine surgery has the obstacle of mobile anatomy due to the many motion segments found throughout the spine and changes in positioning from preoperative imaging (supine vs. prone and changes in anatomy with the progression of the surgery itself [i.e., after osteotomy, screw placement, etc.]).

2.3 Overview of Intraoperative Navigation

Successful application of intraoperative navigation technology requires the execution of four key components: imaging, tracking, registration, and image synthesis/visualization.

2.3.1 Imaging

While MRI and CT imaging techniques have been described for navigation, spine surgical applications require fine detail of bony landmarks and therefore CT is the commonly preferred imaging system. Furthermore, the imaging can be obtained real time, using an integrated CT scanner within the OR allowing for multiple intraoperative scans, or preprocedural scans taken either prior to the OR or obtained using mobile CT scanner technology. The Brainlab Airo is an example of an integrated mobile CT scanner and OR table system, facilitating multiple episodes of intraoperative CT imaging when necessary and minimizing disruptions in workflow.

Due to high radiation doses from multiple CT scans, most surgeons utilize a single preprocedural CT scan. To eliminate confounding variables to imaging fidelity such as prone positioning, mobile CT systems can create intraoperative tomographic imaging that can be utilized for navigation systems. One example is the Medtronic (Minneapolis, MN) O-arm system, a mobile cone-based CT system that can be transported into the OR for intraoperative CT scans. Comparing the use of preoperative and intraoperative CT scans for pedicle screw placement, Costa and colleagues demonstrated no significant difference in accuracy (91.8 vs. 93.5%) but noted decreased registration time (6.5 ± 2 minutes vs. 1.15 ± 0.35 minutes, respectively) with intraoperative CT by avoiding paired-point registration.[11]

Fluoroscopy-based navigation operates similarly to CT-based techniques. Intraoperative fluoroscopy images are obtained in multiple planes and are uploaded to the workstation. Limitations to this technique are based on the quality of the fluoroscopy images; obesity, osteopenia, user error, and rotational deformity can reduce the quality of imaging. Using fluoroscopy-based navigation, Quiñones-Hinojosa reported less than 3 mm accuracy at up to three levels from the registration array and less than 3 mm accuracy up to 120 minutes after registration between 83 and 100%.[12] Newer 3D fluoroscopy machines can re-create CT axial cuts with active rotation around the patient. Siemens and Ziehm are examples of companies that offer fluoroscopy machines that provide 3D imaging.

2.3.2 Tracking

Available tracking technologies utilize either electromagnetic or optical tracking methods, although the majority of the currently utilized intraoperative navigation systems employ the optic camera array technique. Electromagnetic techniques utilize pulsed magnetic fields placed within the OR to localize and triangulate mobile electromagnetic sensors. Although they demonstrate an advantage over optical tracking systems due to small size of mobile sensors and no line-of-sight requirements, the ferromagnetic properties of spinal implants and surgical instruments can interfere with the tracking system, reducing the accuracy of navigation.

Optical systems use two or more cameras placed within the OR at an advantageous position, commonly elevated above the surgical field to improve visualization of the surgical field. Using multiple cameras (camera array) allows for triangulation of the sensors to a discrete position within the OR. Since the cameras require line-of-sight for real-time localization, surgeons and OR staff must avoid obstruction of the cameras.

Optical systems have been developed using either natural or infrared (IR) light systems. Natural light systems use known patterns (commonly black and white checkerboard patterns) that are identified and distinguished by the optical camera array. While these markers are comparatively cheaper than IR sensors, their visualized position can be distorted by variations in OR lighting. IR systems use IR light to track the position of sensors, using either passive (reflective spheres) or active (light-emitting diodes) sensor arrays. Passive sensors reflect emitted IR light commonly from a generator placed adjacent to the camera, whereas active sensors emit IR light for the camera array to receive. The benefit of passive sensors for surgeons is that it allows wireless sensors to be placed on surgical instruments.

Using navigation in place of visualization for spinal procedures requires low tolerances for imaging error. Several studies reviewing error margins for pedicle screws report acceptable parameters as 1 to 3 mm for translation and 4 to 7 mm degrees rotation permissible for pedicle screws.[13,14] Additionally, spine procedures require tracking beyond a discrete location in space, as spatial orientation is critical to understanding trajectories and instrument paths intraoperatively. In order to accomplish this, sensors are placed as arrays on registration and referenced surgical instruments. At least three sensors on each array are required to determine and localize six degrees of freedom (translation and rotation along each of the x-, y-, and z-axes) and each sensor must be continually directly visualized by the camera array. To minimize gaps in real-time tracking, sensor arrays can utilize four or more sensors to ensure at minimum three sensors are continually tracked.

2.3.3 Registration

Registration is the process of associating the preoperative imaging with the navigation tracking system. Spine navigation techniques commonly use a rigid registration system, whereas an "anchor" registration sensory array is either placed on a rigid point of the patient (i.e., iliac crest or spinous process) or rigidly fixed to the table. Brainlab Curve and Medtronic StealthStation are two examples of current navigation systems that utilize optic camera arrays using passive sensors and rigid registration markers. The registration array serves as a fiducial, providing a readily discernable and static position to the patient's anatomy to provide referencing. The Stryker SpineMask Tracker is a surface-based marker offered as an alternative to rigid-registration markers. The SpineMask Tracker is a series of active (LED) sensors adhered to the patient's skin surrounding the surgical incision and can be registered in a similar manner to the rigid-registration systems. It is critical that following registration, the position of the registration array and patient maintain a stable spatial relationship, as any changes in the relationship between the two will malalign the previously coordinated preoperative imaging and intraoperative tracking and will require reregistration.

When intraoperative CBCT scans are utilized, the registration array can be placed prior to the scan, allowing the navigation system to use the tomographic imaging to pair the patient's anatomy to the registration probe. When preoperative CT scans are used or reregistration is required, a paired-point technique is used. Following exposure of the bony anatomy at the proposed surgical levels and placement of the registration probe, a navigated probe is used to first identify the registration array followed by known bony landmarks. Then using the tracking software, visually identifiable bony landmarks are sequentially selected and correlated to the position on the prior CT scan until the system determines the fidelity of the registration is sufficient. There is some concern about increasing distance of the referenced instruments from the registration array (> 3 levels) and increasing duration of surgery (> 1 hour) contributing to inaccuracy of the navigation system.[12,15] To ensure fidelity of the navigation platform following registration and throughout the procedure, users can double-check accuracy touching known observable landmarks and the registration array, verifying fidelity of navigation.

2.3.4 Image Synthesis and Visualization

Following registration, the navigation system can display a real-time overlap of the patient's anatomy with the tracked surgical instruments in the surgical field. Additionally, tracked surgical instruments contain unique sensory arrays that allow for distinguishing the identity of the instruments within the visualized field. Although most navigation systems will provide premade surgical instruments with sensory arrays, some navigation systems will allow placement of sensory arrays on a variety of instruments that can then be secondarily registered. It is critical that tracked instruments are rigid, as the sensory arrays placed on the handles of the instruments will not detect deflection or deformation. Similarly, steep angles encountered intraoperatively at risk for trajectory deflection and skiving or forceful use of instruments causing movement of the patient's anatomy can lead to errors in intraoperative tracking.

The tracked instruments can be viewed on a monitor using 2D axial, sagittal, and coronal images; 3D volume rendering; or simulated anteroposterior and lateral fluoroscopic views, depending on the capabilities of the system and surgeon preferences. Some navigation systems allow for intraoperative implant templating based on the tomographic imaging and provide a visualized target implant position simultaneously with real-time instrument localization.

2.3.5 Outcomes

While it is intuitive that intraoperative navigation can be useful for complex spinal anatomy and pathology, surgeons must determine whether navigation can improve outcomes, reduce complications, and demonstrate cost-effectiveness to justify the costs of implementation. Significant research has been published on this topic, and while subsequent chapters will address specific indications and technical applications, a brief overview is presented below.

Pedicle screw placement using intraoperative navigation has been frequently reported to have very high accuracy.[16] Using intraoperative CT scan with navigation for a total of 1,922 thoracic, lumbar, and sacral screws, Van de Kelft and colleagues reported at 2.5% screw misplacement as determined by postinstrumentation CT scan with 1.8% intraoperative screw revision.[17] Evaluating cervical and upper thoracic screws, Scheufler et al noted acceptable placement of 99.3% of cervical screws and 97.8% of thoracic screws using intraoperative navigation as determined by follow-up CT scans.[15] Furthermore, Yson and colleagues found facet rate violation was significantly lower with navigated versus open techniques (4 vs. 26.5%).[18]

A systematic review by Shin and colleagues reported navigated techniques led to reduced pedicle screw breach rate (6 vs. 15%) when compared to conventional open placement. Furthermore, navigated techniques resulted in zero neurologic complications (4,814 screws in total), whereas open placement resulted in three neurologic complications (3,725 screws in total).[19] A recent meta-analysis of navigation versus fluoroscopic guidance for pedicle screw placement demonstrated significantly lower malposition rate (RR: 0.33, $p < 0.01$), decreased complications (RR: 0.23, $p < 0.01$), and increased operative time (mean: 23.66 minutes, $p < 0.01$).[20] Ughwanogho et al reported significantly lower screw removal for unsafe pedicle screws using navigation compared with free-hand techniques (0.6 vs. 4.9%, respectively).[21]

Despite the widespread support for the utility of navigation for improving accuracy of pedicle screw placement, several studies have suggested no significant improvement over conventional techniques. Comparing fluoroscopic to navigated thoracic and lumbar pedicle screw placement, Shin and colleagues demonstrated no significant difference between techniques in accuracy (91.2 vs. 93.4% with no cortical violation, respectively), but a longer preparation time (4 vs. 19 minutes, respectively).[22] Additionally, Boon Tow and colleagues demonstrated similar accuracy between free-hand and O-arm navigation pedicle screws for single-level lumbar degenerative spondylolisthesis cases (10.53 vs. 14.47%, respectively), while noting a 37.5% breach rate when the registration array was three or more segments from the operative level.[23]

Proponents of navigation propose the cost-effectiveness of navigation is found with improved accuracy of screw placement and subsequently decreased revision surgery rates for screw malposition. Schouten et al noted no revisions for implant malposition in spine trauma applications (27 cases) compared with a 1.2% return to OR for screw revision rate in nonnavigated spine trauma cases.[24] Additionally, Zausinger et al reported a reduction in return to OR for screw revision (0% of 94 navigated cases vs. 4.4% of 182 nonnavigated cases).[25]

Bydon and colleagues suggested that measures taken to improve accuracy of pedicle screw placement might not translate to reduction in reoperation since very few misplaced screws on postoperative imaging require a return to the OR for revision surgery. Their experience using intraoperative CT for confirmation after pedicle screw placement reported an 8.97% intraoperative revision rate of 1,148 cervical, thoracic, and lumbar pedicle screws placed and examined using intraoperative CT.[26] However, they reported a 0.99% return to OR for screw revision for this study compared to a historic cohort of 6,816 screws placed freehand with a return to OR of 0.8%.[26]

Despite the controversy of navigation and the benefits of improved screw accuracy, the few available studies on the economics of intraoperative spine surgical navigation suggest the cost-effectiveness of navigation.[27] Watkins et al reported navigated pedicle screws to decrease revision rates (3 vs. 0%) compared with open techniques, resulting in a proposed cost savings of $71,286 per 100 cases.[28] Dea and colleagues similarly found cost savings for high-volume centers (> 254 instrumented fusions per year) with avoidance of reoperations offsetting the high upfront costs with navigation.[29]

2.4 Conclusion

Building off historical neurosurgical concepts of stereotaxy, the development of intraoperative navigation for spine surgery has the potential to improve surgeons' understanding of complex spine anatomy and pathology. The preponderance of data suggests improved accuracy, reduced complication rate, and a potential for reduced reoperation rate with cost-savings in high-volume spinal fusion centers.

References

[1] Choo AD, Regev G, Garfin SR, Kim CW. Surgeons' perceptions of spinal navigation: analysis of key factors affecting the lack of adoption of spinal navigation technology. SAS J. 2008; 2(4):189–194

[2] Härtl R, Lam KS, Wang J, Korge A, Kandziora F, Audigé L. Worldwide survey on the use of navigation in spine surgery. World Neurosurg. 2013; 79(1): 162–172

[3] Pereira EA, Green AL, Nandi D, Aziz TZ. Stereotactic neurosurgery in the United Kingdom: the hundred years from Horsley to Hariz. Neurosurgery. 2008; 63(3):594–606, discussion 606–607

[4] Foley KT, Smith MM. Image-guided spine surgery. Neurosurg Clin N Am. 1996; 7(2):171–186

[5] Apuzzo ML, Sabshin JK. Computed tomographic guidance stereotaxis in the management of intracranial mass lesions. Neurosurgery. 1983; 12(3):277–285

[6] Enchev Y. Neuronavigation: geneology, reality, and prospects. Neurosurg Focus. 2009; 27(3):E11

[7] Roberts DW, Strohbehn JW, Hatch JF, Murray W, Kettenberger H. A frameless stereotaxic integration of computerized tomographic imaging and the operating microscope. J Neurosurg. 1986; 65(4):545–549

[8] Barnett GH, Kormos DW, Steiner CP, Weisenberger J. Intraoperative localization using an armless, frameless stereotactic wand. Technical note. J Neurosurg. 1993; 78(3):510–514

[9] Reinhardt H, Meyer H, Amrein E. A computer-assisted device for the intraoperative CT-correlated localization of brain tumors. Eur Surg Res. 1988; 20(1): 51–58

[10] Watanabe E, Mayanagi Y, Kosugi Y, Manaka S, Takakura K. Open surgery assisted by the neuronavigator, a stereotactic, articulated, sensitive arm. Neurosurgery. 1991; 28(6):792–799, discussion 799–800

[11] Costa F, Cardia A, Ortolina A, Fabio G, Zerbi A, Fornari M. Spinal navigation: standard preoperative versus intraoperative computed tomography data set acquisition for computer-guidance system: radiological and clinical study in 100 consecutive patients. Spine. 2011; 36(24):2094–2098

[12] Quiñones-Hinojosa A, Robert Kolen E, Jun P, Rosenberg WS, Weinstein PR. Accuracy over space and time of computer-assisted fluoroscopic navigation in the lumbar spine in vivo. J Spinal Disord Tech. 2006; 19(2):109–113

[13] Glossop ND, Hu RW, Randle JA. Computer-aided pedicle screw placement using frameless stereotaxis. Spine. 1996; 21(17):2026–2034

[14] Rampersaud YR, Simon DA, Foley KT. Accuracy requirements for image-guided spinal pedicle screw placement. Spine. 2001; 26(4):352–359

[15] Scheufler KM, Franke J, Eckardt A, Dohmen H. Accuracy of image-guided pedicle screw placement using intraoperative computed tomography-based navigation with automated referencing, part I: cervicothoracic spine. Neurosurgery. 2011; 69(4):782–795, discussion 795

[16] Larson AN, Santos ER, Polly DW, Jr, et al. Pediatric pedicle screw placement using intraoperative computed tomography and 3-dimensional image-guided navigation. Spine. 2012; 37(3):E188–E194

[17] Van de Kelft E, Costa F, Van der Planken D, Schils F. A prospective multicenter registry on the accuracy of pedicle screw placement in the thoracic, lumbar, and sacral levels with the use of the O-arm imaging system and StealthStation Navigation. Spine. 2012; 37(25):E1580–E1587

[18] Yson SC, Sembrano JN, Sanders PC, Santos ER, Ledonio CG, Polly DW, Jr. Comparison of cranial facet joint violation rates between open and percutaneous pedicle screw placement using intraoperative 3-D CT (O-arm) computer navigation. Spine. 2013; 38(4):E251–E258

[19] Shin BJ, James AR, Njoku IU, Härtl R. Pedicle screw navigation: a systematic review and meta-analysis of perforation risk for computer-navigated versus freehand insertion. J Neurosurg Spine. 2012; 17(2):113–122

[20] Meng XT, Guan XF, Zhang HL, He SS. Computer navigation versus fluoroscopy-guided navigation for thoracic pedicle screw placement: a meta-analysis. Neurosurg Rev. 2016; 39(3):385–391

[21] Ughwanogho E, Patel NM, Baldwin KD, Sampson NR, Flynn JM. Computed tomography-guided navigation of thoracic pedicle screws for adolescent idiopathic scoliosis results in more accurate placement and less screw removal. Spine. 2012; 37(8):E473–E478

[22] Shin MH, Ryu KS, Park CK. Accuracy and safety in pedicle screw placement in the thoracic and lumbar spines: comparison study between conventional C-arm fluoroscopy and navigation coupled with O-Arm® guided methods. J Korean Neurosurg Soc. 2012; 52(3):204–209

[23] Boon Tow BP, Yue WM, Srivastava A, et al. Does navigation improve accuracy of placement of pedicle screws in single-level lumbar degenerative spondylolisthesis?: A comparison between free-hand and three-dimensional O-arm navigation techniques. J Spinal Disord Tech. 2015; 28(8):E472–E477

[24] Schouten R, Lee R, Boyd M, et al. Intra-operative cone-beam CT (O-arm) and stereotactic navigation in acute spinal trauma surgery. J Clin Neurosci. 2012; 19(8):1137–1143

[25] Zausinger S, Scheder B, Uhl E, Heigl T, Morhard D, Tonn JC. Intraoperative computed tomography with integrated navigation system in spinal stabilizations. Spine. 2009; 34(26):2919–2926

[26] Bydon M, Xu R, Amin AG, et al. Safety and efficacy of pedicle screw placement using intraoperative computed tomography: consecutive series of 1148 pedicle screws. J Neurosurg Spine. 2014; 21(3):320–328

[27] Al-Khouja L, Shweikeh F, Pashman R, Johnson JP, Kim TT, Drazin D. Economics of image guidance and navigation in spine surgery. Surg Neurol Int. 2015; 6 Suppl 10:S323–S326

[28] Watkins RG, Gupta A, Watkins RG. Cost-effectiveness of image-guided spine surgery. Open Orthop J. 2010; 4:228–233

[29] Dea N, Fisher CG, Batke J, et al. Economic evaluation comparing intraoperative cone beam CT-based navigation and conventional fluoroscopy for the placement of spinal pedicle screws: a patient-level data cost-effectiveness analysis. Spine J. 2016; 16(1):23–31

3 Intraoperative Ultrasound in Spine Surgery: A Versatile and Useful Adjunct

Ralph T. Schär, Howard J. Ginsberg, and Jefferson R. Wilson

Abstract:

Intraoperative ultrasound (IOUS) has been used in spine surgery for more than 30 years. Modern devices are able to provide real-time images of exceptionally high resolution and precise delineation of anatomical structures. This easy-to-use and effective intraoperative tool provides spine surgeons with excellent real-time visualization of the spinal cord and nerve roots as well as of neurocompressive structures. Thus, IOUS is a useful adjunct for guidance and confirmation of adequate surgical interventions in a multitude of spine pathologies such as spinal tumors, spine trauma, degenerative, congenital, and vascular spine disease.

Keywords: intraoperative ultrasound, spinal cord, nerve roots, spinal tumors, degenerative cervical myelopathy, spine surgery

3.1 Introduction

The utility of ultrasound in the field of medicine was first recognized by brothers Karl Theodore and Friederich Dussik in the 1930s and 1940s. These pioneers attempted to scan human brains through the skull by using a 1.5-MHz transmitter and proposed that ultrasound might be able to diagnose brain tumors.[1] Research by Wild led to the use of A-mode imaging with a 15-MHz transducer to visualize and determine bowel wall thickness and gastric cancer in the 1950s.[2] "Amplitude" or A-mode ultrasound was the earliest ultrasound imaging method and described a one-dimensional image displaying the amplitude or strength of a wave along a vertical axis and the time along the horizontal axis. By the late 1940s "brightness" or B-mode ultrasound was developed and was able to obtain two-dimensional (2D) images of tissue where each pixel on a screen represented an individual amplitude spike, relating brightness to the ultrasound wave amplitude. Over the following decades with better physical, physiological, and engineering understanding, the technology of ultrasonography was further improved and advanced. As large and cumbersome ultrasound machines were transformed into smaller and more portable devices, the intraoperative use of ultrasound started to gain popularity. By the 1980s, first reports of intraoperative ultrasound (IOUS) in spine surgery as a valuable adjunct for real-time visualization of various pathologies such as tumors, cysts, and syringomyelia were published.[3,4,5,6] Dohrmann and Rubin recognized that by performing a laminectomy and placing the ultrasound probe directly on the dura, they were able to obtain higher quality images since ultrasound waves were not compromised by impenetrable bone or narrow interlaminar windows.[3,7]

Many spine surgeons today routinely use real-time IOUS to more precisely tailor the extent of bone resection and to more safely guide resection of intradural and intramedullary tumors while preserving normal tissue. Additionally, IOUS can help confirm adequacy of decompression of lesions ventral to the thecal sac such as in the case of calcified thoracic disk herniations or retropulsed bone fragments in spine trauma.[8,9,10] With recent advances in the field of three-dimensional intraoperative computer-assisted navigation, the primacy of IOUS for real-time image guidance has been somewhat supplanted by CT- and/or MRI-based navigation systems in many areas of spine surgery such as for intradural tumors.[11] However, ultrasound still remains the most widely used guidance modality today, due to its availability, relatively low cost, easy operability, and ability to provide real-time visualization with high-spatial resolution.

3.2 Basic Technical Principals of Ultrasound

Ultrasound refers to the transmission of energy as mechanical pressure waves within matter with frequencies above 20 kHz, which is above the human audible range. In order for these waves to propagate, ultrasound essentially requires a physical medium; it cannot be transmitted in a vacuum. In biological tissue with high water content, ultrasound waves propagate mainly longitudinally at an average speed of 1,540 m per second. In medicine, ultrasound frequencies used generally range from 2 to 20 MHz with very short wavelengths allowing for high spatial resolution. As a general rule, the higher the frequency, the higher the spatial resolution and the lower the ultrasound penetration becomes. Conversely, with lower frequencies, spatial resolution is decreased and penetration of the ultrasound beam is increased. Frequencies in the gigahertz (GHz) range can be used for ultrasound microscopy to visualize subcellular structures. The "piezoelectric effect" refers to the capability of quartz crystals or synthetic ceramics within the ultrasound transducer to intermittently deform under pulsatile electrical stimulation. This sudden and rhythmic structural deformation generates mechanical vibration, and ultimately the ultrasound. Piezoelectric transducers are able to transform electrical signals into mechanical waves (ultrasound transmitter), and also to change reflected ("echoing") ultrasound waves back into electrical signals (ultrasound receiver). Ultrasound waves may be partially absorbed by biological tissue and energy is then transformed into heat. As the ultrasound beam propagates across different tissues with different acoustic impedances, interfaces are created. Depending on the acoustic impedance at an interface, the ultrasound waves may be partially or completely reflected, or absorbed and transformed into heat. Only returning echoes are picked up by the transducer, which ultimately constitutes the source of the diagnostic information and contributes to the ultrasound image.

3.3 Ultrasound Modes and Techniques

3.3.1 B-Mode Ultrasound

B-mode ultrasound is certainly one of the most widely used ultrasound applications in medicine. As briefly mentioned earlier, B-mode (brightness-mode) refers to a 2D ultrasound image composed of different dots representing ultrasound echoes. The amplitude of the reflected ultrasound signal (the echo) defines the brightness of each dot. All of these different dots allow for visualization and quantification of anatomical structures as gray scale images.

The intrinsic brightness of these structures is described in terms of their echogenicity, which is compared relative to the surrounding tissue. In general, hyperechoic tissue is brighter, and hypoechoic tissue is darker. If two different tissues are equally bright, they are isoechoic to one another. When the ultrasound beam has no tissue interface to reflect upon, such as within a fluid, the representation of that medium is anechoic and appears dark (black). For instance, pure water will appear black, whereas the presence of red blood cells within the water will appear as bright echogenic specs.

3.3.2 Doppler Ultrasound

Doppler ultrasound is the combination of the Doppler effect with measurement of both direction and velocity by color scale within gray scale (B-mode) images. While the Doppler effect assesses whether objects (usually red blood cells) are moving toward or away from the transducer, color Doppler has the ability to quantify velocity of objects. In spinal surgery, this modality is often used to identify the presence and direction of flow in abnormal vessels and to confirm successful surgical disconnection of dural arteriovenous fistulae (DAVF; see below).

3.3.3 Contrast-Enhanced Ultrasound

Both B-mode and Doppler ultrasound have the limitations of not being able to detect microvasculature. Also, signal detection may often be insufficient due to artifacts and compromised by background noise, especially for deep-seated lesions. Furthermore, with Doppler only one or a few vessels can be studied at a time with the signal changing as soon as the insonation angle is altered. These drawbacks have led to the development of ultrasound contrast media given to the patient intravenously to amplify signals reflected from regions of interest. Contrast

media used today are suspension of microbubbles (mean diameter of 5 μm), which modify the acoustic impedance of tissues and the interaction with the ultrasound beam. This leads to increasing echogenicity and blood backscattering, since the insonated microbubbles themselves will emit ultrasound in a radial fashion. Thus, contrast-enhanced ultrasound delivers high contrast images, and it is a very useful technique for assessing tissue blood perfusion.

3.4 Intraoperative Use of Ultrasound

For the use of IOUS, a mobile ultrasound machine that can easily be operated by the surgeon in a sterile fashion is necessary. Nowadays, specifically designed transducers allow for high-resolution digital imaging of anatomical structures. Depending on the site and extent of bony removal, the spine surgeon may choose from various ultrasound transducers, such as convex or linear probe tips with frequency ranges from 3 to 13.33 MHz. Modern high-frequency transducers up to 18 MHz exist for small or superficial spinal lesions. The linear "hockey stick" spinal cord guidance transducer or the convex transducer with a small footprint of 20 mm is well suited for use in spine surgery (▶ Fig. 3.1).

Following sufficient bony removal through a hemi- or full laminectomy, the dura overlying the surgical region of interest (e.g., the tumor) is exposed. Transdural standard B-mode direct sonography will then confirm sufficient or insufficient bony removal above the lesion of interest before opening of the dura.

To obtain optimal imaging quality, the surgical field is filled with saline for acoustic coupling. Irrigation with a laminar flow will help reduce the accumulation of air bubbles, which can compromise the ultrasound image. Also, bleeding into this fluid bath will lower the image quality since erythrocytes are highly echogenic. An appropriate transducer is then placed just above the dura in the saline bath and images should be obtained in both the axial and sagittal planes by gradually moving the probe across the operative field. Tilting the transducer accordingly within the laminectomy site may be necessary depending

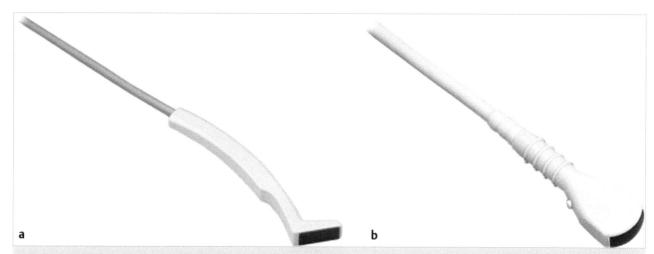

a   b

Fig. 3.1 Hockey-stick spinal cord guidance transducer (UST-536), scan width 19 mm, frequency range 13.33–4.44 MHz **(a)**. Convex guidance transducer (UST-9120), scan with 20 mm radius, 10–4.44 MHz **(b)**. ProSound Alpha 7, Hitachi Aloka Medical America, Inc.

on the extent of bony removal to view adjacent dura and spinal cord underlying bony structures. Holding the transducer directly on the dura may cause an artifact called "near field clutter," since structures in the near field can be obscured due to high amplitude of oscillations by the transducer itself.[12] It is advised to always determine the cranial and caudal, or left and right, orientation of the transducer at the beginning. Depending on the transducer, one side is usually clearly marked and corresponds to the left- or right-hand side of the ultrasound monitor. Structures are most clearly seen by sonography when they are in line or perpendicular with the central acoustical axis.

3.5 Normal Sonographic Anatomy of the Spine

When describing lesions, they are defined as hyperechoic, isoechoic, or hypoechoic relative to the surrounding tissue (e.g., the paraspinal muscles). Other features may have a diffuse or circumscribed appearance; they may be homogeneous or heterogeneous and exhibit the presence of calcifications or cystic areas. Dense calcifications can be extremely hyperechoic and potentially block all propagation of ultrasound.

On ultrasound the bony edges of the laminectomy site are highly reflective and allow only little or no penetration of ultrasound waves. The dura and arachnoid layers are recognized as a single reflective echogenic membrane between the fluid bath and the anechoic subarachnoid space filled with cerebrospinal fluid (CSF). The spinal cord is seen as a relatively homogeneous, low echogenic structure within the CSF, surrounded by an echogenic rim due to the change in physical density from CSF to spinal cord, which creates an acoustical interface.[7,13] The central canal within the spinal cord appears as a bright echogenic line. The dentate ligaments attaching the spinal cord to the dura on either side as well as the spinal nerve roots can also be recognized as echogenic linear structures within the CSF. Ventral to the thecal sac, the vertebral bodies appear hyperechoic and the intervertebral disks appear hypoechoic (▶ Fig. 3.2). The normal spinal cord will exhibit rhythmic pulsations synchronous with the heartbeat and also with the respiratory cycle.[14] Decreased or absence cord pulsations may be indicative of cord compression. Spinal cord contusions will appear as hyperechoic signal within the spinal cord itself. Spinal cord deformation and atrophy are readily detected by ultrasound and are thought to render prognostic information, although this has not been proven.

3.6 Application Areas of Intraoperative Ultrasound in Spine Surgery

3.6.1 Intradural Spinal Tumors

While the surgeon will rely on preoperative MR or CT imaging to identify the surgical level for laminectomy, intraoperative transdural sonography will allow for more accurate and real-time localization of the pathological lesion in question. The extent of bone removal can be optimized for opening the dura precisely above the tumor. For intramedullary tumors, IOUS will safely guide myelotomy and help avoid dissecting through

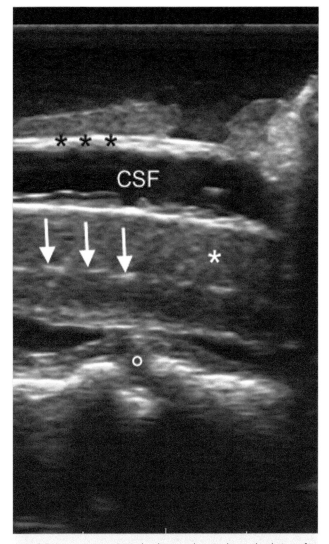

Fig. 3.2 Intraoperative B-mode ultrasound sagittal transdural view of spinal cord (*white asterisk*). The dura (*black asterisks*), cerebrospinal fluid, the spinal cord, the central canal (three *white arrows*), and the intervertebral disk (*white circle*) are easily identified.

healthy tissue. Also, real-time transdural IOUS adds valuable information about the dynamic interactions of the tumor with the surrounding neural and vascular elements. To date, many studies have demonstrated the usefulness of IOUS-guided surgery for spinal tumors.[7,15,16,17]

Intradural Extramedullary Tumors

Schwannomas and meningiomas comprise the vast majority of intradural extramedullary spinal tumors. B-mode real-time IOUS can be very helpful while operating on these intradural tumors.

Schwannomas are benign, slow-growing nerve sheath tumors arising from nerve roots within the spinal canal and are most frequently seen in the cervical and lumbar spine, less commonly in the thoracic spine. They appear as solid and well-circumscribed mildly hyperechoic tumors (▶ Fig. 3.3). However, often they may be less homogeneous as compared to meningiomas. Depending on the level of the tumor, the spinal cord and

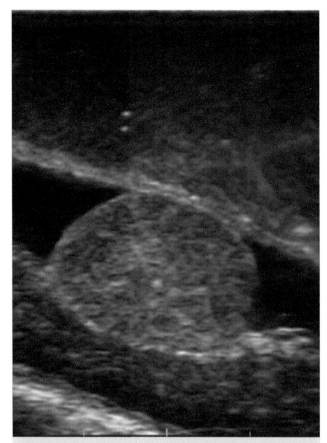

Fig. 3.3 Transdural sagittal view of a thoracic schwannoma. The tumor is well circumscribed and encapsulated. The tumor–spinal cord interface is identified as a fine linear hyperechoic line.

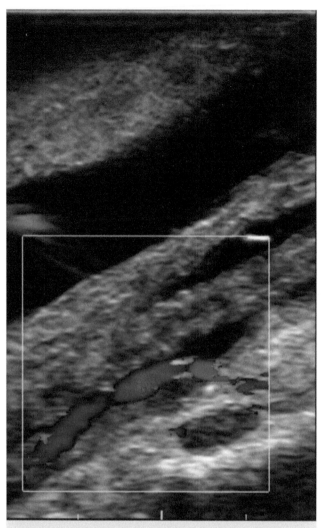

Fig. 3.4 Dural arteriovenous fistula depicted with color Doppler intraoperative ultrasound.

nerve roots are deflected away from the mass lesion. In some cases, schwannomas will display considerable rhythmic cranio-caudal movement, especially in the lumbar spine. In fact, several cases of migratory schwannomas have been previously reported in the literature.[18] Hence, IOUS should be mandatory before dural opening to exclude tumor migration since the time of the preoperative MRI.

Spinal **meningiomas** are most commonly found in the thoracic spine and will typically also appear as well-circumscribed, slightly hyperechoic lesions, relative to the normal spinal cord. The spinal cord and nerve roots are visibly displaced by the tumor, depending on its size and location relative to the neural elements. Dural tails and attachments can be readily visible on ultrasound and can assist in planning of tumor removal.

Intramedullary Tumors

Ependymomas and astrocytomas are the two most common intramedullary spinal tumors. Intramedullary tumors may appear as more or less circumscribed and homogeneously hyperechoic lesions relative to the normal hypoechoic spinal cord, depending on the infiltrative nature of the tumor. In the presence of peritumoral edema, the spinal cord will appear hyperechoic, which makes the distinction between tumor and surrounding spinal cord more challenging.

Intramedullary **ependymomas** are fairly homogeneous and hyperechoic or heteroechoic lesions. They often contain small central cystic components, and occasionally are associated with a syrinx.

Due to their highly infiltrative nature, spinal **astrocytomas** are not easily distinguished from the surrounding spinal cord on IOUS. However, the infiltrated spinal cord may appear thickened and swollen. Tumor margins are blurred and the tumor may have a granular hyperechogenic appearance.

3.6.2 Spinal Dural Arteriovenous Fistulae

For spinal DAVF, intraoperative Doppler ultrasound can be used to verify and localize DAVFs before opening of the dura.[19] The pathologic arterialized vein which can sometimes be challenging to find becomes immediately obvious with the aid of 2D color Doppler ultrasound. The components of this vascular malformation can be further examined with direct recordings of the disturbed flow patterns within the arterialized draining vein and nidus of the fistula (▶ Fig. 3.4). After surgical obliteration of the draining vein, absence of flow within the DAVF on Doppler ultrasound will confirm successful treatment.

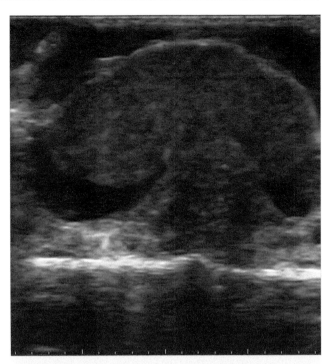

Fig. 3.5 Axial transdural intraoperative ultrasound following laminectomy showing disk herniation with spinal cord compression.

Doppler ultrasound does have some limitations such as artifacts and dependence of the Doppler angle of insonation. More recently, the use of intraoperative contrast-enhanced ultrasound for spinal DAVFs has been described.[20] This method allows real-time visualization before and after obliteration of the draining vein, as well as blood flow changes within the spinal cord and perimedullary plexus. Specifically, following ligation, reduction of spinal cord contrast enhancement confirms restoration of physiologic pressure and flow within the medullary capillary bed.

3.6.3 Thoracic Compression Ventral to the Thecal Sac

IOUS is extremely helpful for visualization of compressive lesions ventral to the spinal cord, such as retropulsed bone fragments in spine trauma or thoracic disk herniations (▶ Fig. 3.5). Under continuous ultrasound guidance, such as with a linear hockey stick probe, angled instruments can be maneuvered beneath the thecal sac from a posterior approach essentially eliminating the need for thecal sac manipulation and large morbid anterolateral approaches to the spine. The extent of decompression of the neural elements can be clearly appreciated on the ultrasound monitor.

Symptomatic **thoracic disk herniations** are very rare and pose a challenge to the treating spine surgeon. A variety of surgical approaches such as posterior (laminectomy, transpedicular, or transfacet pedicle sparing), posterolateral (costotransversectomy), lateral transthoracic, anterolateral transthoracic, or anterior transsternal to these often densely calcified disks have been described. Historically, a direct posterior approach via thoracic laminectomy alone has largely been abandoned because of poor neurological outcome most likely due to iatrogenic

retraction during diskectomy. Recently, an ultrasound-guided thoracic diskectomy by a posterior pedicle-sparing, transfacet approach has been described.[9] After laminectomy through a unilateral or bilateral approach, the diskectomy is performed by reaching a down-angled curette anterior to the thecal sac under continuous intraoperative guidance of transdural ultrasound.

Likewise, in a similar approach, retropulsed bony fragments such as in **thoracolumbar burst fractures** can be accessed and removed under ultrasound guidance avoiding any spinal cord manipulation.[21]

3.6.4 Posterior Cervicothoracic Decompression

As previously mentioned, IOUS is an excellent tool for visualizing anteriorly located compression to the spinal cord and guiding sufficient decompression. The use of IOUS during posterior cervical decompression has been demonstrated for laminoplasty in patients with degenerative cervical myelopathy.[22,23] Residual compression to the cervical spinal cord can lead to poor neurological recovery or deterioration in myelopathic patients.[24] Excessive decompression can lead to iatrogenic instability. The authors of this chapter have been routinely using IOUS for guidance of precise decompression of the cervical spinal cord and nerve roots during posterior cervical laminectomy with or without fusion.[25] Following laminectomy, a linear hockey stick probe is held over the dura and the extent of decompression to the spinal cord and cervical nerve roots especially laterally and in the neuroforamina is assessed (▶ Fig. 3.6 and ▶ Fig. 3.7). With anterior compression to the thecal sac such as with ossification of the posterior longitudinal ligament (OPLL) or calcified cervical disks, the spinal cord will shift posteriorly following sufficient posterior decompression, and this can be verified and documented with IOUS.

3.6.5 Posterior Fossa Decompression for Chiari Malformation Type I

Many studies have described IOUS as a useful tool for guidance of the extent of posterior fossa decompression in patients with Chiari malformation type I, to aid intraoperative decision making with regard to the need of duraplasty, and to assess for restoration of normal CSF flow.[26,27,28] On real-time IOUS, the pathophysiology of this condition with obstruction of the normal CSF pathways can be well studied. Often within the tight subarachnoid space, there is evidence of the distally displaced cerebellar tonsils creating caudally directed, piston-like pulsations. After posterior fossa craniectomy with or without C1 laminectomy and duraplasty, this phenomenon should be resolved signifying adequate decompression.

3.7 Conclusion

IOUS has proven a useful modality to provide real-time imaging for otherwise "unseeable" pathology. It has demonstrated the ability to aid in resection of intradural tumors as well as ventral spinal pathology. Although intraoperative navigated CT and MRI capabilities continue to evolve, currently IOUS still provides the most economic, mobile, and user-friendly experience.

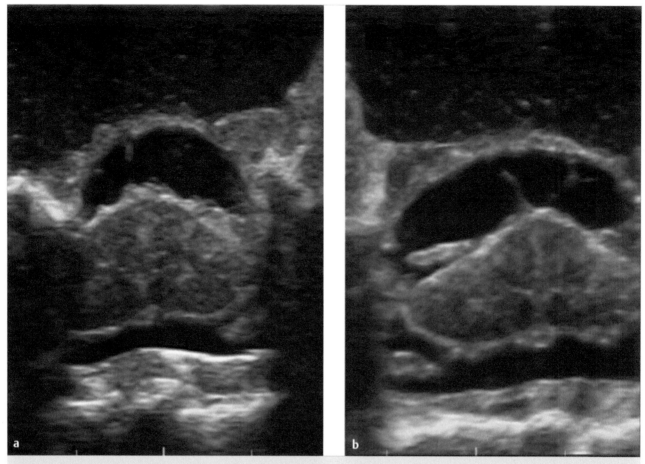

Fig. 3.6 Transdural axial intraoperative ultrasound following cervical laminectomy showing insufficient decompression (a) of the left lateral aspect of the spinal cord and nerve roots. Sufficient decompression (b) is eventually achieved for the spinal cord and both the ventral and dorsal nerve roots.

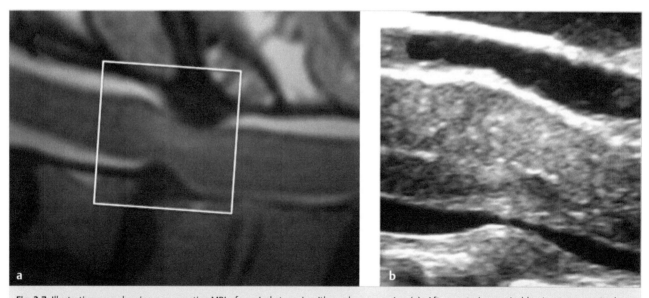

Fig. 3.7 Illustrative case showing preoperative MRI of cervical stenosis with cord compression (a). After posterior cervical laminectomy, sagittal intraoperative ultrasound confirms sufficient decompression (b).

References

[1] Newman PG, Rozycki GS. The history of ultrasound. Surg Clin North Am. 1998; 78(2):179–195

[2] Wild JJ. The use of ultrasonic pulses for the measurement of biologic tissues and the detection of tissue density changes. Surgery. 1950; 27(2):183–188

[3] Dohrmann GJ, Rubin JM. Intraoperative ultrasound imaging of the spinal cord: syringomyelia, cysts, and tumors–a preliminary report. Surg Neurol. 1982; 18(6):395–399

[4] Montalvo BM, Quencer RM. Intraoperative sonography in spinal surgery: current state of the art. Neuroradiology. 1986; 28(5–6):551–590

[5] Raymond CA. Brain, spine surgeons say yes to ultrasound. JAMA. 1986; 255 (17):2258–2259, 2262

[6] Rubin JM, Dohrmann GJ. The spine and spinal cord during neurosurgical operations: real-time ultrasonography. Radiology. 1985; 155(1):197–200

[7] Vasudeva VS, Abd-El-Barr M, Pompeu YA, Karhade A, Groff MW, Lu Y. Use of intraoperative ultrasound during spinal surgery. Global Spine J. 2017; 7(7):648–656

[8] Juthani RG, Bilsky MH, Vogelbaum MA. Current management and treatment modalities for intramedullary spinal cord tumors. Curr Treat Options Oncol. 2015; 16(8):39

[9] Nishimura Y, Thani NB, Tochigi S, Ahn H, Ginsberg HJ. Thoracic discectomy by posterior pedicle-sparing, transfacet approach with real-time intraoperative ultrasonography: clinical article. J Neurosurg Spine. 2014; 21(4):568–576

[10] Lazennec JY, Sailland G, Ramare S, Hansen S. [Intraoperative ultrasound study of thoracolumbar spinal fractures with spinal canal fragments. Determining canal width and anatomic control of decompression: comparative analysis with CT]. Unfallchirurg. 1998; 101(5):353–359

[11] Overley SC, Cho SK, Mehta AI, Arnold PM. Navigation and robotics in spinal surgery: where are we now? Neurosurgery. 2017; 80 3S:S86–S99

[12] Bertrand PB, Levine RA, Isselbacher EM, Vandervoort PM. Fact or artifact in two-dimensional echocardiography: avoiding misdiagnosis and missed diagnosis. J Am Soc Echocardiogr. 2016; 29(5):381–391

[13] Quencer RM, Montalvo BM. Normal intraoperative spinal sonography. AJR Am J Roentgenol. 1984; 143(6):1301–1305

[14] Jokich PM, Rubin JM, Dohrmann GJ. Intraoperative ultrasonic evaluation of spinal cord motion. J Neurosurg. 1984; 60(4):707–711

[15] Regelsberger J, Fritzsche E, Langer N, Westphal M. Intraoperative sonography of intra- and extramedullary tumors. Ultrasound Med Biol. 2005; 31(5):593–598

[16] Ivanov M, Budu A, Sims-Williams H, Poeata I. Using intraoperative ultrasonography for spinal cord tumor surgery. World Neurosurg. 2017; 97:104–111

[17] Prada F, Vetrano IG, Filippini A, et al. Intraoperative ultrasound in spinal tumor surgery. J Ultrasound. 2014; 17(3):195–202

[18] Friedman JA, Atkinson JL, Lane JI. Migration of an intraspinal schwannoma documented by intraoperative ultrasound: case report. Surg Neurol. 2000; 54 (6):455–457

[19] Iacopino DG, Conti A, Giusa M, Cardali S, Tomasello F. Assistance of intraoperative microvascular Doppler in the surgical obliteration of spinal dural arteriovenous fistula: cases description and technical considerations. Acta Neurochir (Wien). 2003; 145(2):133–137, discussion 137

[20] Prada F, Del Bene M, Faragò G, DiMeco F. Spinal dural arteriovenous fistula: is there a role for intraoperative contrast-enhanced ultrasound? World Neurosurg. 2017; 100:712.e15–712.e18

[21] Lerch K, Völk M, Heers G, Baer W, Nerlich M. Ultrasound-guided decompression of the spinal canal in traumatic stenosis. Ultrasound Med Biol. 2002; 28 (1):27–32

[22] Kimura A, Seichi A, Inoue H, et al. Ultrasonographic quantification of spinal cord and dural pulsations during cervical laminoplasty in patients with compressive myelopathy. Eur Spine J. 2012; 21(12):2450–2455

[23] Seichi A, Chikuda H, Kimura A, et al. Intraoperative ultrasonographic evaluation of posterior decompression via laminoplasty in patients with cervical ossification of the posterior longitudinal ligament: correlation with 2-year follow-up results. J Neurosurg Spine. 2010; 13(1):47–51

[24] Seichi A, Takeshita K, Ohishi I, et al. Long-term results of double-door laminoplasty for cervical stenotic myelopathy. Spine. 2001; 26(5):479–487

[25] Schär RT, Wilson JR, Ginsberg HJ. Intraoperative ultrasound-guided posterior cervical laminectomy for degenerative cervical myelopathy. World Neurosurg. 2019; 121:62–70

[26] McGirt MJ, Attenello FJ, Datoo G, et al. Intraoperative ultrasonography as a guide to patient selection for duraplasty after suboccipital decompression in children with Chiari malformation Type I. J Neurosurg Pediatr. 2008; 2 (1):52–57

[27] Milhorat TH, Bolognese PA. Tailored operative technique for Chiari type I malformation using intraoperative color Doppler ultrasonography. Neurosurgery. 2003; 53(4):899–905, discussion 905–906

[28] Yeh DD, Koch B, Crone KR. Intraoperative ultrasonography used to determine the extent of surgery necessary during posterior fossa decompression in children with Chiari malformation type I. J Neurosurg. 2006; 105 (1) Suppl:26–32

4 Magnetic Resonance Imaging–Based Navigation

Jonathan G. Seavey and Langston T. Holly

Abstract:

Magnetic resonance imaging (MRI) provides high-resolution imaging of soft tissues via the excitation of hydrogen nuclei placed within a large external magnetic field. By varying scanning parameters, different aspects of the anatomic area of interest can be emphasized. Advantages over computed tomography include improved soft-tissue resolution and lack of ionizing radiation; however, these are balanced by increased image acquisition times and need for RF shielding. MRI can be integrated into surgical workflows in several ways: (1) coregistration of a preoperative MRI with intraoperative imaging, (2) colocation of the MRI suite and surgical suite (or gantry-mounted MRI scanners that can enter/exit the surgical field), and (3) performance of surgery within an open bore or double-donut scanner using MR-compatible instruments and equipment. Cost, engineering, and operative time constraints have largely limited utilization of true intraoperative MRI to the treatment of intracranial pathology and spine tumor resection. However, as the demand for minimally invasive surgery grows and technology improves, the role of MRI-based surgical navigation will continue to evolve.

Keywords: magnetic resonance imaging, MRI navigation, intraoperative MRI

4.1 Introduction

Magnetic resonance imaging (MRI) utilizes nuclear magnetic resonance spectra produced by radiofrequency (RF) excitation of tissue hydrogen nuclei within a strong external magnetic field to generate detailed, volumetric imaging representations of the target structures. It can provide unparalleled soft-tissue image quality for defining normal anatomic structures as well as detecting and delineating pathology. By varying scanning parameters, different output variables (anatomic detail, tissue edema, neural structures, etc.) can be emphasized. Fundamentally MRI differs significantly from fluoroscopy, plain film, and computed tomographic (CT) scanning which all utilize the attenuation of ionizing radiation as it passes through the target tissue to generate an image. In addition to superb image quality, images can be captured independently along multiple axes (as compared to CT where coronal and sagittal images are generated from the natively acquired axial images) with no exposure to ionizing radiation.

Image quality in MRI is a function of signal-to-noise ratio, and in general, better images can be obtained with larger external magnetic fields. Most modern MRI scanners use a cooled superconducting magnet to generate a magnetic field with a strength ranging from 1.5 to 3.0 Tesla (for comparison, Earth's magnetic field at the surface is 25–65 microteslas) which necessitates exclusion of ferromagnetic materials from proximity to the system. Generated RF signal reception can be improved by proximity of the receiver coils to imaged structures, frequently by use of anatomic region–specific coils (i.e., shoulder or knee) placed on the body surface. Minimization of background noise

can be accomplished by utilizing an RF-shielded environment for signal acquisition.

Given some of the physical constraints associated with MRI, real-time incorporation of MRI into surgical workflow presents technical and engineering challenges not encountered with fluoroscopy, intraoperative CT scanning, or visual/infrared navigation. MRI-based navigation in spine surgery can roughly be broken into three different genera: (1) Preoperative MR images are coregistered with intraoperative CT scanning or ultrasound and/or input into an image-based navigation or robotics system. (2) Surgery is performed in an operative suite collocated with an MRI suite allowing for intraoperative transfer of the patient from a traditional operating room (OR) to the MRI scanner and back. (3) True intraoperative MRI, with creation of a surgical field in a double-donut or open bore MRI scanner allowing for near real-time imaging during surgery.

MRI-based navigation allows for surgeon "visualization" of surgical instruments in relation to normal and pathologic anatomy, an effect which is most pronounced where there are narrow approach corridors or where local anatomy precludes dissection and direct visualization. Much of the early literature on the use of MRI in surgery reflects this and describes use of the technology to address intracranial pathology. The goals of this chapter are to provide a background on MRI technology and describe the development of MRI-based surgical navigation, and how it is currently utilized in spine surgery.

4.2 Magnetic Resonance Imaging Basics

MRI has gained widespread use since its introduction as a medical diagnostic tool in the late 1970s. It allows for excellent soft-tissue definition and contrast and can be used to define and distinguish normal anatomy from pathological processes and their sequelae. MRI, as medical imaging modality, emerged from nuclear magnetic resonance (NMR) spectroscopy, a technology developed in the 1940s.

NMR spectroscopy was originally developed as a research tool which utilized the behavior of certain types of atomic nuclei within a strong magnetic field to provide information about the atomic and molecular structure of studied compounds. The resolution of NMR spectroscopy is such that it can distinguish not only between different functional groups in organic compounds but also between identical functional groups which have different neighboring atoms.[1,2,3]

MRI and NMR both rely on a physical property of certain atomic nuclei, called *spin*, which is the result of interactions between the subatomic particles, namely, gluons and quarks, which compose protons and neutrons. Depending on the number and ratio of protons and neutrons, atomic nuclei may possess spin values from 0 to 8 in half-integer increments. For the purposes of most medical MRI, the abundant hydrogen nucleus, composed of a single proton with spin value ½, is used.

A charged, spinning proton generates a magnetic field parallel to the axis of rotation, and is often stylized as a small bar magnet (▶ Fig. 4.1a). Under normal circumstances, the spin axes of protons within tissue are not coordinated (▶ Fig. 4.1b); however, when placed within a large external magnetic field (such as the bore of an MRI scanner), designated as B_0, the spin axis aligns with the north–south (longitudinal or z) axis of the external magnetic field, B_0 (▶ Fig. 4.1c). Radiofrequency (RF) energy can then be applied at the resonant frequency of nuclear precession,* which tips the spin axis away from the longitudinal axis of the external field. Typically, RF energy is applied to tip the spin axis 90 degrees to the longitudinal axis, into the xy or transverse plane (▶ Fig. 4.1d). (*The resonant frequency of precession, f, is determined by the Larmor equation: $f = \gamma B_0$, where γ is a constant, the gyromagnetic ratio [characteristic of each type of nuclei], and B_0 is the main magnetic field strength.)

Cessation of the external RF energy pulse allows time-dependent relaxation of the nuclei spin axes back to their resting state parallel to the longitudinal axis of B_0 (▶ Fig. 4.1e). This time-dependent relaxation is tissue specific, and differences in relaxation times can be used to differentiate between tissue types.[4,5,6,7,8] During relaxation, the nuclei precess (or wobble, like a child's top) around the longitudinal/z-axis defined by B_0. As the nuclei precess, they continue to generate small magnetic fields parallel to their internal spin axis, and these fields can be resolved into z and xy components: when all spin axes are aligned with B_0, the z-component of the magnetic field is maximized, and the xy-component is minimized. Conversely, after an RF pulse that tips the spin axes into the transverse plane, the z-component is minimized, and the xy-component is maximized. Imaging sequences that emphasize differences in the longitudinal (z-axis) component of relaxation are described as T1 weighted (▶ Fig. 4.1f), while imaging sequences that emphasize differences in transverse plane decay are described as T2-weighted (▶ Fig. 4.1g).

Signal generation occurs because precessing nuclei are functionally small, spinning magnets: their precession induces small electrical currents in receiver coils. These induced currents encode information about the structural arrangement and composition of the imaged tissue and are used to generate the visual representation of the imaged structures.[4,5,6,7] Manipulation of imaging parameters, RF pulse sequences, and processing algorithms allows different aspects to the imaged structures to be emphasized; most frequently in spine surgery, fat-suppressed T2-weighted images are used to identify pathologic processes and provides good contrast between cerebrospinal fluid (CSF; hyperintense) and disk material (hypointense; ▶ Fig. 4.2). For oncologic or infectious workups, T1-weighted images obtained before and after administration of intravenous gadolinium contrast can be useful in identifying the extent of tumors and defining cystic structures.

4.3 Uses of Magnetic Resonance Imaging in Spine Surgery

4.3.1 Traditional Uses: Identifying Pathology and Preoperative Planning

MRI is frequently used in conjunction with plain radiographs as part of the planning process prior to spine surgery. Radiographs provide fine bony detail, can demonstrate dynamic instability with flexion/extension and bending radiographs, and can be used to define overall spinopelvic alignment such as lumbar lordosis, pelvic incidence, and coronal and sagittal vertical axes and are frequently obtained under physiologic load. MRI provides soft-tissue delineation of tissue planes, pathology and neurovascular structures, and their proximity to approach corridors. In combination, these modalities can be used to develop a holistic surgical plan which includes the safest approach that allows access to pathology, potential risks (e.g., aberrant nerve root origination, the location of the lumbar plexus in the psoas), as well as target spinopelvic parameters in spinal arthrodesis.[9,10,11]

4.3.2 Intraoperative Integration of Magnetic Resonance Imaging in Spine Surgery

There are several basic requirements for new technologies to gain widespread implementation in the surgical suite. First, the technology must provide some tangible benefit either in improved accuracy and/or outcomes, time or cost savings, and improved workflow/ease of use or in increasing the minimally invasive nature of a procedure. Frequently, new technologies improve on one of these aspects, at the expense of others. Intraoperative navigation may improve accuracy, but it typically increases cost, and may increase operative times, especially during the initial learning curve.

One such example of the cost–benefit interplay is the use of navigation and/or intraoperative CT scanning for the placement of pedicle screws: purported benefits of this technology include improved pedicle screw placement, decreased risk to adjacent neural elements, and improved intraoperative recognition of screws requiring revision. Some studies have shown improved accuracy with intraoperative CT scanning,[12,13,14] while other studies have not shown a statistically significant difference.[15,16,17] Given the lack of consensus as to the benefits of intraoperative CT scan compared to freehand technique, many surgeons utilize selective employment of this technology in cases where there is an underlying anatomic reason (dysmorphic vertebral anatomy, narrow pedicles) or to verify freehand pedicle screw placement in a long construct prior to wound closure.

Similarly, the implementation and use of MRI as part of a spine surgery procedure must provide some tangible benefit: in safety, efficacy, cost, or time, which is not easily achievable by more conventional means. It is unsurprising then that the primary area for integration of MRI with spine surgery has occurred when dealing with tumors of the spine and spinal cord. In tumor resections, precise localization of the tumor, identification of the blood supply, and assessment of the spatial relationship between the tumor and surrounding critical structures can often make the difference between a curative resection and a catastrophic complication. Therefore, MRI, which can provide unparalleled soft-tissue resolution, is well suited to this application.

4.3.3 Preoperative MRI Coregistration with Other Intraoperative Navigation Modalities

One of the least technically challenging means of introducing the soft-tissue resolution and definition of MRI into the operative suite is through coregistration of preoperative MRI scans

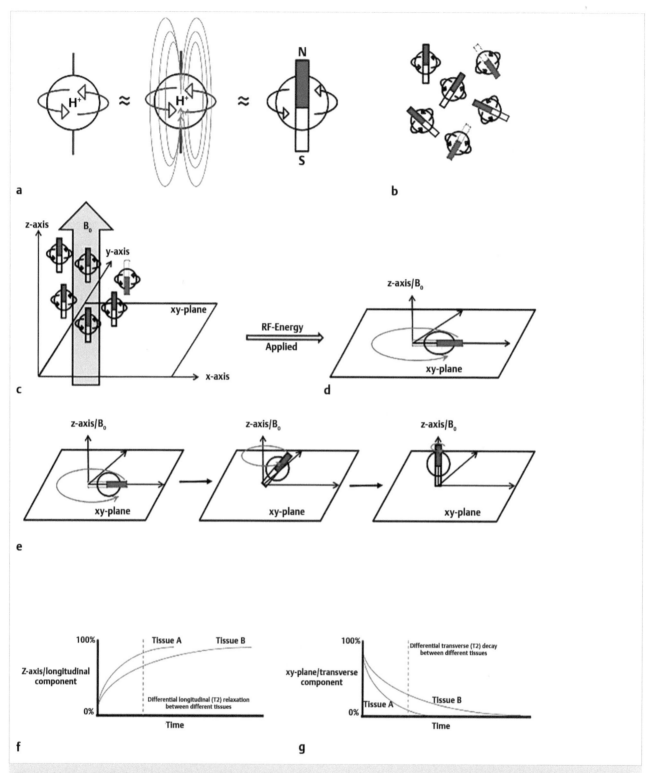

Fig. 4.1 (a) A spinning hydrogen nucleus (proton) produces a magnetic field and can be thought of schematically as a small bar magnet. (b) Under normal conditions, the magnetic axes of different protons are not coordinated. (c) After application of a large external magnetic field B_0, the magnetic axes of the protons align. The axis of the magnetic field is designated the longitudinal or z-axis and the transverse or xy-plane is perpendicular to the longitudinal axis. (d) RF energy is applied which causes the spin axes to flip from longitudinal to transverse. The proton continues to spin around its internal spin axis, but also precesses (*blue curved arrow*) around the magnetic axis defined by the internal field. (e) Following cessation of the RF energy pulse, the nuclear spin axis relaxes from the transverse plane to the longitudinal axis. (f,g) Relaxation to the longitudinal axis (f) and decay from the transverse plane (g) are time dependent in a tissue-specific manner and can be used to differentiate between tissue types.

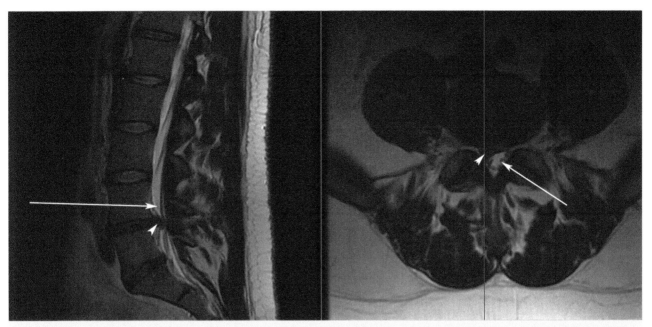

Fig. 4.2 Sagittal and axial T2-weighted MRI of the lumbar spine demonstrating a right-sided paracentral L4–L5 disk herniation. The disk is hypointense (*white arrowheads*), while the CSF is hyperintense (*white arrows*).

with intraoperative O-arm or fluoroscopy images. Merging of the imaging can be accomplished by both automatic and manual methods, typically by aligning the bony anatomy of the vertebral bodies on the preoperative and intraoperative imaging. This method of MRI incorporation avoids most of the engineering challenges and electromagnetic shielding requirements necessitated by true intraoperative MRI use. However, there are limitations to this system: most preoperative MRIs are obtained with the patient supine in the MRI scanner, whereas most spine surgeries are performed in the prone position. Over short segments, differences are minimal, but over longer distances, the angular differences in vertebral alignment can cause significant spatial discrepancies between the pre- and intraoperative imaging. Therefore, most authors recommend, merging the imaging over short segments only, centered on the pathology to be addressed. Additionally, 1- to 2-mm slices through the area of interest and modification of patient positioning during the preoperative MRI (e.g., scan in the lateral decubitus for lateral approach surgeries) have been recommended.[18,19,20,21,22]

There have been case series reported in the literature over the past several years describing this technology in the treatment of intramedullary and paraspinal tumors of the cervical, thoracic, and lumbar spine, as well as the sacrum. The benefits of merged MRI/intraoperative navigation include accurate placement of laminectomies and durotomies as well as identification and avoidance of normal neurovascular structures during resection and validate both the benefits and feasibility of merged imaging in the treatment of spinal tumors.[18,19,20,21,22]

4.3.4 Intraoperative Magnetic Resonance Imaging

In comparison to the previous examples of preoperative MRI merged with intraoperative CT scan–based navigation, true intraoperative MRI (iMRI) has more significant barriers to wide-spread utilization in spine surgery. Utilizing iMRI for the management of intracranial pathology has been described for more than 20 years. [23,24,25,26] The ability of iMRI to provide detailed visualization and delineation of normal and pathologic brain and spinal cord tissue can provide near real-time feedback on the placement of instruments, adequacy of resection, and the presence of complications such as hematoma. iMRI images can also be utilized to update navigational software and account for brain shift caused by CSF leaks.[24]

However, incorporation of an MRI scanner into the operative suite poses some significant engineering challenges including exclusion of ferromagnetic items from the large static field produced by the scanner and RF shielding the receiver coils in order to minimize background noise and improve image quality. Early pioneers of intraoperative MRI circumvented some of these challenges by creating twin OR setup, whereby a normal neurosurgical OR suite was collocated next to an RF-shielded OR suite containing the MRI scanner.[23,25,26] In this setup, patients are transferred from the normal surgical suite to the imaging suite and back intraoperatively. Depending on the design of the scanner (i.e., open MRI), limited instrumentation with MR-compatible devices (cannulas, needles, probes) may be performed while the patient is in the scanner. Similarly, other surgeons have utilized a system which allows a mobile ceiling-mounted MR scanner to move in and out of the operative field as required for imaging during surgery.[24,27] Utilization of an RF-shielded, 1.5-T gantry-based MRI system to lesions of the craniovertebral junction has been described.[28,29,30]

Use of co-located MRI and surgical suites or mobile scanners allows for integration of MRI into the surgical workflow, but the ability to obtain near real-time intraoperative imaging and navigation within an active surgical field required an evolution in MRI scanner design as well as development of an array of

MRI-compatible surgical instrumentation and OR equipment. Open-bore and double-donut scanners which allowed creation of the operative field within the imaging system were developed, mated to conventional navigation systems and combined with newly developed MRI-compatible surgical instrumentation and anesthesia machines.[25,31,32,33,34]

In addition to providing excellent spatial resolution between tissues of different types and/or normal/pathological tissue, MRI can also be utilized to measure small differences in tissue temperature, a valuable capability when ablating tumors in close proximity to neural structures. MR thermography has been utilized to guide thermal therapy by assessing the adequacy of treatment in the area of interest, while minimizing deleterious effects on surrounding nontarget tissues.[35,36,37] MR thermography combined with stereotactic surgical navigation and iMRI have been described for interstitial laser ablation of cranial tumors with good results. In these cases, fixed, bone-based fiducial markers and/or bolt placement was performed and used to guide the placement of laser probes. Local temperature gradients around the probes were measured using iMRI to assess the adequacy of ablation and effects on surrounding tissue.[38,39]

More recently, iMRI and MR thermography have been combined with optical surgical navigation systems and fluoroscopy for ablation of metastatic spinal masses causing compression of the neural elements. In this system, fiducial markers are placed on the anesthetized patient's back, and a plastic cradle is placed over the back and used to support the MRI coil. Preoperative T2-weighted images are obtained using iMRI, and the images are exported to surgical navigation software. Utilizing a reference array sutured to the patient, Jamshidi needles are positioned and advanced using navigation software and the coregistered T2-weighted images. Position of the Jamshidi needles is confirmed with fluoroscopy and then the needles are exchanged for MRI-compatible cannulas. iMRI is then used to confirm the final position of the cannulas in relation to the target tissue prior to laser probe implantation, followed by use of MR thermography to assess the adequacy of the subsequent ablation.[40]

4.4 Future Directions

The use of MRI technology for spinal surgical navigation continues to evolve as MR-compatible instrumentation is developed and integration of scanners into the operative field progresses. Currently, surgical resection or ablation of spinal tumors, especially those with narrow approach corridors and distorted regional anatomy, seems to be the most promising area for implementation and utilization of this technology. At this point, it is unclear whether the potential benefits of iMRI will be worth the additional cost and likely increased operative times in other realms of spine surgery. However, as more minimally invasive procedures are developed, the demand for better intraoperative imaging is likely to continue to grow: it remains to be seen, however, if this demand will be filled by MRI or some other imaging modality.

References

[1] Hinds MG, Norton RS. NMR spectroscopy of peptides and proteins. Practical considerations. Mol Biotechnol. 1997; 7(3):315–331

[2] Nelson FA, Weaver HE. Nuclear magnetic resonance spectroscopy in superconducting magnetic fields. Science. 1964; 146(3641):223–232

[3] Ferguson RC, Phillips WD. High-resolution nuclear magnetic resonance spectroscopy. Advances in instrumentation in this field are leading to new applications in chemistry and biology. Science. 1967; 157(3786):257–267

[4] Bitar R, Leung G, Perng R, et al. MR pulse sequences: what every radiologist wants to know but is afraid to ask. Radiographics: a review publication of the Radiological Society of North America. Inc. 2006; 26:513–537

[5] de Figueiredo EH, Borgonovi AF, Doring TM. Basic concepts of MR imaging, diffusion MR imaging, and diffusion tensor imaging. Magn Reson Imaging Clin N Am. 2011; 19(1):1–22

[6] Jacobs MA, Ibrahim TS, Ouwerkerk R. AAPM/RSNA physics tutorials for residents: MR imaging: brief overview and emerging applications. Radiographics: a review publication of the Radiological Society of North America. Inc. 2007; 27:1213–1229

[7] Pooley RA. AAPM/RSNA physics tutorial for residents: fundamental physics of MR imaging. Radiographics: a review publication of the Radiological Society of North America. Inc. 2005; 25:1087–1099

[8] Nelson TR, Hendrick RE, Hendee WR. Selection of pulse sequences producing maximum tissue contrast in magnetic resonance imaging. Magn Reson Imaging. 1984; 2(4):285–294

[9] Menezes CM, de Andrade LM, Herrero CF, et al. Diffusion-weighted magnetic resonance (DW-MR) neurography of the lumbar plexus in the preoperative planning of lateral access lumbar surgery. Eur Spine J. 2015; 24(4):817–826

[10] Quinn JC, Fruauff K, Lebl DR, et al. Magnetic resonance neurography of the lumbar plexus at the L4-L5 disc: development of a preoperative surgical planning tool for lateral lumbar transpsoas interbody fusion (LLIF). Spine. 2015; 40(12):942–947

[11] Galbusera F, Lovi A, Bassani T, Brayda-Bruno M. MR imaging and radiographic imaging of degenerative spine disorders and spine alignment. Magn Reson Imaging Clin N Am. 2016; 24(3):515–522

[12] Shin MH, Hur JW, Ryu KS, Park CK. Prospective comparison study between the fluoroscopy-guided and navigation coupled with O-arm-guided pedicle screw placement in the thoracic and lumbosacral spines. J Spinal Disord Tech. 2015; 28(6):E347–E351

[13] Ling JM, Dinesh SK, Pang BC, et al. Routine spinal navigation for thoraco-lumbar pedicle screw insertion using the O-arm three-dimensional imaging system improves placement accuracy. J Clin Neurosci. 2014; 21(3):493–498

[14] Knafo S, Mireau E, Bennis S, Baussart B, Aldea S, Gaillard S. Operative and perioperative durations in O-arm vs C-arm fluoroscopy for lumbar instrumentation. Oper Neurosurg (Hagerstown). 2018; 14(3):273–278

[15] Laudato PA, Pierzchala K, Schizas C. Pedicle screw insertion accuracy using O-arm, robotic guidance or freehand technique: a comparative study. Spine. 2017; 4; 3(6):E373::E378

[16] Boon Tow BP, Yue WM, Srivastava A, et al. Does navigation improve accuracy of placement of pedicle screws in single-level lumbar degenerative spondylolisthesis?: A comparison between free-hand and three-dimensional O-arm navigation techniques. J Spinal Disord Tech. 2015; 28(8):E472–E477

[17] Fan Y, Du J, Zhang J, et al. Comparison of accuracy of pedicle screw insertion among 4 guided technologies in spine surgery. Med Sci Monit. 2017; 23: 5960–5968

[18] Costa F, Ortolina A, Cardia A, et al. Preoperative magnetic resonance and intraoperative computed tomography fusion for real-time neuronavigation in intramedullary lesion surgery. Oper Neurosurg (Hagerstown). 2017; 13(2): 188–195

[19] D'Andrea K, Dreyer J, Fahim DK. Utility of preoperative magnetic resonance imaging coregistered with intraoperative computed tomographic scan for the resection of complex tumors of the spine. World Neurosurg. 2015; 84(6): 1804–1815

[20] Hlubek RJ, Theodore N, Chang SW. CT/MRI fusion for vascular mapping and navigated resection of a paraspinal tumor. World Neurosurg. 2016; 89:732.e7–732.e12

[21] Stefini R, Peron S, Mandelli J, Bianchini E, Roccucci P. Intraoperative spinal navigation for the removal of intradural tumors: technical notes. Oper Neurosurg (Hagerstown). 201 8; ; 15(1):54–59

[22] Yang YK, Chan CM, Zhang Q, Xu HR, Niu XH. Computer navigation-aided resection of sacral chordomas. Chin Med J (Engl). 2016; 129(2): 162–168

[23] Steinmeier R, Fahlbusch R, Ganslandt O, et al. Intraoperative magnetic resonance imaging with the Magnetom open scanner: concepts, neurosurgical indications, and procedures: a preliminary report. Neurosurgery. 1998; 43 (4):739–747, discussion 747–748

[24] Sutherland GR, Louw DF. Intraoperative MRI: a moving magnet. CMAJ. 1999; 161(10):1293

[25] Tronnier VM, Wirtz CR, Knauth M, et al. Intraoperative diagnostic and interventional magnetic resonance imaging in neurosurgery. Neurosurgery. 1997; 40(5):891–900, discussion 900–902

[26] Bohinski RJ, Kokkino AK, Warnick RE, et al. Glioma resection in a shared-resource magnetic resonance operating room after optimal image-guided frameless stereotactic resection. Neurosurgery. 2001; 48(4):731–742, discussion 742–744

[27] Hoult DI, Saunders JK, Sutherland GR, et al. The engineering of an interventional MRI with a movable 1.5 Tesla magnet. J Magn Reson Imaging. 2001; 13 (1):78–86

[28] Kaibara T, Hurlbert RJ, Sutherland GR. Intraoperative magnetic resonance imaging-augmented transoral resection of axial disease. Neurosurg Focus. 2001; 10(2):E4

[29] Kaibara T, Hurlbert RJ, Sutherland GR. Transoral resection of axial lesions augmented by intraoperative magnetic resonance imaging. Report of three cases. J Neurosurg. 2001; 95(2) Suppl:239–242

[30] Dhaliwal PP, Hurlbert RJ, Sutherland GS. Intraoperative magnetic resonance imaging and neuronavigation for transoral approaches to upper cervical pathology. World Neurosurg. 2012; 78(1–2):164–169

[31] Black PM, Moriarty T, Alexander E, III, et al. Development and implementation of intraoperative magnetic resonance imaging and its neurosurgical applications. Neurosurgery. 1997; 41(4):831–842, discussion 842–845

[32] Alexander E, III, Moriarty TM, Kikinis R, Black P, Jolesz FM. The present and future role of intraoperative MRI in neurosurgical procedures. Stereotact Funct Neurosurg. 1997; 68(1–4, Pt 1):10–17

[33] Alexander E, III. Optimizing brain tumor resection. Midfield interventional MR imaging. Neuroimaging Clin N Am. 2001; 11(4):659–672

[34] Tomanek B, Foniok T, Saunders J, Sutherland G. An integrated radio frequency probe and cranial clamp for intraoperative magnetic resonance imaging: technical note. Neurosurgery. 2007; 60(2) Suppl 1:E179–E180, discussion E180

[35] Denis de Senneville B, Quesson B, Moonen CT. Magnetic resonance temperature imaging. International Journal of Hyperthermia: the official journal of European Society for Hyperthermic Oncology. North American Hyperthermia Group. 2005; 21:515–531

[36] Quesson B, de Zwart JA, Moonen CT. Magnetic resonance temperature imaging for guidance of thermotherapy. J Magn Reson Imaging. 2000; 12(4):525–533

[37] Rieke V, Butts Pauly K. MR thermometry. J Magn Reson Imaging. 2008; 27(2): 376–390

[38] Chan AY, Tran DK, Gill AS, Hsu FP, Vadera S. Stereotactic robot-assisted MRI-guided laser thermal ablation of radiation necrosis in the posterior cranial fossa: technical note. Neurosurg Focus. 2016; 41(4):E5

[39] Tovar-Spinoza Z, Choi H. MRI-guided laser interstitial thermal therapy for the treatment of low-grade gliomas in children: a case-series review, description of the current technologies and perspectives. Childs Nerv Syst. 2016; 32(10):1947–1956

[40] Tatsui CE, Nascimento CNG, Suki D, et al. Image guidance based on MRI for spinal interstitial laser thermotherapy: technical aspects and accuracy. J Neurosurg Spine. 2017; 26(5):605–612

5 Shared Control Robotics

Elvis L. Francois and Arjun S. Sebastian

Abstract

Shared control robotics is a system in which the user maintains some degree of direct or indirect control over an automated system. While semiautomated systems require user intervention, in a shared control system, both the user and the robot are capable of acting independently from one another toward a shared surgical goal. Ideally, this design allows the qualities of the user to be enhanced through robotic automation. In the field of spine surgery, the goal of controlled robotics has been used to augment the surgeon's tactile processes while refining intraoperative judgment. The ideal use of shared control robotics allows for reduction in human error, increased efficiency, reproducibility, and geometric precision. The goal of this chapter is to provide a focused analysis of the most common indications for shared controlled robotics as well as a purview of the most common robotic systems in use.

Keywords: shared control robotics, transpedicular fixation, learning curve, radiation exposure

5.1 Introduction

In 1992, the ROBODOC system (Integrated Surgical Systems, Sacramento, CA) was the first machine to partake in a human-robotic surgery. Since then, many surgical subspecialties including urology, general surgery, and gynecology have worked to continue to expand robotic use. Robotics has been increasingly utilized in spine surgery in an effort to mitigate some of the surgical risk.

The advantages of technology and robotics to the surgeon has been consistently demonstrated in the form of fatigue reduction, increased surgical precision, and even decreased postoperative pain.[1] Shared-control robots have been used to assist in varying spine procedures including pedicle screw placement, tumor resections, and vertebroplasty.

Kosmopoulos and Shizas performed a meta-analysis of 16,717 pedicle screws placed in the lumbar spine in vivo and found that 86.7% were accurately positioned. Specifically, navigated pedicle screw placement improved screw accuracy by a mean of 5% when compared to traditional freehand techniques.[2] Automation of surgery via robotics has provided promising results and as more studies emerge, its benefits have become more evident.

5.2 Robotic Surgery for Transpedicular Fixation

Transpedicular fixation has been the primary, and most widely practiced and studied use, for shared control robots. Robotics and navigation can help mitigate some of the challenges of pedicle screw placement, including pedicle fracture, pedicle screw misplacement, and radiation in the setting of fluoroscopic assistance.

One of the original descriptions of shared control robotics for spine application was by Sautot et al in Grenoble, France, in 1992,[3] who adapted an industrial robot to assist in transpedicular fixation. Preoperative planning employed computed tomographic (CT) scans to generate three-dimensional (3D) images of segmentation of a particular vertebra which served as a guide for pedicle screw trajectory. Intraoperatively, two X-ray devices formatted a 2D projection. The robot carrying a laser optical guide was then employed to superimpose a laser beam in the preoperatively planned surgical trajectory. The authors subsequently demonstrated a drilling experiment on plastic vertebrae, with reported submillimeter accuracy.[3]

From 2002 to 2012, eight out of 18 novel spine surgical robots developed had a particular focus on transpedicular screw insertion.[4] In 2003, a team of Israeli investigators developed the Miniature Robot for Surgical Procedures (MARS),[5,6] which ultimately became the SpineAssist/Renaissance system, currently commercialized by Mazor Robotics (Caesarea, Israel). The revolutionary innovation of MARS/SpineAssist was a significant reduction in size and weight which allowed for direct attachment to the patient. These miniature robotic systems allowed for a drastic simplification of the process where the surgical robot interpreted the spatial reference points directly based on the patient's bony landmarks.

5.3 SpineAssist Mazor Robotics

The SpineAssist robot/Mazor system (MAZOR Robotics Inc, Orlando, FL) has been the most widely studied of all shared control robots utilized in spine surgery. Conceptually utilizing three separate outrigger arms with an accommodating drill guide sleeve, the robotic software, in sync with a computer-assisted navigation, predicts which arm allows for the most accurate pathway for pedicle instrumentation determined by the implant and relative location of the SpineAssist robot to the predetermined entry point and screw trajectory. The robot may be attached and positioned directly onto a spinous process or it may be affixed to a frame triangulated by percutaneously placed guide wires (e.g., one Kirschner wire [K-wire] attached to the spinous process and two Steinmann pins in the posterior superior iliac spines) in the setting of minimally invasive spine (MIS) procedures.[7]

In the preoperative period, the SpineAssist software creates a virtual spinal map by procuring and registering CT images of the operative spinal levels. Subsequently, templating of the desired screw entry point, trajectory, screw diameter, and length can be performed. The templating process may be done preoperatively or intraoperatively and is derived from the 3D spinal map prepared by the software and transferred into the intraoperative SpineAssist workstation. After the virtual template for the desired instrumentation has been created, a secondary verification procedure is performed, where tracked K-wire inserted into the mounted robot act to cross verify the accuracy of the template system. This secondary verification process assures an accuracy of less than 1.5 mm of deviation from the actual implant and the preoperative template.[7]

The terminal point of registration occurs by obtaining six static fluoroscopic images utilized for calibration and registration. After registration and calibration have been completed, the SpineAssist software selects the optimal position of the selected arm for insertion of the drill sleeve and a cannulated drill guide is inserted into the arm which is automatically aligned along the predetermined trajectory. The drill then creates a cortical breach at the designated entry point and a guide wire is inserted into the vertebral body to allow a screw pilot hole to be drilled along the trajectory of the guide wire. A screw with an ideal length and diameter is then inserted into the pilot hole after pedicle probing and final confirmation of accuracy by the surgeon.[7,8]

Early cadaveric studies of this novel robotic-assisted technique have reported average deviations from preoperative templates to actual implant position to be 1 mm or less.[6,8] Togawa et al sought to evaluate the accuracy of bone-mounted miniature robotic systems for the percutaneous placement of pedicle and translaminar facet screws in a cadaveric series including 35 instrumented spinal levels. Using reconstructed 3D virtual X-rays of each vertebra, preoperative optimal entry points, and trajectories for screws were templated. A miniature robot was then mounted on to a clamp and the robotic system controlled the cannulated drill guide along the planned trajectory. K-wires were then advanced through the same cannulated guide trajectory and remained in the cadaver. Twenty-nine of 32 K-wires were found to be placed less than 1.5 mm of deviation, thus verifying the system's accuracy and lending support for its use in MIS surgery.[6]

Several clinical studies have attempted to determine the accuracy and efficacy of the SpineAssist robot (MAZOR Robotics Inc) in the clinical setting.[9,10] Roser et al demonstrated a 99% accuracy rate for lumbosacral pedicle screw instrumentation when utilizing the SpineAssist robot compared to 98 and 92% utilizing fluoroscopic and navigation techniques, respectively.[11] Utilizing the SpineAssist system, Schizas et al demonstrated a 95% accuracy rate in robot-assisted lumbosacral pedicle screw instrumentation compared to 92% accuracy rate with conventional fluoroscopy.[12] Kantelhardt et al demonstrated similar results with a 95% accuracy versus 92% accuracy when utilizing SpineAssist compared to conventional fluoroscopy.

Alternatively, some studies have found decreased screw accuracy rates. A randomized controlled trial by Ringel et al found a diminished accuracy rate of lumbosacral pedicle screw instrumentation with SpineAssist robot at 85% compared to 93% in fluoroscopy-guided screws ($p = 0.019$).[10] The authors identified several points which may have led to their inferior robotic accuracy. The authors noted that utilization of a percutaneous means of fixation with one K-wire attached to the spinous process and two Steinmann pins inserted into the posterior superior iliac spines may have been insufficient. The authors also identified potential lateral deflection (slippage) of the cannula during screw insertion which could have contributed to the malpositioning of screws (which, when found, were laterally deviated). In turn, the authors have recommended superior fixation for the hover T K-wire (mounting system for Mazor) and utilization of a more lateral entry point, increasing screw medicalization and potentially avoiding "slippage" down the side of hypertrophic facets.

5.4 Renaissance Robotic System

Introduced in the market in June 2011, the Renaissance Robotic System acts as the second-generation platform of the SpineAssist robotic system manufactured by Mazor Robotics. This newer generation robot further reduced dimensions and weight, and was engineered with enhanced ergonomic design, sensitivity of positioning, and significantly faster software transaction time. Furthermore, technological advances, primarily in the 2D C-arm output with 15-second manual scan providing 3D modeling, has allowed for the Renaissance Robotic system to be usable in real-time intraoperative implant corrections (C-OnSite).

Surgical Workflow of the Renaissance Robotic System

1. Preoperative planning stage:
   Spinal CT images are uploaded into the robotic software. These images are required to be compatible with vertebral anatomy and must have 0.4 to 1 mm of cross-sectional interval. The software subsequently converts CT images into a 3D representation which the surgeon utilizes to determine the spatial properties of the instrumentation in the form of screw diameter, length, and type of intervention. The system allows for precise fine tuning of inserted instrumentation in the 3D sagittal, coronal, and axial planes. These plans are then uploaded into the robot in the operating room via portable memory units.

2. Intraoperative determination of disposable clamp kit:
   There are a number of platform systems and percutaneous versus open surgery options from which the surgeon may select. The surgeon selects among options including T, lumbar, and thoracic clamp kits for the procedure.

3. Registration of clamp position:
   The system necessitates that the robot recognizes the appropriate coordinates of a clamp inserted into the vertebra in a 3D plane by matching preoperative planning information with preoperative X-rays. A disposable 3D marker kit is placed onto the clamp and anterior, posterior, and oblique X-ray images are obtained and uploaded into the robot. The software then provides results to the surgeon along with proposed margin of errors with acceptable margin of errors being between 0 and 1 mm. The surgeon must accept and confirm the results to continue.

4. Robot assembly and motion:
   A disposable kit is then stabilized on a suitable intraoperative platform on the patient with the aid of a clamp. The stability of the platform can be augmented by a second stabilizer onto the sacrum which avoids swift changes in the position of the robot due to possible unexpected movement of the table or of the patient. The surgeon then identifies specific coordinates on the patient and these coordinates are uploaded to the robot to facilitate localization.

5. Manual application: At this point, screws can be inserted down the predetermined path by means of a K-wire allowing for the execution of the planned surgical intervention.

5.5 ROSA Robot Medtech

The ROSA robot by Medtech (Medtech S.A., Montpellier, France) was originally designed for cranial neurosurgical applications, but was noted to have translational characteristics which could potentially address some of the technical flaws noted by Ringel et al[10] in spine applications. The ROSA robot design potentially mitigates the variability that comes with inadequate fixation of the robot onto the patient's bony anatomy. By design, the ROSA robot acts as a freestanding robotic assistant with a base that is stationary and fixed to the floor connected to a rigid robotic arm. Furthermore, the ROSA robot has a robotic arm that moves in a 3D plane in sync with the patient, guided by tracking camera monitoring and real-time, percutaneously placed tracking pins on the patient's bony anatomy which move in concordance with tracking spheres attached on the robot arm.[7] Lonjon et al reported a screw accuracy rate of 97.3% for screws placed with ROSA compared to 92% accuracy for a freehand technique.[13] To date, this robotic platform has yet to be validated for use in spinal pedicle instrumentation. As such, additional data are required to assess the clinical utility of the ROSA robot.

5.6 da Vinci Robotic System

The da Vinci robot system was approved by the Food and Drug Administration (FDA) in 2000 for general laparoscopic procedures. The da Vinci robot is functionally designed via the telesurgical model and although discussed more thoroughly in the telesurgical robotic chapter, a brief overview of its shared control features will be discussed herein. The telesurgical model is designed to allow a surgeon to visualize the operative field on a 3D vision screen while stationed in a telesurgical booth. The surgeon executes the operative procedure in the telesurgical booth and operates the robot as an extension of his or her arm to execute complex surgical techniques. Benefits of this model include limitless range of motion, tremor filtering, fatigue reduction, and stereoscopic vision with magnification.[14]

As an extension of its laparoscopic use, the da Vinci surgical system (Intuitive Surgical) has been extrapolated for use in laparoscopic anterior lumbar interbody fusion (ALIF) and has demonstrated promising clinical results. The increased visualization, magnification, and added dexterity afforded by the da Vinci surgical system can help avoid the morbidity of vascular or neurologic injury.[15,16]

The first laparoscopic ALIF was reported in 1991, utilizing the da Vinci robot via an MIS approach with the goal of reduction in vascular complications, retrograde ejaculation, postoperative pain, and improvements in recovery time, hospital stay, and incision size.[17] Early studies failed to demonstrate any technical or clinically significant advantage of the da Vinci robot over open ALIF[18,19,20] which lead to the dormancy of this technology for the next two decades. Recent changes to the usability of the da Vinci system prompted renewed interest in its role for spine surgery and over the past 5 years, a series of small case reports have demonstrated effective and safe surgical dissection in the approach of ALIF with good early fusion results.[21,22] To date the da Vinci robot is not yet FDA approved for the implantation of spinal instrumentation and more data are required to validate its use in spine surgery.

Applications for the da Vinci surgical system have also been extended to include transoral surgeries. In 2006, O'Malley was the first to present a series of robot-assisted transoral surgeries for squamous cell tumors where patients were demonstrated to subsequently report improved swallowing function with robotic surgery.[23] In the field of spine surgery, use of da Vinci for craniocervical cases requiring an anterior approach where a narrow surgical corridor (transoral) is utilized may lessen the technical difficulty and requisite dexterity in these cases.

In fact, several cadaveric studies have been performed exploring the potential utility of the da Vinci surgical system in the transoral approach of the craniocervical spine.[24] Lee et al utilized the da Vinci system to perform an odontoidectomy for a patient with basilar invagination and severe myelopathy.[25] Although the odontoid resection was successfully executed, the authors encountered significant difficulty with robotic use of the Kerrison punch and bone drilling, both of which will require further adjustments for future use. In 2012, the da Vinci surgical system obtained FDA clearance for use in transoral approaches in the setting of severe myelopathy and basilar invagination.

5.7 Broad Considerations

5.7.1 Radiation Exposure

Radiation exposure to operative staff during MIS procedures conducted using fluoroscopic guidance[26] has become a growing concern among the spine community. Shared controlled robotics offers the opportunity to greatly reduce radiation exposure with such procedures. A systematic review of the literature by Joseph et al evaluated radiation exposure in conjunction with robotic spinal instrumentation in 10 separate studies and found that robotic-assisted surgery consistently results in a lower amount of radiation exposure when compared to fluoroscopy-guided techniques.[27]

Kantelhardt et al demonstrated that robotically placed screws had a mean fluoroscopy time (FT) of 34 seconds per screw compared to a mean FT of 77 seconds for screws placed using conventional fluoroscopy.[9] Furthermore, in that series, there was no difference in fluoroscopic time whether screws were robotically placed open or percutaneously. Hyun et al showed a mean robotic FT per screw of 3.5 seconds compared to 13.3 for non-robotic screw insertion.[28] Ringel et al demonstrated similar results when comparing intraoperative FT in robotic and freehand pedicle groups and Schizas et al also noted radiation times to be similar between both groups.[10,12] Roser et al compared radiation exposure during freehand, standard navigation, and robotically placed screws. FT and total radiation dosage was lowest in the standard navigation group with the greatest FT found among the freehand cohort.[11]

5.7.2 Learning Curve

The introduction and implementation of novel surgical techniques, specifically robotics, carries its own learning curve. Devito et al assessed the ability to place screws via a shared control robotics system and found a success rate of 83.7% in their total cohort which subsequently increased to 90.8% when assessing more recent procedures performed later in their robotic experience.[29] Many studies also demonstrate expected increases in intraoperative efficiency overtime. Hu et al assessed the learning curve of robotic-assisted pedicle screw placement and demonstrated that after 30 procedures, the surgical success rate significantly increased with a commensurate decrease in conversion to open cases.[30]

To demonstrate the improvement in screw accuracy with increasing robotic experience, Schatlo et al assessed the accuracy of screw placement among 13 surgeons and graded accuracy by five-case increments. The authors found that the rate of misplacement peaked between 5 and 25 surgeries and steadily declined with surgeries beyond that point.[31] The authors postulated that this could be explained by a transition from decreased supervision to increased confidence of the surgeon when adopting new techniques prior to actually mastering them. The investigators further recommended ensuring competent supervision for new surgeons during the first 25 robotic spine procedures to optimize overall accuracy.[31]

5.8 Conclusion and Future Directions

Currently, the placement of pedicle screws via shared control robotic systems is supported in the literature as being safe and accurate in comparison to freehand techniques. The promise of improved outcomes must be tempered by potential limitations. These include a lack of high-quality prospective studies assessing operative times, cost–benefit, and overall patient outcomes.

From a workflow and design perspective, the success of these technologies ultimately depends on more widespread adoption by surgeons. Some barriers to use have been the potential for increased surgical time (at least early on), the potential for an inefficient workflow, and cumbersome machines in potentially limited operative room space.[10] With increasing use, demonstration of added efficiency may become more manifest and may lead to a paradigm shift where incorporation of spine robotics becomes more mainstream. As technology continues to advance, the applications of shared control robotics will likely continue to evolve.

References

[1] Kazemi N, Crew LK, Tredway TL. The future of spine surgery: new horizons in the treatment of spinal disorders. Surg Neurol Int. 2013; 4 Suppl 1:S15–S21

[2] Kosmopoulos V, Schizas C. Pedicle screw placement accuracy: a meta-analysis. Spine. 2007; 32(3):E111–E120

[3] Sautot P, Cinquin P, Lavallée S, Troccaz J. Computer assisted spine surgery: a first step toward clinical, application in orthopaedics. Paper presented at the 1992 14th Annual International Conference of the IEEE Engineering in Medicine and Biology Society, Paris; 1992:1071–1072

[4] Bertelsen A, Melo J, Sánchez E, Borro D. A review of surgical robots for spinal interventions. Int J Med Robot. 2013; 9(4):407–422

[5] Shoham M, Lieberman IH, Benzel EC, et al. Robotic assisted spinal surgery–from concept to clinical practice. Comput Aided Surg. 2007; 12(2):105–115

[6] Togawa D, Kayanja MM, Reinhardt MK, et al. Bone-mounted miniature robotic guidance for pedicle screw and translaminar facet screw placement: part 2–Evaluation of system accuracy. Neurosurgery. 2007; 60(2) Suppl 1: ONS129–ONS139, discussion ONS139

[7] Overley SC, Cho SK, Mehta AI, Arnold PM. Navigation and robotics in spinal surgery: where are we now? Neurosurgery. 2017; 80(3S):S86–S99

[8] Lieberman IH, Togawa D, Kayanja MM, et al. Bone-mounted miniature robotic guidance for pedicle screw and translaminar facet screw placement: Part I–Technical development and a test case result. Neurosurgery. 2006; 59(3): 641–650, discussion 641–650

[9] Kantelhardt SR, Martinez R, Baerwinkel S, Burger R, Giese A, Rohde V. Perioperative course and accuracy of screw positioning in conventional, open robotic-guided and percutaneous robotic-guided, pedicle screw placement. Eur Spine J. 2011; 20(6):860–868

[10] Ringel F, Stüer C, Reinke A, et al. Accuracy of robot-assisted placement of lumbar and sacral pedicle screws: a prospective randomized comparison to conventional freehand screw implantation. Spine. 2012; 37(8):E496–E501

[11] Roser F, Tatagiba M, Maier G. Spinal robotics: current applications and future perspectives. Neurosurgery. 2013; 72 Suppl 1:12–18

[12] Schizas C, Thein E, Kwiatkowski B, Kulik G. Pedicle screw insertion: robotic assistance versus conventional C-arm fluoroscopy. Acta Orthop Belg. 2012; 78(2):240–245

[13] Lonjon N, Chan-Seng E, Costalat V, Bonnafoux B, Vassal M, Boetto J. Robot-assisted spine surgery: feasibility study through a prospective case-matched analysis. Eur Spine J. 2016; 25(3):947–955

[14] Lanfranco AR, Castellanos AE, Desai JP, Meyers WC. Robotic surgery: a current perspective. Ann Surg. 2004; 239(1):14–21

[15] Quah HM, Jayne DG, Eu KW, Seow-Choen F. Bladder and sexual dysfunction following laparoscopically assisted and conventional open mesorectal resection for cancer. Br J Surg. 2002; 89(12):1551–1556

[16] Than KD, Wang AC, Rahman SU, et al. Complication avoidance and management in anterior lumbar interbody fusion. Neurosurg Focus. 2011; 31(4):E6

[17] Obenchain TG. Laparoscopic lumbar discectomy: case report. J Laparoendosc Surg. 1991; 1(3):145–149

[18] Chung SK, Lee SH, Lim SR, et al. Comparative study of laparoscopic L5-S1 fusion versus open mini-ALIF, with a minimum 2-year follow-up. Eur Spine J. 2003; 12(6):613–617

[19] Inamasu J, Guiot BH. Laparoscopic anterior lumbar interbody fusion: a review of outcome studies. Minim Invasive Neurosurg. 2005; 48(6):340–347

[20] Liu JC, Ondra SL, Angelos P, Ganju A, Landers ML. Is laparoscopic anterior lumbar interbody fusion a useful minimally invasive procedure? Neurosurgery. 2002; 51(5) Suppl:S155–S158

[21] Lee JY, Bhowmick DA, Eun DD, Welch WC. Minimally invasive, robot-assisted, anterior lumbar interbody fusion: a technical note. J Neurol Surg A Cent Eur Neurosurg. 2013; 74(4):258–261

[22] Lee Z, Lee JY, Welch WC, Eun D. Technique and surgical outcomes of robot-assisted anterior lumbar interbody fusion. J Robot Surg. 2013; 7(2):177–185

[23] Weinstein GS, O'Malley BW, Jr, Snyder W, Hockstein NG. Transoral robotic surgery: supraglottic partial laryngectomy. Ann Otol Rhinol Laryngol. 2007; 116(1):19–23

[24] Lee JY, O'Malley BW, Jr, Newman JG, et al. Transoral robotic surgery of the skull base: a cadaver and feasibility study. ORL J Otorhinolaryngol Relat Spec. 2010; 72(4):181–187

[25] Lee JY, Lega B, Bhowmick D, et al. Da Vinci Robot-assisted transoral odontoidectomy for basilar invagination. ORL J Otorhinolaryngol Relat Spec. 2010; 72 (2):91–95

[26] Yu E, Khan SN. Does less invasive spine surgery result in increased radiation exposure? A systematic review. Clin Orthop Relat Res. 2014; 472(6):1738–1748

[27] Joseph JR, Smith BW, Liu X, Park P. Current applications of robotics in spine surgery: a systematic review of the literature. Neurosurg Focus. 2017; 42(5): E2

[28] Hyun SJ, Kim KJ, Jahng TA, Kim HJ. Minimally invasive robotic versus open fluoroscopic-guided spinal instrumented fusions: a randomized controlled trial. Spine. 2017; 42(6):353–358

[29] Devito DP, Kaplan L, Dietl R, et al. Clinical acceptance and accuracy assessment of spinal implants guided with SpineAssist surgical robot: retrospective study. Spine. 2010; 35(24):2109–2115

[30] Hu X, Ohnmeiss DD, Lieberman IH. Robotic-assisted pedicle screw placement: lessons learned from the first 102 patients. Eur Spine J. 2013; 22(3):661–666

[31] Schatlo B, Martinez R, Alaid A, et al. Unskilled unawareness and the learning curve in robotic spine surgery. Acta Neurochir (Wien). 2015; 157(10):1819–1823, discussion 1823

6 Telesurgical Robots

Kyle W. Mombell and Patrick B. Morrissey

Abstract

Telesurgical robots are machines that allow for the completion of complex and delicate surgical tasks under direct control of an operative surgeon. These robots are indefatigable, capable of performing precise maneuvers in confined spaces, and controlled through a remote workstation that can be positioned anywhere, from beside the patient to another operating room around the world. Several telerobotic systems have been developed, with proven applications in cardiac, general surgical, urologic, gynecologic, and laparoscopic procedures. More recently, applications in spinal surgery have begun to emerge with procedures such as anterior lumbar interbody fusion and paraspinal tumor excision demonstrating successful integration of telesurgical technologies. This chapter outlines the evolution of telesurgical robot technology and provides an overview of current and future surgical capabilities of the most commonly used system, da Vinci, particularly as it relates to applications in spinal surgery.

Keywords: telesurgical robots, robotic spine surgery, robot-assisted surgery, anterior lumbar interbody fusion, ZEUS, da Vinci

6.1 Introduction

Telerobotic surgery has its origins in battlefield medicine. After successful demonstration of telesurgical open bowel anastomosis with the system created by Phil Green and colleagues with the Stanford Research Institute (SRI), the United States Army utilized Department of Defense grants and collaboration with the Defense Advanced Research Projects Agency (DARPA) to prototype a mechanism to allow surgeons to operate on combat casualties at a site remote from the battlefield.[1] Their vision was to deploy robotic arms to casualties via armored vehicles to the site of the battlefield injury while the surgeon remained at the forward surgical hospital controlling the robot remotely. This was performed for the first time in 1994 when a porcine intestinal anastomosis was performed via wireless microwave connection.

6.2 ZEUS Robotic System

Commercially available modern telesurgical robots began with the implementation of the ZEUS system (Computer Motion, Santa Barbara, CA) in 1998. ZEUS introduced the concept of master–slave telepresence surgery with the surgeon at a console remote from the patient.[2] The ZEUS robot consists of a Storz 3D imaging system (Karl Storz Endoscopy, Santa Barbara, CA) and three arms, two of which are surgical and the third an automated imaging arm. The ZEUS robot achieved success in closed chest beating heart cardiac surgery and successfully performed a telerobotic cholecystectomy on a patient in Strasbourg, France, with the surgeon and console in New York.[3,4,5,6,7] The ZEUS robot was produced until 2003 when its parent company merged with Intuitive Surgical. It was subsequently phased out in favor of the now commonplace da Vinci Telesurgical System (▶ Fig. 6.1).

6.3 da Vinci Robotic System

Following the successful trials of the Department of Defense and DARPA prototypes, the surgeon and entrepreneur Frederick H. Moll created Intuitive Surgical, a company founded on the goal of solving the limitations of conventional endoscopic surgery by advancing the concept of telerobotic surgery.[1,8]

The da Vinci robotic system (Intuitive Surgical, Sunnyvale, CA) is currently the only Food and Drug Administration (FDA)-approved robot for laparoscopic surgery and the most well-known with over 1,400 units deployed in the United States as of 2011 and the number of telesurgical procedures increasing 400% over the preceding 4 years.[9] In 1997, the first telesurgical robotic cholecystectomy was performed and in the following year, the first cardiac revascularization procedure was performed with early versions of the da Vinci. While the initial development of the system focused on the potential role for cardiac revascularization, results in this field lagged behind those in general surgery and the device was first FDA-approved in 2000 for general laparoscopic abdominal surgeries.[10,11,12,13] In the same year, the first robotic prostatectomy was performed utilizing the da Vinci which heralded the beginning of the robot's widespread use in urologic and gynecologic surgeries (▶ Fig. 6.2).[14,15]

6.3.1 Design

The da Vinci is a master–slave style robotic system with separate surgical and control consoles. The control console is composed of a computer and 3D imaging system and is responsible for remotely controlling the robotic arms. The surgical tower is deactivated by an infrared sensor when the surgeon's eyes exit the binoculars, thus acting as a safety mechanism to prevent inadvertent movements. The robot is able to imitate the human wrist with seven degrees of freedom and two planes of axial rotation, providing maximal dexterity within the tight confines of the surgical space. Limited haptic feedback is available to the surgeon through resistance of movement, when tensioning suture, for example; however, the majority of tactile information is derived from visual clues.[7] The da Vinci employs binocular endoscopic vision to immerse the surgeon in a 3D experience, enhancing depth perception and special awareness.[16] This is created by two independent scopes within the 12-mm telescope whose images are transmitted to separate but synchronized screens inside the surgeon's console.[17]

6.3.2 Technical Advantages

Traditional laparoscopic surgery has several fundamental limitations. These are related to the length and lack of articulation of laparoscopic instruments, which decrease precision and limit

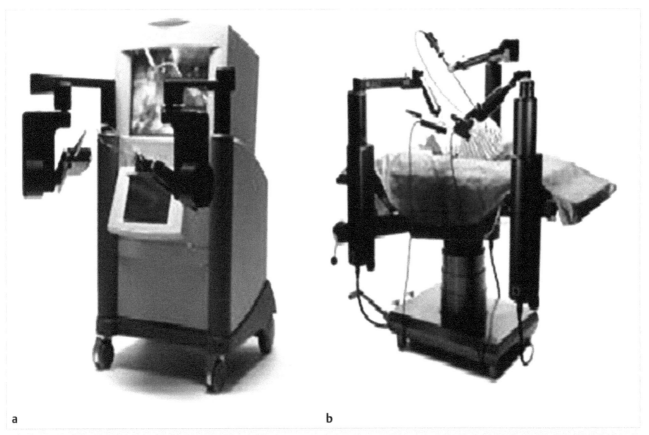

a   b

Fig. 6.1 (a,b) ZEUS Robotic Surgical System. (Reproduced with permission from Ghezzi TL, Corleta OC. 30 years of robotic surgery. World J Surg 2016;40:2550–2557.)

motion due to the fulcrum effect of the body wall. By adding articulation to the endoscopic instruments, placing the sensors near the tips and creating software to eliminate tremor and enhance fine movements, the da Vinci system has multiple theoretical advantages over laparoscopic surgery both technically and ergonomically.[7] Clinical outcome studies for robotic surgery are currently limited but show at least equivalent results to similar laparoscopic general surgery procedures. Promising results for robotic procedures have been shown in randomized controlled trials exhibiting lower risk of viscus perforation, improved postoperative quality of life, and shorter hospital stays with robotic Heller myotomy, bariatric surgery, and cholecystectomy, among other procedures, when compared to their laparoscopic equivalent. Disadvantages of increased cost, increased surgical time, and conversion to open procedures are common, but not particularly problematic in today's healthcare environment.[18]

6.3.3 Applications in Spine Surgery

Applications of telesurgical robotics with the da Vinci system are evolving but remain limited in spine surgery. Currently, most applications are theoretical or cadaver/animal-based models; however, several case reports and case series exist regarding demonstrated utility of the da Vinci system in real-world spinal procedures.

Anterior Lumbar Interbody Fusion

Case reports and a small case series demonstrate the safety and feasibility of early application of the da Vinci robot for anterior lumbar interbody fusion. The largest case series describes a single institution's experience with utilizing the da Vinci for access to the ventral lumbar spine in 11 patients. This was performed by a urologist and the robot was undocked for the diskectomy and fusion portion of the case which was performed laparoscopically. There were no complications in the series related to the approach.[19] Case reports and operative techniques exist for performing the diskectomy and fusion in a porcine model. Advantages of careful dissection of the retroperitoneal space including great vessels, ureters, and hypogastric plexus are cited, while lack of procedure-specific instrumentation and a significant learning curve for the surgeon and team is acknowledged.[20,21]

Robotic-Assisted Transoral Odontoidectomy

At present, cadaveric and case report evidence exists for robotic-assisted transoral odontoidectomy for decompression of the craniocervical junction.[22,23] The authors of these reports propose use of the da Vinci robot for careful dissection of delicate structures in a tight space. No notable cord or adjacent tissue injuries were reported despite the lack of tactile feedback the da Vinci offers.

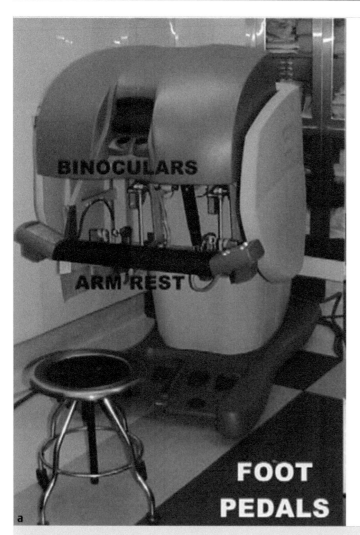
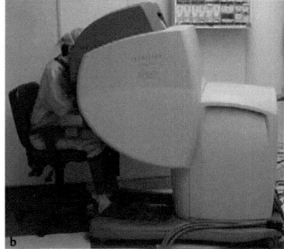
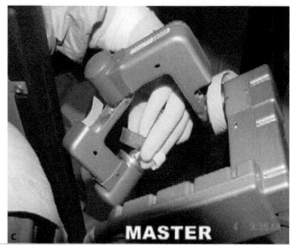

Fig. 6.2 The surgeon's master control console for the da Vinci system. (a) The surgeon places his eyes in the binoculars. (b) The console is adjustable and ergonomic. (c) The master controls the movement of the telesurgical instruments. (Reproduced with permission from Ballantyne GH, Moll F. The da Vinci telerobotic surgical system: the virtual operative field and telepresence surgery. Surg Clin North Am 2003;83:1293–304, vii.)

Tumor Surgery

Case reports detail the use of the da Vinci telesurgical robot in resection of complex paraspinal schwannomas.[24] First, a laminectomy and facetectomy was carried out with a posterolateral approach with minimally invasive retractors (Nuvasive, San Diego, CA). Next, a minimally invasive thoracoscopy was performed with the da Vinci system for resection of the intrathoracic portion of the schwannoma. Both patients in the case report had complete gross resections of the tumor without complication and a 3-day or less hospital stay while avoiding the morbidity of an open thoracotomy.

Future Directions

Animal model experiments support the use of the da Vinci system for robotic approaches to the posterior spine. Citing improved ergonomics for the surgeon and indefatigability of the robot, Ponnusamy et al proposed utilizing the da Vinci for routine posterior lumbar surgery including laminotomy and laminectomy.[25] The authors acknowledged the present lack of purposefully designed instrumentation for these procedures but showed encouraging results with improved surgeon stamina and precise soft-tissue handling. Translation to clinical research is warranted to assess whether these advantages result in improved patient outcomes, lowered blood loss, and reduced durotomy rates as suggested in the investigation.

6.4 Conclusion

As spine surgeons continue to explore the capabilities of telerobotic surgery, it is likely that the field undergoes a similar period of rapid growth similar to that of other surgical specialties. This is particularly true with respect to the evolution of minimally invasive technologies and techniques, where the spatial limitations of the human hand and the visualization difficulties of current minimally invasive access systems provide the most significant barriers to progress. Telesurgical robots offer solutions to these problems through their compact end effector units and videoscopic capabilities.

In addition to the technical benefits, as telesurgical equipment and techniques become more mainstream, the potential for remote surgery, with surgeon and patient separated by hundreds or even thousands of miles, will increase, expanding the reach of spine surgery experts outside their local populations to more remote locations with previously limited access to the skills of a surgical subspecialist.

References

[1] Ballantyne GH, Moll F. The da Vinci telerobotic surgical system: the virtual operative field and telepresence surgery. Surg Clin North Am. 2003; 83(6): 1293–1304, vii

[2] Kalan S, Chauhan S, Coelho RF, et al. History of robotic surgery. J Robot Surg. 2010; 4(3):141–147

[3] Reichenspurner H, Damiano RJ, Mack M, et al. Use of the voice-controlled and computer-assisted surgical system ZEUS for endoscopic coronary artery bypass grafting. J Thorac Cardiovasc Surg. 1999; 118(1):11–16

[4] Boehm DH, Reichenspurner H, Gulbins H, et al. Early experience with robotic technology for coronary artery surgery. Ann Thorac Surg. 1999; 68(4):1542–1546

[5] Boehm DH, Reichenspurner H, Detter C, et al. Clinical use of a computer-enhanced surgical robotic system for endoscopic coronary artery bypass grafting on the beating heart. Thorac Cardiovasc Surg. 2000; 48(4):198–202

[6] Boyd WD, Rayman R, Desai ND, et al. Closed-chest coronary artery bypass grafting on the beating heart with the use of a computer-enhanced surgical robotic system. J Thorac Cardiovasc Surg. 2000; 120(4):807–809

[7] Marescaux J, Leroy J, Gagner M, et al. Transatlantic robot-assisted telesurgery. Nature. 2001; 413(6854):379–380

[8] Satava RM. Surgical robotics: the early chronicles: a personal historical perspective. Surg Laparosc Endosc Percutan Tech. 2002; 12(1):6–16

[9] Carreyrou J. Annual report. Intuitive surgical. 2011.Available at: http://phx.corporate-ir.net/phoenix.zhtml? c=122359&p=irol-irhome. Accessed September 24, 2012

[10] Himpens J, Leman G, Cadiere GB. Telesurgical laparoscopic cholecystectomy. Surg Endosc. 1998; 12(8):1091

[11] Hagen ME, Stein H, Curet MJ. Introduction to the robotic system. In: Kim CH, ed. Robotics in General Surgery. New York, NY: Springer; 2014:9–16

[12] Hashizume M, Sugimachi K. Robot-assisted gastric surgery. Surg Clin North Am. 2003; 83(6):1429–1444

[13] Leal Ghezzi T, Campos Corleta O. 30 years of robotic surgery. World J Surg. 2016; 40(10):2550–2557

[14] Binder J, Kramer W. Robotically-assisted laparoscopic radical prostatectomy. BJU Int. 2001; 87(4):408–410

[15] Ficarra V, Cavalleri S, Novara G, Aragona M, Artibani W. Evidence from robot-assisted laparoscopic radical prostatectomy: a systematic review. Eur Urol. 2007; 51(1):45–55, discussion 56

[16] Byrn JC, Schluender S, Divino CM, et al. Three-dimensional imaging improves surgical performance for both novice and experienced operators using the da Vinci Robot System. Am J Surg. 2007; 193(4):519–522

[17] Sung GT, Gill IS. Robotic laparoscopic surgery: a comparison of the DA Vinci and Zeus systems. Urology. 2001; 58(6):893–898

[18] Maeso S, Reza M, Mayol JA, et al. Efficacy of the Da Vinci surgical system in abdominal surgery compared with that of laparoscopy: a systematic review and meta-analysis. Ann Surg. 2010; 252(2):254–262

[19] Lee Z, Lee JY, Welch WC, Eun D. Technique and surgical outcomes of robot-assisted anterior lumbar interbody fusion. J Robot Surg. 2013; 7(2):177–185

[20] Kim MJ, Ha Y, Yang MS, et al. Robot-assisted anterior lumbar interbody fusion (ALIF) using retroperitoneal approach. Acta Neurochir (Wien). 2010; 152(4): 675–679

[21] Yang MS, Yoon DH, Kim KN, et al. Robot-assisted anterior lumbar interbody fusion in a Swine model in vivo test of the da Vinci surgical-assisted spinal surgery system. Spine. 2011; 36(2):E139–E143

[22] Yang MS, Yoon TH, Yoon DH, Kim KN, Pennant W, Ha Y. Robot-assisted transoral odontoidectomy : experiment in new minimally invasive technology, a cadaveric study. J Korean Neurosurg Soc. 2011; 49(4):248–251

[23] Lee JY, Lega B, Bhowmick D, et al. Da Vinci Robot-assisted transoral odontoidectomy for basilar invagination. ORL J Otorhinolaryngol Relat Spec. 2010; 72 (2):91–95

[24] Perez-Cruet MJ, Welsh RJ, Hussain NS, Begun EM, Lin J, Park P. Use of the da Vinci minimally invasive robotic system for resection of a complicated paraspinal schwannoma with thoracic extension: case report. Neurosurgery. 2012; 71(1) Suppl Operative:209–214

[25] Ponnusamy K, Chewning S, Mohr C. Robotic approaches to the posterior spine. Spine. 2009; 34(19):2104–2109

7 Supervisory-Controlled Robotics

Sohrab Pahlavan and Nathan H. Lebwohl

Abstract:

Supervisory-controlled robotics involves a semiautomated process executed by a robotic application that is actively supervised by a human operator. It is derived from supervisory-controlled theory and has been widely applied in vehicular and infrastructural processes prior to its introduction to surgery. Supervisory-controlled robotics in surgery involves the combination of process control and vehicle control into a manipulator system. It generally involves three stages: planning, registration, and navigation. Planning involves image acquisition, registration applies this to the surgical field, and navigation involves executing the physical work of performing the procedure. Various iterations of supervisory-controlled systems have been developed for surgery. The applications for spine surgery have mainly involved assisting in spinal instrumentation. Future developments are aimed toward safer and less invasive execution of other components of procedures such as decompression. The potential advantages of supervisory systems are improved precision and a less invasive approach. Potential pitfalls are failing to recognize errors in data interpretation and execution, especially between registration and execution stages. While future applications of robotic surgery may eventually seek full automation, supervisory-controlled systems offer precision and improved and less invasive surgical trajectories while having the safety of human supervision.

Keywords: supervisory control, vehicle control, process control, manipulator system, robotic spine surgery

7.1 Introduction

In medicine, robotic applications are generally divided into three different categories.[1] The first is shared control systems, where the surgeon provides the input and guidance for actions as the robot gives feedback and input on the actions, usually in the form of movement enhancement or stabilization. The second is the telesurgery system where the surgeon remotely controls the robot movements as in the da Vinci surgical system. The third is the supervisory-controlled robotic systems, which are the focus of this chapter.

7.2 Supervisory-Controlled Theory

Supervisory-controlled robotics is derived from supervisory-controlled theory,[2] which in general takes two forms. One is where an automated process is directly supervised by human control and, when needed, has its algorithm modified to better meet the needs of the operator's goals. The alternative form involves a preprogrammed machine process, which completes a smaller task, provides feedback on the result, and then awaits further instructions from a human operator in how to proceed. Essentially, it is a process in which the human operator, on a continuous basis, is programming (i.e., instructing) the robot, which in turn continuously relays information back regarding the operating environment. In one respect, it takes a step back from a fully automated environment that requires the ability to sense and respond to every possible combination of problems and challenges that can arise. The supervisory system instead leaves any problems that arise during the automated process to the human operator to respond to and solve.

Supervisory control has been a dominant element in process control and vehicle control for over half a century, playing major roles in improving safety, efficacy, and overall capabilities in several sectors of industry and infrastructure.[2] Process control is integral to the operations of power plants and water management systems to name a few large-scale processes. Vehicle control has had a large role in aerospace systems, underwater exploration, and industrial manufacturing with famous examples including the Apollo spacecraft, modern air traffic control, and underwater submarines. More pertinent to robotic surgery, however, is the combination of process and vehicle control into a manipulator system such as a robotic arm or display system that expands the human operator's capabilities.

The manipulator system application of a supervisory-controlled system is what underlies the modern robotic surgery system. Compared to an assembly line system, where each task is predetermined, applications requiring supervisory control of manipulators consist of unpredictable tasks and environments. The human operator (i.e., surgeon) must program the manipulator (i.e., robot) in order to deal with each new situation. This may even include merely initiating predetermined tasks at the correct time.

7.3 Supervisory-Controlled Surgery Elements and Applications

In general, supervisory-controlled robotic surgery consists of three steps—planning, registration, and navigation. The planning stage consists of gathering imaging data of the patient. This may consist of X-rays, computed tomography (CT) scans, magnetic resonance imaging (MRI), or ultrasound images. The imaging collected is usually limited to the anatomical area pertinent to the procedure to be performed. It can either be collected preoperatively or intraoperatively using newer generation imaging acquisition systems. The registration phase involves identifying the pertinent anatomical points on the patient and match them to their corresponding imaging sequences from the planning stage. Finally, the navigation stage is where the operator (i.e., surgeon) verifies the planning stage and positions the robot according to the registered points followed by execution of the supervised protocol.

One of the first supervisory surgical systems was the Probot, developed in the late 1980s at Imperial College of London. Its application was in prostatic surgery and allowed the surgeon to predetermine the volume of prostatic tissue to be cut and would then automatically proceed to do so without active control of the surgeon. Another system was the ROBODOC from Integrated Surgical Systems, developed in 1992, designed to improve implant placement during total hip arthroplasty.[3,4]

Early applications of supervisory-controlled systems in spinal surgery were focused on enhancement of precision and accuracy of placement of spinal instrumentation. One of the best-known systems is the SpineAssist (MAZOR Surgical Technologies, Caesarea, Israel) that uses a mounted robotic arm to guide the surgeon in placing instrumentation for spinal stabilization.[4]

7.4 Advantages and Pitfalls of Supervisory Control

Potential advantages of supervisory control include the potential to improve quality and productivity with the ability to enable automation and execution of the surgical trajectory.[5] While the technology for implant placement now is widely available, newer applications including cauterization, dissection, decompression, and closure could also be made available. This is especially valuable in operations involving areas with highly constrained space and limited approach trajectory options.[6] Hence, the great benefit of supervisory-controlled systems is the precision they offer, which in the case of spine surgery theoretically entails less tissue trauma and lower rates of instrumentation malpositioning.

Potential disadvantages of supervisory control mainly relate to the inability of the system itself to recognize error in the data collection phase prior to execution. If, during planning and registration phases, there is some form of discrepancy between the input and the desired output, catastrophic injury could occur. An example is if a navigation registration marker is somehow erroneously altered between the registration and the navigation phase of a procedure. In such a case, instrumentation, for example, could be placed in an erroneous path, potentially causing harm. Due to the potential for such error, it is imperative that all supervisory-controlled systems have an actively engaged and vigilant operator.

7.5 Conclusion

Supervisory-controlled robotics has a long track record of safe and efficient use in the industrial sector and with further development of surgical robotics it will extend into more widespread use in medicine as well. While there may ultimately be an evolution into fully automated systems, safety and technological limits will, for the time being, leave supervisory control as a safer and more efficient approach to robotic surgery. It allows the reproducibility and augmented mechanical ability that robots provide with the safety and real-time vigilance of human supervision.

References

[1] Nathoo N, Cavuşoğlu MC, Vogelbaum MA, Barnett GH. In touch with robotics: neurosurgery for the future. Neurosurgery. 2005; 56(3):421–433, discussion 421–433

[2] Sheridan TB. Telerobotics, Automation, and Human Supervisory Control. MIT Press; 1992

[3] Satava RM. Surgical robotics: the early chronicles: a personal historical perspective. Surg Laparosc Endosc Percutan Tech. 2002; 12(1):6–16

[4] Ryan H, Tsuda S. Essentials of Robotic Surgery. In: Kroh M, Chalikonda S, eds. Springer; 2015

[5] Karas CS, Chiocca EA. Neurosurgical robotics: a review of brain and spine applications. J Robot Surg. 2007; 1(1):39–43

[6] Chop WW, Green B, Levi A. Fluoroscopic guided targeting system with a robotic arm for pedicle screw insertion. Neurosurgery. 2000; 47:872–878

8 Radiation Exposure and Navigated Spinal Surgery

Scott C. Wagner

Abstract:

Ionizing radiation exposure during instrumented spinal surgery may be associated with increased long-term risks to the surgeon, operating room staff, and patient. Advances in computerized navigation techniques allow for improved accuracy of instrumentation placement and may be associated with decreased intra-operative fluoroscopy requirements. These new technologies may also be associated with increased radiation exposure to individual patients, increased upfront costs, and are thus far without any proven decrease in perioperative complications. However, as the technology improves, these navigation systems may yield cost-effective techniques to minimize the need for continuous fluoroscopy during minimally invasive spine surgery and reduce overall radiation exposure to the operating team.

Keywords: navigation, ionizing radiation, fluoroscopy, robotics

8.1 Introduction

As spinal surgeons continue to strive for increasingly minimally invasive surgical techniques for various spinal interventions, a trend toward reliance on various intraoperative image-guidance systems to aid in achieving minimal access goals has developed.[1] Such systems include traditional fluoroscopy, computer-assisted navigation (CAN), and various robotic platforms. However, the cumulative ionizing radiation dose to spinal surgeons secondary to this increasing reliance on intraoperative fluoroscopy has also become an area of significant interest and research, as there may be an increased risk of certain types of malignancies to spinal surgeons related to this lifetime exposure.[2,3] Strategies to mitigate, or at least reduce, the cumulative radiation exposure have begun to gain widespread traction in the spine surgery community, and advances in navigation and robotics may have some theoretical advantages in this regard.

Since the first pedicle screw was implanted via CAN in 1995, three-dimensional navigation and robotic systems continue to transform the landscape of spine surgery.[4,5,6] These systems have been shown to improve pedicle screw accuracy throughout the literature.[7,8,9,10] There is also an increasing awareness of the impact these systems may have on radiation exposure to the patient, surgeon, and operating room team.[11] Some studies have attempted to examine the radiation dose to individual patients with regard to the use of navigation, as there is some concern regarding additional preoperative or intraoperative computed tomography (CT).[12] Hypothetically, however, CAN may decrease or altogether obviate the necessity of intraoperative fluoroscopy, thereby reducing surgeon exposure to radiation, particularly when compared to traditional fluoroscopic image guidance. The benefits to the surgeon and operating room team must be considered in the context of potential risks to the patient, and vice versa. In this chapter, studies evaluating the effects of various CAN and robotic platforms on radiation exposure to the patient, surgeon, and operating room team will be explored. However, it is important to clearly note that the literature directly comparing radiation exposure to patients and surgical teams in navigated and nonnavigated spinal instrumentation cohorts is relatively limited, and major recommendations have not yet been established.

8.2 Patient Exposure

Many studies, including a relatively recent meta-analysis, have demonstrated the precision and accuracy with which pedicle screws can be placed with CAN.[13,14,15] In addition, other spinal procedures such as vertebral body augmentation for fractures[1] or intradiscal electrothermal treatments[16] can also be performed with the use of navigation. While no obvious clinical benefit has been demonstrated with regard to more accurate pedicle screw placement,[17] concerns have been raised with regard to potentially increased radiation exposure to the patient secondary to either pre- or intraoperative CT scan.[12]

Mendelsohn et al[18] performed a retrospective cohort study examining CAN versus fluoroscopic-guided pedicle screw instrumentation. The authors found that for 73 patients in the CAN group, "intraoperative CT-based navigation increased the radiation dose emitted to the patient by 2.77 times compared with conventional fluoroscopy-guided cases." However, the authors note that the cumulative dose to the patient intraoperatively was less than a traditional CT scan, such as would be obtained for preoperative CAN systems. In contrast, Urbanski et al[19] compared traditional freehand pedicle screw placement versus placement with intraoperative 3D navigation in patients with idiopathic scoliosis and assessed the radiation dose received by patients with both techniques. The authors found no difference in accuracy between techniques in 49 consecutive patients, though the only pedicle breaches greater than 4 mm occurred in the upper thoracic spine in the freehand group. Most alarming, however, was their finding that patients undergoing CAN pedicle screws received almost 700 mGy/cm more than the freehand group, which was statistically significant.

In contrast, however, Villard et al[11] conducted a randomized prospective trial of CAN versus fluoroscopy-guided pedicle screw placement in 21 patients undergoing lower thoracic and/or transforaminal lumbar interbody fusion (TLIF) to determine patient radiation exposure risk. They identified instances of radiation exposure occurring at several different points during the navigated procedures, namely (1) when marking the spinal level initially; (2) positioning of the C-arm after exposure prior to running the 3D scan; (3) implantation of the interbody devices; and (4) final 3D images to confirm screw position prior to wound closure. Cumulative radiation dose to the patient was obtained from the imaging system and was found to be reduced in the navigated group (888 vs 1,884 cGy/cm^2, respectively), though this finding did not reach statistical significance. The authors concluded that despite failing to show any statistically significant reduction in patient radiation exposure, the trend toward decreased total dose should be considered. Further corroborating these findings in a comparative cohort study,

Fomekong et al[20] found that the radiation exposure to patients undergoing percutaneous pedicle screw implantation was significantly reduced with intraoperative three-dimensional fluoroscopy: the average radiation dose per patient was 571.9 mGy/m2 in the nonnavigated group, compared with 365.6 mGy/m2 in the navigated group. Zhang et al[21] had similar findings when using intraoperative CT-based navigation during lateral interbody fusion: radiation exposure to the patient was significantly lower in the intraoperative CT scan group compared to the conventional fluoroscopy group (9.38 vs. 44.59 mGy, respectively).

In a study examining patient radiation exposure during navigated vertebral body augmentation with kyphoplasty or vertebroplasty, Barzilay et al[1] reported that the use of robotic assistance initially increased radiation exposure to the patient by the nature of the requirements for high-kV preoperative CT scan; however, they were able to alter the preoperative protocol and reduce the preoperative dose to the patient by 75%. When compared to the published literature on navigated vertebral augmentation, they found a reduction of over 50% in radiation exposure with the use of surgical robotics. However, they noted that in patients with osteoporosis, a higher power preoperative CT scan may be required to successfully navigate such procedures.[1] Based on this study, it may be likely that the tradeoff for decreased intraoperative radiation exposure may increase preoperative exposure, but may vary from patient to patient. A systematic review examining this question concludes that the use of intraoperative CT to facilitate CAN results in increased radiation exposure to the patient, specifically when compared with standard fluoroscopy, but the authors found that in general it is a lower dose than preoperative CT.[22]

8.3 Operating Team Exposure

While radiation dose to the patient is of high concern, it is the cumulative effect on the surgeon and the operating team that must also be considered. While some authors argue that alterations in radiation exposure to the patient are limited to a single operation, a surgeon and the circulating nurse, scrub technician, and other members of the surgical team are often exposed over the course of hundreds or thousands of surgeries throughout many years. In fact, some literature has associated intraoperative radiation exposure with the occurrence of some malignancies in providers performing some image-guided spinal procedures. Harstall et al[23] found that during fluoroscopy-guided percutaneous vertebroplasty, average annual exposure to the lens of the eye was roughly 8% of the cumulative dose related to the development of cataracts, while the incidence of thyroid malignancy leading to death was 25 times greater than in the general population.

A recent prospective, randomized comparison of navigated versus freehand transforaminal lumbar spinal instrumentation measured surgeon radiation exposure by placing dosimeters on the dominant forearm and at the levels of the thorax and eyes.[11] They found that the accumulated radiation dose was significantly higher for the surgeon in the nonnavigated group. Specifically, exposure to the thorax, the eyes, and the forearm was 9.96, 5.06, and 6.53 times higher with fluoroscopy, respectively.[11] These differences were due to fluoroscopy use during pedicle screw insertion, as fluoroscopy was utilized during the interbody cage placement portion of the procedures in both groups. Similarly, the retrospective cohort study by Mendelsohn et al[18] examined 73 navigated spinal instrumentation procedures that utilized intraoperative CT scan, comparing radiation exposure (defined as the effective dose, a risk-weighted measure of radiation compared with background radiation) to historical controls. The authors found that the overall effective dose to the surgical team was decreased compared to exposure levels reported for conventional fluoroscopy-guided procedures, though a lack of control group limited the applicability of the findings. Kraus et al,[24] using a retrospective analysis of cervical spine trauma, found that three-dimensional computer navigation decreased the overall radiation emitted during surgery, despite increasing the operative time. A recently published systematic review concluded that using advanced imaging, such as CT and/or three-dimensional C-arm imaging with computer-assisted navigation, can overall lead to a decrease in radiation exposure to operating room personnel and surgeons, rather than conventional fluoroscopy.[22]

Overall, the available literature appears to support the conclusion that utilization of intra- or preoperative CT and computer-assisted navigation can decrease the amount of radiation to which the operating team is exposed. Typically, most surgical teams leave the operating room during intraoperative CT and use of preoperative CT may obviate intraoperative radiation completely. When compared to standard intraoperative imaging, such as traditional fluoroscopy, the differences appear to be substantial.

8.4 Cost Considerations

While there may be benefits in terms of radiation exposure with the use of CAN, other considerations also exist that may influence the decision to pursue navigation: in particular, CAN and robotics systems are expensive. One study evaluated the cost-effectiveness of these systems for use in pedicle screw placement: Dea et al[25] published an observational case–control study that compared pedicle screw placement with conventional fluoroscopy and CAN, assessing the number of reoperations for screw misplacement in both groups. The study also compared the cost of obtaining and maintaining an intraoperative CAN system to the cost of reoperations. A total of 502 patients (5,132 pedicle screws) were included, and the authors found that the pedicle screw accuracy rate was lower, and the revision rate was higher, in the conventional control group, and the CAN system was cost-effective based on the number of reoperations that were avoided.

8.5 Conclusion

The demand for less invasive spinal surgery continues to rise. Various imaging tools have been developed to allow for decreasing access and incision requirements, but the burden of increased radiation exposure associated therewith is not without problems. Careless or nonjudicious use of ionizing radiation can lead to long-term, harmful effects on both patients and providers, and as such techniques and strategies to minimize radiation exposure are becoming more important. The advent of computer-assisted navigation systems, including intraoperative

CT and robotics, may be part of those strategies. Despite the increased upfront costs of obtaining such navigation systems, improved screw accuracy and decreased radiation exposure may make these systems cost-effective in the long term. By reducing the need for continuous radiation exposure during minimally invasive spinal surgery, the surgeon can positively impact the delayed and immediate effects of ionizing radiation exposure to the entire operating room staff.

References

[1] Barzilay Y, Schroeder JE, Hiller N, et al. Robot-assisted vertebral body augmentation: a radiation reduction tool. Spine. 2014; 39(2):153–157

[2] Mastrangelo G, Fedeli U, Fadda E, Giovanazzi A, Scoizzato L, Saia B. Increased cancer risk among surgeons in an orthopaedic hospital. Occup Med (Lond). 2005; 55(6):498–500

[3] Dewey P, Incoll I. Evaluation of thyroid shields for reduction of radiation exposure to orthopaedic surgeons. Aust N Z J Surg. 1998; 68(9):635–636

[4] Nolte L-P, Visarius H, Arm E, Langlotz F, Schwarzenbach O, Zamorano L. Computer-aided fixation of spinal implants. J Image Guid Surg. 1995; 1(2):88–93

[5] Nolte LP, Zamorano LJ, Jiang Z, Wang Q, Langlotz F, Berlemann U. Image-guided insertion of transpedicular screws. A laboratory set-up. Spine. 1995; 20(4):497–500

[6] Nolte LP, Zamorano L, Visarius H, et al. Clinical evaluation of a system for precision enhancement in spine surgery. Clin Biomech (Bristol, Avon). 1995; 10 (6):293–303

[7] Han W, Gao ZL, Wang JC, et al. Pedicle screw placement in the thoracic spine: a comparison study of computer-assisted navigation and conventional techniques. Orthopedics. 2010; 33(8):33

[8] Ishikawa Y, Kanemura T, Yoshida G, Ito Z, Muramoto A, Ohno S. Clinical accuracy of three-dimensional fluoroscopy-based computer-assisted cervical pedicle screw placement: a retrospective comparative study of conventional versus computer-assisted cervical pedicle screw placement. J Neurosurg Spine. 2010; 13(5):606–611

[9] Kelleher MO, McEvoy L, Nagaria J, Kamel M, Bolger C. Image-guided transarticular atlanto-axial screw fixation. Int J Med Robot. 2006; 2(2):154–160

[10] Ughwanogho E, Patel NM, Baldwin KD, Sampson NR, Flynn JM. Computed tomography-guided navigation of thoracic pedicle screws for adolescent idiopathic scoliosis results in more accurate placement and less screw removal. Spine. 2012; 37(8):E473–E478

[11] Villard J, Ryang YM, Demetriades AK, et al. Radiation exposure to the surgeon and the patient during posterior lumbar spinal instrumentation: a prospective randomized comparison of navigated versus non-navigated freehand techniques. Spine. 2014; 39(13):1004–1009

[12] Flynn JM, Sakai DS. Improving safety in spinal deformity surgery: advances in navigation and neurologic monitoring. Eur Spine J. 2013; 22 Suppl 2:S131–S137

[13] Verma R, Krishan S, Haendlmayer K, Mohsen A. Functional outcome of computer-assisted spinal pedicle screw placement: a systematic review and meta-analysis of 23 studies including 5,992 pedicle screws. Eur Spine J. 2010; 19(3):370–375

[14] Zhang W, Takigawa T, Wu Y, et al. Accuracy of pedicle screw insertion in posterior scoliosis surgery: a comparison between intraoperative navigation and preoperative navigation techniques. Eur Spine J. 2016

[15] Tian NF, Huang QS, Zhou P, et al. Pedicle screw insertion accuracy with different assisted methods: a systematic review and meta-analysis of comparative studies. Eur Spine J. 2011; 20(6):846–859

[16] Ohnsorge JA, Salem KH, Ladenburger A, Maus UM, Weisskopf M. Computer-assisted fluoroscopic navigation of percutaneous spinal interventions. Eur Spine J. 2013; 22(3):642–647

[17] Wagner SC, Morrissey PB, Kaye ID, Sebastian A, Butler JS, Kepler CK. Intraoperative pedicle screw navigation does not significantly affect complication rates after spine surgery. J Clin Neurosci. 2018; 47:198–201

[18] Mendelsohn D, Strelzow J, Dea N, et al. Patient and surgeon radiation exposure during spinal instrumentation using intraoperative computed tomography-based navigation. Spine J. 2016; 16(3):343–354

[19] Urbanski W, Jurasz W, Wolanczyk M, et al. Increased radiation but no benefits in pedicle screw accuracy with navigation versus a freehand technique in scoliosis surgery. Clin Orthop Relat Res. 2018; 476(5):1020–1027

[20] Fomekong E, Pierrard J, Raftopoulos C. Comparative cohort study of percutaneous pedicle screw implantation without versus with navigation in patients undergoing surgery for degenerative lumbar disc disease. World Neurosurg. 2018; 111:e410–e417

[21] Zhang YH, White I, Potts E, Mobasser JP, Chou D. Comparison perioperative factors during minimally invasive pre-psoas lateral interbody fusion of the lumbar spine using either navigation or conventional fluoroscopy. Global Spine J. 2017; 7(7):657–663

[22] Yu E, Khan SN. Does less invasive spine surgery result in increased radiation exposure? A systematic review. Clin Orthop Relat Res. 2014; 472(6):1738–1748

[23] Harstall R, Heini PF, Mini RL, Orler R. Radiation exposure to the surgeon during fluoroscopically assisted percutaneous vertebroplasty: a prospective study. Spine. 2005; 30(16):1893–1898

[24] Kraus M, von dem Berge S, Perl M, Krischak G, Weckbach S. Accuracy of screw placement and radiation dose in navigated dorsal instrumentation of the cervical spine: a prospective cohort study. Int J Med Robot. 2014; 10(2):223–229

[25] Dea N, Fisher CG, Batke J, et al. Economic evaluation comparing intraoperative cone beam CT-based navigation and conventional fluoroscopy for the placement of spinal pedicle screws: a patient-level data cost-effectiveness analysis. Spine J. 2016; 16(1):23–31

Part II
Techniques for Navigation-Assisted Spine Surgery

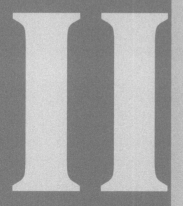

9 Outcomes in Navigated Spinal Surgery

Brian T. Sullivan, Alex A. Johnson, Nicholas Theodore, Jeff Jacobson, and A. Jay Khanna

Abstract:

This chapter reviews the major outcomes observed in modern spine surgery using navigated technologies. The aim of this chapter is to critically analyze current radiographic, clinical, surgical, patient-reported, and financial outcomes in computer-assisted navigated spine surgery compared with conventional fluoroscopic techniques. Another chapter will describe outcomes in robotic spine surgery. Navigation in spine surgery may be considered as an adjunct for optimizing surgical outcomes. However, a firm understanding of the anatomy and surgical skills needed for more conventional techniques remains important to the modern spine surgeon. Pedicle screw insertion with navigation has largely been shown to be more accurate and requires less time than conventional freehand techniques. Navigated spinal surgery decreases radiation exposure to the surgical team. Operative times in navigated spine surgery have shown noninferiority metrics when compared to conventional methods. Perioperative complications and patient-reported outcomes may require additional studies to better understand the complex interaction of navigation techniques and associated outcomes. Early comparative studies indicate less blood loss and the potential for decreased neurovascular intraoperative complications resulting from more accurate instrumentation placement. Some of the limitations and challenges seen in navigated spine surgery include high acquisition costs of the equipment, the learning curve for surgeon and healthcare team, and unique risks associated with the technology.

Keywords: navigated spine surgery, pedicle screw accuracy, operative times, learning curve, complications, freehand technique, fluoroscopy

9.1 Introduction

Spine surgery requires meticulous dissection, a comprehensive understanding of spinal anatomy, and constant focus by the surgeon, especially when working near-critical neurovascular structures. Technological advances, including navigated and robotic spine surgery, were developed to reduce the chance for human error and improve three-dimensional (3D) visualization of anatomy in the setting of more minimally invasive approaches. Historically, spine surgeons relied on experience and open approaches with direct visualization of anatomical landmarks throughout the case to insert implants and used serial radiographic evaluation to confirm proper placement of spinal instrumentation.[1,2,3] This cumbersome process and high pedicle screw malposition rate ranging from 8 to 50%[4,5,6,7] led to the development of image-guided surgery, aiming to expedite the operation and improve the accuracy and precision of implant insertion. Over time, computer-assisted navigation and robotic-assisted techniques have become commonplace in spine surgery.

Computer-assisted navigation technology relies on computed tomography (CT) or fluoroscopic imaging in combination with specialized cameras and tracked surgical equipment that are processed to create a 3D visualization to guide the surgeon intraoperatively (▶ Fig. 9.1). Often, CT-based navigation requires preoperative registration and preparation when compared to fluoroscopy-based navigation (▶ Fig. 9.2). The theoretical advantages of computer-assisted navigation include real-time 3D assessment of anatomy, reduction in intraoperative fluoroscopic use and radiation, decreased operative time, and improved accuracy and precision of implant placement.

Robotic spine surgery, an extension of navigation techniques, is a broad term that encompasses any operation that partially or completely utilizes robotic devices or artificial intelligence. Robotic surgery offers the advantage of improved precision of movement beyond the capacity of human physiology.[8,9] Robotic surgery is introduced fully in Chapter 2 and explored throughout the remainder of this book.

Although the technology available in the modern era of navigated spine surgery is exciting and shows promising clinical and radiographic potential, it is of paramount importance for spine surgeons to understand the efficacy and limitations of this technology in terms of clinical outcomes compared to traditional unguided methods. This is particularly true in an age when cost and quality of care are increasingly scrutinized. The aim of this chapter is to critically analyze current radiographic, clinical, surgical, patient-reported, and financial outcomes in computer-assisted navigated spine surgery compared with conventional techniques. The merits and downfalls of specific computer-assisted navigation platforms are beyond the scope of this discussion and have been discussed elsewhere.[10]

9.2 Discussion

The following discussion explores some of the key outcomes in navigated spine surgery, including, but not limited to, pedicle screw accuracy rates, radiation exposure to the patient and operating room personnel, operative time, perioperative complications, and patient-reported outcomes (PRO). The limitations of navigated spine surgery, such as initial acquisition costs, learning curve, and unique risks, are reviewed thereafter.

9.2.1 Pedicle Screw Accuracy Rates

Pedicle screws are now a mainstay in spine surgery due to the structural integrity offered with three-column fixation, rotational control, and increased pullout strength. Correctly positioned pedicle screws avoid high-risk intraoperative complications including vascular injury, devastating neurological sequelae, and the need for revision surgery associated with other implants. Evaluation of pedicle screw placement is one of the most studied aspects in the navigated spine surgery literature.

In a systematic review of 30 studies, Mason et al found 3D fluoroscopic navigation-guided (96%) modalities to be more accurate than two-dimensional (2D) navigation-guided (84%) and conventional fluoroscopy counterparts (68%).[6] In a meta-analysis of 10 studies comparing 3D CT-based navigation and

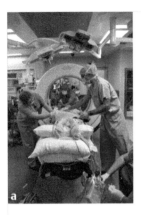
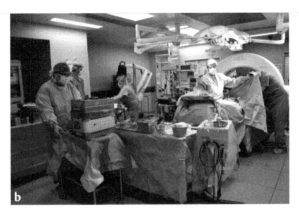
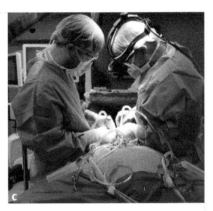
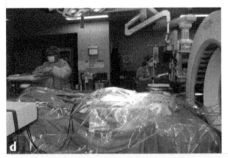
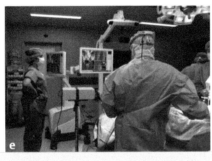
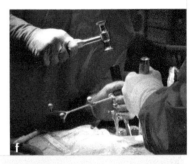

Fig. 9.1 Operating room setup and workflow for a 79-year-old female with history of thoracolumbar scoliosis, multilevel lumbar stenosis, and L4–L5 spondylolisthesis who underwent a T10 to pelvis posterior spinal arthrodesis with instrumentation, L2 to L5 laminectomies, and L5–S1 transforaminal lumbar interbody fusion using intraoperative CT-based navigation (Brainlab navigation system) in partnership with orthopaedic surgery and neurosurgical colleagues at our institution. (**a**) The surgical team carefully places the patient in the prone position with appropriate supports and padding on the adjustable, image-guidance table. (**b**) The large operating room is shown, which supports the numerous personnel and equipment needed for appropriate workflow using navigated techniques. (**c**) The surgeon and his first assistant perform the initial exposure to mount the anatomic reference array and identify key anatomy in standard fashion. (**d**) The patient undergoes an intraoperative CT using the Airo Mobile scanner after the wound site and sterile field are draped with clear, plastic covering (to allow for visualization of the reference array during the scan). These images were used for intraoperative navigation and image guidance after accuracy and precision of image acquisition was confirmed on the Brainlab stereotactic workstation. (**e**) The surgeons use the intraoperative guidance for pedicle screw insertion with the stereotactic video monitor displayed in the upper field. (**f**) After placement of all of the pedicle screws, the surgeons begin the decompression portion of the procedure; in this case, the surgeons use an osteotome during the initial portion of the decompression. Note that an array is still attached on the S1 spinous process. A final CT scan was performed intraoperatively, and position of the instrumentation was noted to be excellent.

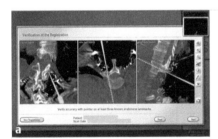
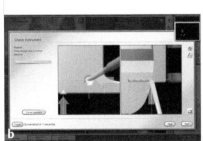
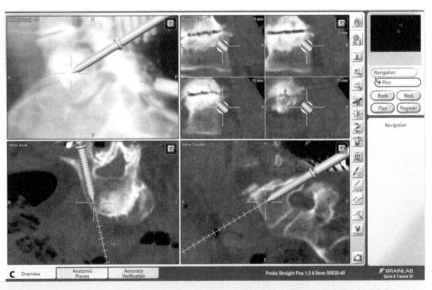

Fig. 9.2 Steps required for accurate and precise image registration along with the planned trajectories of instrumentation using the Brainlab navigation system. (**a**) The coronal, axial, and sagittal views are shown to verify the registration accuracy based on comparison with known anatomical markers by the surgeon. (**b**) Each instrument has three attached reference points and is calibrated for use in image-guided surgery. This displays the calibration process for a navigated probe with reference markers to confirm accuracy. (**c**) Once the image registration and instrument calibration are confirmed, the planned trajectory for instrumentation is available in real time with multiplanar views via stereotactic guidance.

Table 9.1 Recent meta-analysis and systematic review studies investigating pedicle screw position accuracy rates in spine surgery using conventional freehand surgery (fluoroscopy) versus navigated techniques

Study, author (year published)	Conventional (%)	Navigated 2D or 3D fluoroscopy (%)	Navigated CT (%)
Kosmopoulos and Schizas (2007)[13]	90.3	NR	95.2
Tian and Xu (2009)[14]	NR	85.5	90.8
Verma et al (2010)[15]	84.7	NR	93.3
Shin et al (2012)[7]	85.0	NR	94.0
Mason et al (2014)[6]	68.1	2D: 84.3 3D: 95.5	NR
Bourgeois et al (2015)[4]	86.9	NR	99.7
Meng et al (2016)[16]	84.9	NR	94.6

Abbreviation: NR, not reported.

2D- and 3D-fluoroscopy-based navigation techniques, Du et al found significant improvements in the screw placement accuracy with the 3D fluoroscopy navigated group when compared to the CT navigation group (relative risk [RR] 95%, CI: 0.4–0.9, $p = 0.01$) and 2D navigation group (RR: 95%, CI: 0.2–0.6, $p < 0.01$).[11]

Several additional meta-analyses using mostly individual cohort studies along with prospective and randomized controlled trials to evaluate pedicle screw accuracy rates found improved accuracy rates with navigation techniques over non-navigated counterparts (▶ Table 9.1). However, not all studies agree with the result, as one study found no difference in 3D CT-based navigation pedicle screw accuracy (96%) compared with freehand placement (96%) in a retrospective review of 49 subjects with idiopathic scoliosis who underwent placement of a total of 835 pedicle screws.[12]

Despite the overall increase in accuracy when compared to freehand techniques, Uehara et al[17] showed in a review of 359 subjects that CT-based navigation may be more accurate in the lumbar spine than in the cervical spine in which they reported significantly higher pedicle screw breach rates. Similarly, in the thoracic spine region, Kosmopoulos and Schizas[13] found no differences in pedicle screw accuracy rates in a meta-analysis and subgroup analysis comparing navigation with nonnavigated techniques, despite an overall improvement in the navigated group. These findings suggest that navigation techniques remain as a surgical adjunct, and an exquisite understanding of the anatomy is paramount for successful spine surgery. Confounders in comparing accuracy rates across studies may be limited by the surgeon's experience level, open versus minimally invasive approaches, patients' body habitus among other clinical variables, and the criteria or diagnostic tools used to identify pedicle screws in malposition.[18]

Unique Populations

1. *Congenital scoliosis*: In this group of pediatric disorders which are frequently associated with challenging anatomy, one study reviewing pedicle screw placement in 14 consecutive children with congenital spine deformity found that CT-based navigated screw placement resulted in a 99.3% accuracy rate and offered the benefits of identifying missing or dysmorphic pedicles intraoperatively.[19]

2. *Tumor*: Image guidance has largely become standard of care for cranial oncology surgeries. As oncology surgeries often require complete resection of tumor across multiple tissue planes, intraoperative image guidance has been shown to improve accuracy of resection in spinopelvic regions.[20,21,22] D'Andrea and colleagues[23] reported on a unique technique which combines preoperative MRI with intraoperative CT-based navigation to optimize visualization of tumor burden and surrounding neurovascular structures in the spine. This co-registered navigation technique effectively permitted the complete resection of tumor burden at 1-year follow-up but was limited by the small case series size ($n = 4$) and heterogeneous group of pathology.

3. *Minimally invasive spine surgery (MISS)*: In MISS, the surgeon has limited direct visualization of the relevant anatomy and landmarks and must rely more on visual and radiographic adjuncts. Three-dimensional spine navigation uniquely aids the surgeon by providing visualization with limited exposure. The surgeon has real-time feedback and unlimited degrees of freedom with his or her tools, and several studies indicate improved instrumentation accuracy rates in the setting of MISS with 3D navigation guidance.[4,24,25] In addition, the benefit in terms of radiation dose reduction is greatest in minimally invasive spine surgical procedures given the greater amounts of radiation that are typically required with conventional fluoroscopic guidance.

9.2.2 Radiation Exposure

Another important consideration in spine surgery is both the radiation exposure to patient and occupational hazards for the surgical team. Spine surgeons are commonly exposed to radiation from fluoroscopy and may be at a higher risk for malignancy and cataracts when compared to the general population.[26,27,28,29,30] This topic is discussed fully in Chapter 8. In brief, several studies[31,32] indicate that the radiation exposure in navigated spinal surgery is decreased for the surgical team but may be slightly increased or similar for the patient when compared to traditional fluoroscopic techniques. Intraoperative navigation systems permit the surgical team to step away from the surgical field to minimize exposure to occupational hazard risks. The increase in radiation exposure to the patient is thought to remain within tolerated limits.[31,33] Also, there is commonly no need for an immediate postoperative CT scan in navigated surgery to confirm position of instruments. Therefore, advocates of navigation suggest the patient may have a potential lower total exposure in the long term, especially if the increased pedicle screw accuracy affords a decreased requirement for revision surgery. Exciting advances, such as using low-dose protocols in CT cone beam–navigated techniques, were shown in a prospective study to significantly decrease radiation levels to the patient while having no decrease in accuracy of implant placement.[34] Other advances, including ultrasound- and MRI-guided navigation, may permit similar visualization while decreasing irradiation levels to the patient.[35,36]

9.2.3 Surgical Time

Concern for increased surgical time related to operating room preparation and image registration is a factor why many spine surgeons have not transitioned to navigation.[37] Although some reports show navigated surgery may decrease operative times,[38] many studies indicate no significant differences between conventional freehand and navigated methods in terms of operative time.

In a meta-analysis comparing pedicle screw insertion in all spinal regions, no significant differences were found in operative times in the navigation group when compared to the non-navigated counterparts.[7] A retrospective study investigating the total operative times and time associated with surgical room preparation in single-level lumbar fusions found an overall decreased operative time, by a mean of 23 minutes, in CT-based navigated surgeries versus traditional freehand technique, but a greater surgical room preparation time in the navigated operations that trended toward significance.[38] The total operative time in the navigation group decreased over the course of the study, which may be attributed to a learning curve as the freehand preparation time showed no difference at the beginning versus the end of the study duration.[38] Knafo et al[39] retrospectively compared 3D fluoroscopy-based navigation with freehand techniques using conventional fluoroscopy focusing on operative times. The authors found that imaging techniques did not independently predict operative times and that surgeon performance and operative indications were the main predictors of surgical duration. Similarly, in a review of spine tumor cases, no differences in operative time were observed in cases with 3D fluoroscopy-based navigation (193 minutes) versus conventional fluoroscopy (201 minutes; $p = 0.6$).[40] In a meta-analysis, Tian et al[41] found that overall surgical time was not different when comparing navigation and freehand techniques; however, the authors noted that individual pedicle screw insertion time was less in the navigation group.

Total operative time may be noninferior in navigated versus freehand techniques. Navigated spine surgery shows potential to decrease operative times as optimization of registration and other processes required for successful navigation occur in the future. Simple initiatives, including workflow checklists,[42] may help reduce operative times in the setting of navigated spine surgery.

In the authors' experience, the greatest benefit in terms of decreases in surgical time using intraoperative navigation (rather than conventional landmarks with or without fluoroscopy) tends to occur with larger thoracolumbar and cervicothoracic instrumentation and fusion cases, especially with significant spinal deformity. In these cases, navigation allows for more rapid and reproducible localization of pedicle and other anatomic structures for screw insertion relative to conventional techniques. Conversely, the least benefit is seen in smaller and more simple cases such as one-level lumbar fusion cases where the time for room setup and image acquisition may exceed the minimal time required to localize levels and perhaps check starting points for four lumbar pedicle screws.

9.2.4 Perioperative Complications

While increased implant accuracy and decreased radiation exposure to the surgical team are recognized advantages in navigated spinal surgery, perioperative complication rates are important to consider when determining surgical approach.

Although accuracy rates of instrumentation have improved with navigated techniques, one must consider the clinical sequelae of pedicle screws placed incorrectly which are, primarily, the need for revision surgery and neurological and vascular complications. In a retrospective review comparing the rates of revision surgery due to pedicle screw malposition in posterior instrumentation of the thoracic and lumbar spine, Fichtner et al[43] found that 3D fluoroscopy-based navigated surgery was associated with a significantly decreased risk for revision surgery (1.4%) when compared to freehand with conventional fluoroscopy techniques (4.4%; odds ratio: 3.4). In a systematic review, Shin et al[7] found a 0.39 decreased odds ratio for pedicle screw malposition in navigated spinal surgery when compared to nonnavigated techniques but did not observe a difference in revision rates per screw (navigated surgery = 1.4% and nonnavigated = 2.0%, $p = 0.1$). Some studies suggest a lack of significant differences in perioperative complications (e.g., neurological complications) when reviewing pedicle screw accuracy.[44]

Wagner et al[45] sought to determine the differences in perioperative complications in navigated versus nonnavigated multilevel spinal fusions for adult deformity using the American College of Surgeons National Surgical Quality Improvement Project (ACS NSQIP) dataset. The authors found no significant differences in the reoperation rates, intraoperative surgical complications, or postoperative complications. This study is limited by the lack of spine-specific variables and outcome measures in the ACS NSQIP registry along with the absence of long-term outcomes but provides one of the first comparisons of complications on this important topic. In another study[46] using the ACS NSQIP registry to review perioperative complications in single-level posterior lumbar fusions, no differences were found in surgical site infections, reoperations, or readmissions in navigated and nonnavigated groups.

In the thoracic region of the spine, Meng et al[16] observed decreased blood loss and fewer complications in navigated spinal surgery when compared to conventional fluoroscopy-guided techniques. Similarly, in the cervical region, decreased blood loss in the setting of stabilization of C1–C2 was observed in a retrospective review of 3D navigation versus direct visualization and conventional fluoroscopic techniques.[47] Shin et al[7] noted a trend in decreased estimated blood loss in a meta-analysis comparing those who underwent navigation with controls (freehand technique). The decrease in blood loss with navigated techniques may be attributed to smaller incisions, more precise pedicle screw insertion resulting in less damage to nearby soft tissues and blood vessels, and decreased insertion time for the pedicle screws.

9.2.5 Patient-Reported Outcomes

In navigated spine surgery, it is recognized that instruments can be placed more accurately and potentially with less complication than conventional fluoroscopic techniques. However, it is important to consider if navigated techniques improve overall PROs in spine surgery, as measured by standard outcome metrics, such as SF-36, Oswestry Disability Index (ODI), and visual analog score (VAS). PROs can successfully identify pain relief, quality of life, and restoration of function in spine surgery, which is frequently viewed as a corollary to the efficacy of the procedure to treat a particular condition.[48] As navigated spine surgery is still in its infancy, PROs are limited but a few early studies have reviewed these important metrics.

Zhang et al[49], in a retrospective review of subjects who underwent minimally invasive oblique lumbar interbody fusion for lumbar degenerative disease using CT-based navigated and conventional fluoroscopic techniques, found no differences in outcomes between the groups using the Smiley-Webster scale. This study was limited by reviewing 42 subjects with only medium-term follow-up (range: 6–24 months) available. Khanna et al[50] found that ODI, back VAS, and leg VAS significantly improved in subjects who underwent minimally invasive transforaminal lumbar interbody fusion with conventional fluoroscopy and CT-based navigated techniques at 6 months postoperative. These differences slightly favored the navigated group but did not reach significance. In a prospective cohort study reviewing single level transforaminal lumbar interbody fusion in spondylolisthesis, Wu et al[51] found VAS decreased most in MISS with CT-based navigation when compared to conventional open surgery and MISS with conventional fluoroscopy. However, no significant differences were found in ODI or overall patient satisfaction between groups. Overall, there is a paucity of literature focusing on PRO associated with navigated spine surgery[15] and many of the positive clinical outcomes have been extrapolated from other benchmarks, such as improved accuracy offering better fixation and less need for revision surgery.

9.3 Limitations of Navigated Spine Surgery

Navigated spine surgery is not without disadvantages. One of the major challenges with incorporating any new technology involves learning to use the technology in an efficient and safe manner. Additionally, the initial startup costs associated with training the operating team and acquiring new equipment can be substantial. In a survey of spine surgeons in 2008, at a time when many responded they had limited experience with navigated spine surgery, the authors found that navigated spine surgery was frequently limited by a perception of lack of need, the potential for high acquisition costs, and the inherent risks for intraoperative user errors with potential catastrophic consequences associated with the technology.[52]

9.3.1 Costs and Economic Impact

The cost associated with the acquisition of capable, computer-assisted navigated spine surgery software and equipment is high and may be limiting to smaller surgical centers. Additionally, the software and equipment are rapidly evolving, making a routine maintenance and its associated expenses a reality that centers must consider. In a cost-effective analysis, one referral center observed in subjects with adult spine deformity undergoing surgical correction with CT-based navigation methods that a center would be economically advantaged if it performed more than 254 operations in a fiscal year due to the decreased

risk for reoperation in the study group when compared to conventional fluoroscopic methods.[53] These cost effects were due to the high costs associated with reoperation and may extend beyond economic value to improve PRO.[53] More research is needed to elucidate whether modern navigation techniques may result in decreased costs across navigated spine surgery.[54] Additional advances and expansion of the uses of the intraoperative navigation equipment beyond spine surgery may help mitigate the high acquisition costs.

9.3.2 Learning Curve

In addition to economic considerations, a learning curve exists when employing navigation in spine surgery. One prospective study stratified 145 subjects who underwent 3D fluoroscopy-based navigated spine surgery by the time of implementation of the technology into four periods (first or reference period through fourth period over 18-month enrollment time). The study observed significant decreasing trends in time for pedicle screw placement and pedicle screw malposition rates when analyzed over the study period.[55] Rivkin and Yocom noted a significantly higher rate (13.2%) of pedicle screw breach in the first 30 patients who underwent CT-based navigated thoracic and lumbar pedicle screw insertion when compared to the subsequent 30 patients (5.6%), which was attributed to a learning curve.[56] The aforementioned single-center studies may be limited by specific procedure types and surgeon experience when generalizing the finding to all navigated spine surgery techniques. However, these examples showcase the importance of acknowledging the potential of navigated spine surgery and encourage novel methods to rapidly train surgical teams with the goal to provide the best clinical outcomes possible. The learning curve may be mitigated for surgeons transitioning to navigated spine surgery through mentorship models or cadaveric workshops led by experts in the technology. Exciting new training systems are being developed and incorporated for surgical trainees to master anatomy and improve manual dexterity using simulated models.[57] Further information and tips can be found in Chapter 31. Once the learning curve is surpassed, the improved 3D visualization and real-time feedback may offer superior learning opportunities to trainees than those available with traditional freehand techniques.

9.3.3 Intraoperative Risks Specific to Navigated Techniques

As navigation techniques in spine surgery require additional equipment and preparation, there are inherent risks specific to its use in spine surgery. Theoretical complications may include infection or fracture associated with fiducial array placement within the bone, unrecognized registration failure with catastrophic malposition of implants, sterility issues with incorporation of imaging equipment into the surgical field, among others. Although largely unreported in the literature, the authors recommend consideration of potential pitfalls with navigated techniques and constant quality improvement to prevent patient morbidity as navigation methods continue to evolve and gain popularity in spine surgery.

9.4 Conclusion and Future Directions

- Navigation and its use in spine surgery can be considered as an adjunct for optimizing surgical outcomes. However, a firm understanding of the anatomy and surgical skills needed for more conventional techniques remain important to the modern spine surgeon.
- Pedicle screw insertion with navigation has largely been shown to be more accurate and require less time than conventional freehand techniques in several meta-analysis studies, particularly in the setting of complex deformity or regions of challenging anatomy (e.g., cervical vertebrae).
- Navigated spinal surgery decreases radiation exposure to the surgical team.
- Operative times in navigated spine surgery have shown noninferiority metrics when compared to conventional methods and offer the potential to decrease over time as the surgeon and operating room staff move beyond the learning curve.
- Perioperative complications may require additional studies to better understand the complex interaction of navigation techniques and associated outcomes. Early comparative studies indicate less blood loss and the potential for decreased neurovascular intraoperative complications resulting from more accurate instrumentation placement.
- Navigated spine surgery has a high acquisition cost. In the high-volume surgical center, these initial costs can be overcome largely through a decreased rate of reoperation and its associated costs and patient morbidity. More cost-effective analysis studies are suggested to elucidate the trends in economics of spine surgery using navigated techniques.
- As with most new technologies, there is a learning curve with navigated spine surgery. Surgeons can overcome the learning curve by having a thorough understanding of the anatomy and technology along with using innovative training platforms.

9.4.1 Future Directions

Clinical outcomes such as pseudoarthrosis rates, patient satisfaction, and functional outcomes will take more time and larger studies to better understand their differences in navigated versus conventional spine surgery. As navigated spine surgery is still a relatively new technology, long-term studies evaluating methods to decrease the learning curve and reduce costs are warranted. It is important to consider the limitations of navigated spine surgery to guide advancements in technology and improve patient safety. The future of spine surgery is bright with further optimization of navigation technologies, particularly when coupled with the continued advances in robotic-assisted devices. Finally, there is an overall paucity of randomized controlled trials comparing navigated spinal surgery with traditional counterparts.

References

[1] Foley KT, Smith MM. Image-guided spine surgery. Neurosurg Clin N Am. 1996; 7(2):171–186

[2] Holly LT, Foley KT. Intraoperative spinal navigation. Spine. 2003; 28(15) Suppl:S54–S61

[3] Verma K, Boniello A, Rihn J. Emerging techniques for posterior fixation of the lumbar spine. J Am Acad Orthop Surg. 2016; 24(6):357–364

[4] Bourgeois AC, Faulkner AR, Bradley YC, et al. Improved accuracy of minimally invasive transpedicular screw placement in the lumbar spine with 3-dimensional stereotactic image guidance: a comparative meta-analysis. J Spinal Disord Tech. 2015; 28(9):324–329

[5] Hicks JM, Singla A, Shen FH, Arlet V. Complications of pedicle screw fixation in scoliosis surgery: a systematic review. Spine. 2010; 35(11):E465–E470

[6] Mason A, Paulsen R, Babuska JM, et al. The accuracy of pedicle screw placement using intraoperative image guidance systems. J Neurosurg Spine. 2014; 20(2):196–203

[7] Shin BJ, James AR, Njoku IU, Härtl R. Pedicle screw navigation: a systematic review and meta-analysis of perforation risk for computer-navigated versus freehand insertion. J Neurosurg Spine. 2012; 17(2):113–122

[8] Joseph JR, Smith BW, Liu X, Park P. Current applications of robotics in spine surgery: a systematic review of the literature. Neurosurg Focus. 2017; 42(5):E2

[9] Roser F, Tatagiba M, Maier G. Spinal robotics: current applications and future perspectives. Neurosurgery. 2013; 72 Suppl 1:12–18

[10] Nooh A, Lubov J, Aoude A, et al. Differences between manufacturers of computed tomography-based computer-assisted surgery systems do exist: a systematic literature review. Global Spine J. 2017; 7(1):83–94

[11] Du JP, Fan Y, Wu QN, Wang DH, Zhang J, Hao DJ. Accuracy of pedicle screw insertion among 3 image-guided navigation systems: systematic review and meta-analysis. World Neurosurg. 2018; 109:24–30

[12] Urbanski W, Jurasz W, Wolanczyk M, et al. Increased radiation but no benefits in pedicle screw accuracy with navigation versus a freehand technique in scoliosis surgery. Clin Orthop Relat Res. 2018; 476(5):1020–1027

[13] Kosmopoulos V, Schizas C. Pedicle screw placement accuracy: a meta-analysis. Spine. 2007; 32(3):E111–E120

[14] Tian NF, Xu HZ. Image-guided pedicle screw insertion accuracy: a meta-analysis. Int Orthop. 2009; 33(4):895–903

[15] Verma R, Krishan S, Haendlmayer K, Mohsen A. Functional outcome of computer-assisted spinal pedicle screw placement: a systematic review and meta-analysis of 23 studies including 5,992 pedicle screws. Eur Spine J. 2010; 19(3):370–375

[16] Meng XT, Guan XF, Zhang HL, He SS. Computer navigation versus fluoroscopy-guided navigation for thoracic pedicle screw placement: a meta-analysis. Neurosurg Rev. 2016; 39(3):385–391

[17] Uehara M, Takahashi J, Ikegami S, Kuraishi S, Futatsugi T, Kato H. Screw perforation rates in 359 consecutive patients receiving computer-guided pedicle screw insertion along the cervical to lumbar spine. Eur Spine J. 2017; 26(11):2858–2864

[18] Aoude AA, Fortin M, Figueiredo R, Jarzem P, Ouellet J, Weber MH. Methods to determine pedicle screw placement accuracy in spine surgery: a systematic review. Eur Spine J. 2015; 24(5):990–1004

[19] Larson AN, Polly DW, Jr, Guidera KJ, et al. The accuracy of navigation and 3D image-guided placement for the placement of pedicle screws in congenital spine deformity. J Pediatr Orthop. 2012; 32(6):e23–e29

[20] Laitinen MK, Parry MC, Albergo JI, Grimer RJ, Jeys LM. Is computer navigation when used in the surgery of iliosacral pelvic bone tumours safer for the patient? Bone Joint J. 2017; 99-B(2):261–266

[21] Nasser R, Drazin D, Nakhla J, et al. Resection of spinal column tumors utilizing image-guided navigation: a multicenter analysis. Neurosurg Focus. 2016; 41(2):E15

[22] Rajasekaran S, Kamath V, Shetty AP. Intraoperative iso-C three-dimensional navigation in excision of spinal osteoid osteomas. Spine. 2008; 33(1):E25–E29

[23] D'Andrea K, Dreyer J, Fahim DK. Utility of preoperative magnetic resonance imaging coregistered with intraoperative computed tomographic scan for the resection of complex tumors of the spine. World Neurosurg. 2015; 84(6):1804–1815

[24] Kim TT, Drazin D, Shweikeh F, Pashman R, Johnson JP. Clinical and radiographic outcomes of minimally invasive percutaneous pedicle screw placement with intraoperative CT (O-arm) image guidance navigation. Neurosurg Focus. 2014; 36(3):E1

[25] Moses ZB, Mayer RR, Strickland BA, et al. Neuronavigation in minimally invasive spine surgery. Neurosurg Focus. 2013; 35(2):E12

[26] Falavigna A, Ramos MB, Iutaka AS, et al. Knowledge and attitude regarding radiation exposure among spine surgeons in Latin America. World Neurosurg. 2018; 112:e823–e829

[27] Giordano BD, Rechtine GR, II, Morgan TL. Minimally invasive surgery and radiation exposure. J Neurosurg Spine. 2009; 11(3):375–376, author reply 376–377

[28] Hayda RA, Hsu RY, DePasse JM, Gil JA. Radiation exposure and health risks for orthopaedic surgeons. J Am Acad Orthop Surg. 2018; 26(8):268–277

[29] Mastrangelo G, Fedeli U, Fadda E, Giovanazzi A, Scoizzato L, Saia B. Increased cancer risk among surgeons in an orthopaedic hospital. Occup Med (Lond). 2005; 55(6):498–500

[30] Srinivasan D, Than KD, Wang AC, et al. Radiation safety and spine surgery: systematic review of exposure limits and methods to minimize radiation exposure. World Neurosurg. 2014; 82(6):1337–1343

[31] Mendelsohn D, Strelzow J, Dea N, et al. Patient and surgeon radiation exposure during spinal instrumentation using intraoperative computed tomography-based navigation. Spine J. 2016; 16(3):343–354

[32] Riis J, Lehman RR, Perera RA, et al. A retrospective comparison of intraoperative CT and fluoroscopy evaluating radiation exposure in posterior spinal fusions for scoliosis. Patient Saf Surg. 2017; 11:32

[33] Noriega DC, Hernández-Ramajo R, Rodríguez-Monsalve Milano F, et al. Risk-benefit analysis of navigation techniques for vertebral transpedicular instrumentation: a prospective study. Spine J. 2017; 17(1):70–75

[34] Pireau N, Cordemans V, Banse X, Irda N, Lichtherte S, Kaminski L. Radiation dose reduction in thoracic and lumbar spine instrumentation using navigation based on an intraoperative cone beam CT imaging system: a prospective randomized clinical trial. Eur Spine J. 2017; 26(11):2818–2827

[35] Jolesz FA. Intraoperative imaging in neurosurgery: where will the future take us? Acta Neurochir Suppl (Wien). 2011; 109:21–25

[36] Moiyadi AV. Intraoperative ultrasound technology in neuro-oncology practice-current role and future applications. World Neurosurg. 2016; 93:81–93

[37] Härtl R, Lam KS, Wang J, Korge A, Kandziora F, Audigé L. Worldwide survey on the use of navigation in spine surgery. World Neurosurg. 2013; 79(1):162–172

[38] Khanna AR, Yanamadala V, Coumans JV. Effect of intraoperative navigation on operative time in 1-level lumbar fusion surgery. J Clin Neurosci. 2016; 32:72–76

[39] Knafo S, Mireau E, Bennis S, Baussart B, Aldea S, Gaillard S. Operative and perioperative durations in O-arm vs C-arm fluoroscopy for lumbar instrumentation. Oper Neurosurg (Hagerstown). 2018; 14(3):273–278

[40] Miller JA, Fabiano AJ. Comparison of operative time with conventional fluoroscopy versus spinal neuronavigation in instrumented spinal tumor surgery. World Neurosurg. 2017; 105:412–419

[41] Tian W, Zeng C, An Y, Wang C, Liu Y, Li J. Accuracy and postoperative assessment of pedicle screw placement during scoliosis surgery with computer-assisted navigation: a meta-analysis. Int J Med Robot. 2017; 13(1)

[42] Rahmathulla G, Nottmeier EW, Pirris SM, Deen HG, Pichelmann MA. Intraoperative image-guided spinal navigation: technical pitfalls and their avoidance. Neurosurg Focus. 2014; 36(3):E3

[43] Fichtner J, Hofmann N, Rienmüller A, et al. Revision rate of misplaced pedicle screws of the thoracolumbar spine-comparison of three-dimensional fluoroscopy navigation with freehand placement: a systematic analysis and review of the literature. World Neurosurg. 2018; 109:e24–e32

[44] Gelalis ID, Paschos NK, Pakos EE, et al. Accuracy of pedicle screw placement: a systematic review of prospective in vivo studies comparing free hand, fluoroscopy guidance and navigation techniques. Eur Spine J. 2012; 21(2):247–255

[45] Wagner SC, Morrissey PB, Kaye ID, Sebastian A, Butler JS, Kepler CK. Intraoperative pedicle screw navigation does not significantly affect complication rates after spine surgery. J Clin Neurosci. 2018; 47:198–201

[46] Bovonratwet P, Nelson SJ, Ondeck NT, Geddes BJ, Grauer JN. Comparison of 30-day complications between navigated and conventional single-level instrumented posterior lumbar fusion: a propensity score matched analysis. Spine. 2018; 43(6):447–453

[47] Hitti FL, Hudgins ED, Chen HI, Malhotra NR, Zager EL, Schuster JM. Intraoperative navigation is associated with reduced blood loss during C1-C2 posterior cervical fixation. World Neurosurg. 2017; 107:574–578

[48] McCormick JD, Werner BC, Shimer AL. Patient-reported outcome measures in spine surgery. J Am Acad Orthop Surg. 2013; 21(2):99–107

[49] Zhang YH, White I, Potts E, Mobasser JP, Chou D. Comparison perioperative factors during minimally invasive pre-psoas lateral interbody fusion of the lumbar spine using either navigation or conventional fluoroscopy. Global Spine J. 2017; 7(7):657–663

[50] Khanna R, McDevitt JL, Abecassis ZA, et al. An outcome and cost analysis comparing single-level minimally invasive transforaminal lumbar interbody fusion using intraoperative fluoroscopy versus computed tomography-guided navigation. World Neurosurg. 2016; 94:255–260

[51] Wu MH, Dubey NK, Li YY, et al. Comparison of minimally invasive spine surgery using intraoperative computed tomography integrated navigation, fluoroscopy, and conventional open surgery for lumbar spondylolisthesis: a prospective registry-based cohort study. Spine J. 2017; 17(8):1082–1090

[52] Choo AD, Regev G, Garfin SR, Kim CW. Surgeons' perceptions of spinal navigation: analysis of key factors affecting the lack of adoption of spinal navigation technology. SAS J. 2008; 2(4):189–194

[53] Dea N, Fisher CG, Batke J, et al. Economic evaluation comparing intraoperative cone beam CT-based navigation and conventional fluoroscopy for the placement of spinal pedicle screws: a patient-level data cost-effectiveness analysis. Spine J. 2016; 16(1):23–31

[54] Al-Khouja L, Shweikeh F, Pashman R, Johnson JP, Kim TT, Drazin D. Economics of image guidance and navigation in spine surgery. Surg Neurol Int. 2015; 6 Suppl 10:S323–S326

[55] Ryang YM, Villard J, Obermüller T, et al. Learning curve of 3D fluoroscopy image-guided pedicle screw placement in the thoracolumbar spine. Spine J. 2015; 15(3):467–476

[56] Rivkin MA, Yocom SS. Thoracolumbar instrumentation with CT-guided navigation (O-arm) in 270 consecutive patients: accuracy rates and lessons learned. Neurosurg Focus. 2014; 36(3):E7

[57] Lorias-Espinoza D, Carranza VG, de León FC, Escamirosa FP, Martinez AMA. A low-cost, passive navigation training system for image-guided spinal intervention. World Neurosurg. 2016; 95:322–328

10 Navigated Subaxial Cervical Spine Pedicle Screw Instrumentation

John A. Buza III and Peter G. Passias

Abstract:
Computer navigation increases the accuracy of pedicle screw placement in the cervical spine, but further studies must elucidate clear proof of benefit to the patient before more widespread adoption of this technology. Cervical pedicle screw placement is technically difficult, and computer navigation has been employed as a means of increasing the accuracy of this procedure. Computer navigation is generally classified by the associated imaging modality, and may utilize either CT scan or fluoroscopy. CT scans may now be obtained either preoperatively or intraoperatively. Traditional fluoroscopy was two-dimensional, but newer technology has allowed for three-dimensional fluoroscopy to be obtained intraoperatively. The process of intraoperative registration is vitally important, and should be performed at each spinal segment individually. The major advantage of computer-assisted navigation is increased accuracy and reliability, and a decreased rate of major pedicle cortical violations. This would in theory decrease the rate of vascular or neurological injuries, although this is yet to be shown. The major disadvantages of navigation are increased operating room time and cost. No studies have demonstrated a clear clinical benefit to the patient from the adoption of this technology. Future high-level studies are required demonstrating a clear clinical benefit. The available series has demonstrated that while navigation-assisted cervical pedicle screw placement may increase accuracy and reliability, there is still a relatively high rate of major cortical violations. Therefore, it is critically important to take great care when placing cervical pedicle screws, even with the use of this technology.

Keywords: cervical pedicle screws, navigation, CT scan, fluoroscopy, registration

10.1 Introduction

Pedicle screw placement in the cervical spine is challenging, and the rate of cervical pedicle screw misplacement varies from 2.5 to 29.1% in the literature.[1,2,3,4,5,6] There are a number of possible reasons for the relatively high rate of pedicle screw misplacement in the cervical spine. The anatomy is smaller in size compared to the lumbar spine. There are frequently three-dimensional (3D) deformities, and a number of vital anatomic structures lie in close proximity to the pedicle, including the spinal cord, cervical nerve roots, and vertebral artery. There is extremely limited space for deviation of a pedicle screw from the ideal trajectory between the spinal canal medially and the vertebral artery laterally between C3 and C7, and therefore a significant risk of neurovascular injury by inaccurate screw position. The standard posterior approach to the cervical spine allows a two-dimensional (2D) visualization of a complex 3D structure. Conventional orientation to the spine is achieved by identifying this surface anatomy, in combination with 2D

fluoroscopy. However, several situations can make identification of surface anatomy more challenging. Minimally invasive approaches to the spine limit the exposure of surface anatomy, decreasing the number of known landmarks. The aging population typically presents with advanced degenerative changes in the cervical spine, which may also mask the surface anatomy. Instrumentation of the cervical spine is therefore very complex and requires significant spatial awareness and experience.

Due to the inherent challenges and higher precision required in the cervical spine, intraoperative navigation has been developed in an effort to provide the surgeon with spatial information to enhance the accuracy of screw placement. This has the potential to significantly increase screw accuracy and limit the amount of intraoperative radiation exposure.

10.2 Intraoperative Techniques

Several techniques are available for navigation in cervical pedicle screw placement, which differ in both the imaging modality and registration method. The imaging modality may be broadly classified as CT imaging, 2D fluoroscopy, or intraoperative 3D fluoroscopy. While CT-based methods were frequently used in the development of spinal navigation, intraoperative imaging and, in particular, 3D fluoroscopy are being used with increasing frequency. The registration method has largely changed from surface matching methods to automatic registration of the intraoperative fluoroscopy imaging dataset.

There are advantages and disadvantages to these techniques, which will be further reviewed below.

10.2.1 CT-Based Navigation

CT-based navigation was the first imaging modality for image-guided spinal navigation. CT-based navigation traditionally requires that the patient undergo a preoperative CT scan with a special protocol acquiring consecutive axial images of 1.5 mm thickness. Screw entry point and screw direction are then determined using surgical software planning to minimize potential risk to surrounding neurovascular structures. Both screw length and diameter can be determined using this software.

At the beginning of the surgical case, intraoperative landmarks are mapped and then correlated with the virtual data obtained by CT scan (▸ Fig. 10.1, ▸ Fig. 10.2). This process is known as "registration." There are three different methods by which registration may occur, including paired-point matching, region matching, and CT-fluoro matching. In paired-point matching, anatomically distinct points are identified in the CT scan and these points are "presented" to the navigation system by surgeon with the use of a pointer after attachment of a reference array to the spine. Region matching is a similar process, but the navigation system constructs a 3D model of the spine,

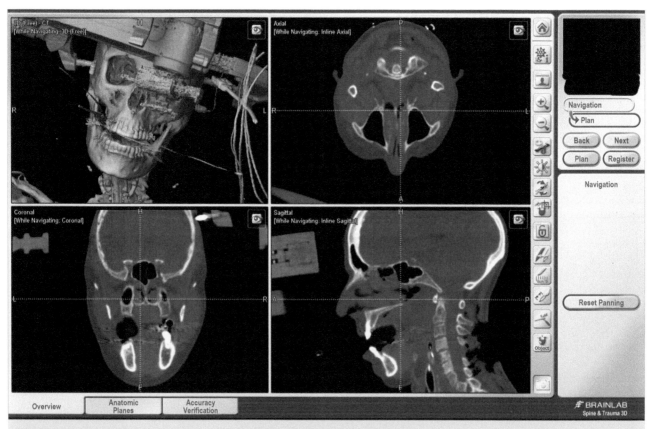

Fig. 10.1 Intraoperative CT scan is performed using the Brainlab Airo Mobile Intraoperative CT.

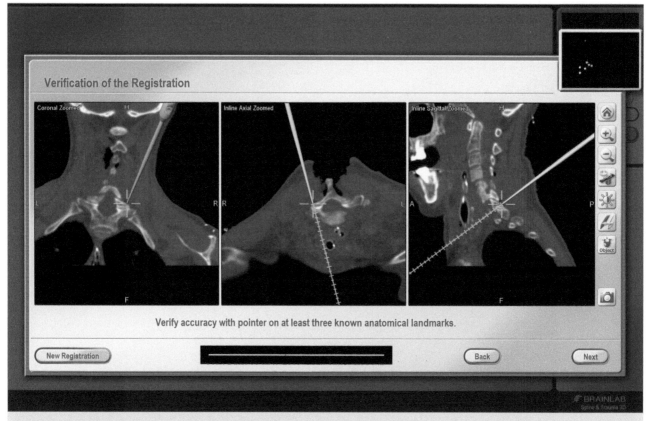

Fig. 10.2 Intraoperative registration is performed by verifying the accuracy of the pointer on three known anatomical landmarks (Brainlab Airo Mobile Intraoperative CT).

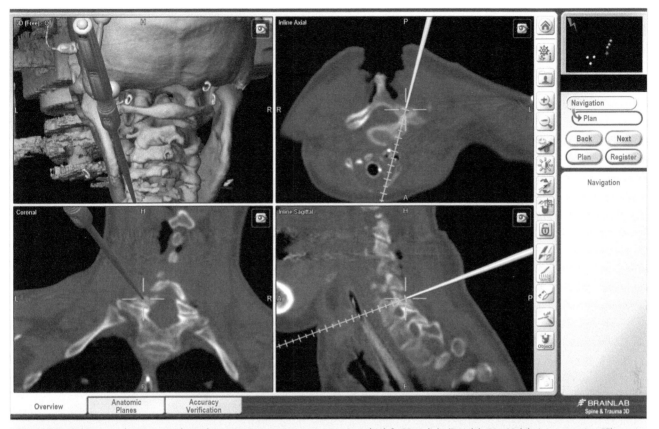

Fig. 10.3 Pedicle screw placement is planned using intraoperative navigation into the left C6 pedicle (Brainlab Airo Mobile Intraoperative CT).

and a random cloud of surface anatomy points is correlated by the surgeon with that 3D model. The third method of registration is CT-fluoro matching, in which the preoperative CT scan is matched with intraoperative 2D fluoro images taken from multiple angles.

This process of registration is the key influencing factor for the accuracy of any navigation-based technology. The patient's anatomy must be carefully and accurately registered to the imaging data set. When using CT-based navigation, the spatial relation between vertebral segments may change greatly as the patient goes from a supine position during CT scan to the prone position during a posterior surgery. Therefore, a careful and repeated control of registration accuracy using distinct anatomic points is necessary during surgery, particularly for instrumentation at more than one level. Tauchi et al demonstrated this in a retrospective study of 46 patients undergoing CT-based navigated pedicle screw placement.[7] The authors found that the pedicle screw misplacement rate for single-time multilevel registration was 23.4%, compared to 6.2% for separate registration times.[7] The inaccuracy of single-time registration was most pronounced for patients with increased preoperative cervical range of motion, and the authors concluded that it is particularly important to perform separate registrations in this patient population.[7]

Regardless of the registration method used, each method allows for identification of the surgical instruments in relation to the surgical field. The surgeon can then use the virtual field to achieve precise positioning of all instruments, which allows

for entry point identification and screw trajectory (▶ Fig. 10.3). A reference frame attached to the patient can also track any movement of the patient, such as excursion of the thorax caused by breathing, which may alter the relation of the virtual field to the surgical field.

Given some of the limitations surrounding the use of preoperative CT scans for navigation-based pedicle screw placement, the use of intraoperative CT scan has been advocated. In a study of 129 pedicle screws placed in the cervicothoracic junction (C5–T3), Barsa et al found that the use of intraoperative CT scan resulted in a relatively low rate of pedicle screw misplacement (5 of 129, 3.9%).[8] The authors used a 32-slice portable CT-scanner (BodyTom; NeuroLogical, Danvers). While the imaging quality is less than a traditional helical CT-scan, the authors concluded that the quality of intraoperative CT imaging sufficient for navigation was obtained at all spinal segments regardless of patient's habitus or positioning. The authors did report a higher radiation exposure for the patient, and an average increase of 27 minutes of operative time for this technique.[8]

10.2.2 Two-Dimensional Fluoroscopy-Based Navigation

Fluoroscopy-based navigation does not require any preoperative imaging. In this technique, a number of 2D fluoroscopic views of the cervical spine are taken and processed in the navigation computer. Registration occurs automatically by tracking the C-arm during image acquisition. The navigation computer then correlates the position of the image intensifier with the surgical instruments, so that the entry point and trajectory can be virtually determined. Unlike CT-based navigation, however, the third dimension of depth cannot be determined virtually, so the surgeon must judge screw length intraoperatively.

10.2.3 Three-Dimensional Fluoroscopy-Based Navigation

With the invention of 3D fluoroscopy, 3D-fluoro-based navigation was applied to the cervical spine. A virtual 3D model of a spinal region of interest is created by a rotating C-arm. This creates a 3D virtual model of the spine that is similar in nature to that created by CT-based technology, a definite advantage over 2D-based fluoroscopy. Unlike CT-based navigation, however, 3D-flouro-based navigation is not limited by the problem of changing spatial relationships between adjacent vertebral segments. Registration is performed automatically during the imaging scan, so spinal navigation is immediately possible after verification of the registration accuracy. This eliminates time-consuming registration steps, and makes re-registration for adjacent vertebral bodies unnecessary. This technology avoids many of the limitations of both CT-based navigation and traditional 2D-based fluoroscopy.

10.3 Advantages

Navigation-based pedicle screw placement has been shown to increase the accuracy of screw position in the subaxial cervical spine. In one of the earliest studies on this topic, Ludwig et al used a cadaver model to compare the accuracy of pedicle screw implantation using three different techniques: (1) using surface landmarks alone, (2) performing laminotomies to provide additional visual and tactile control, and (3) using a computer-assisted surgical guidance system.[9] The authors found that the use of the computer-assisted surgical guidance system provided the highest rate of accurate screw positions, and lowest rate of critical perforations compared to the other methods.[9] Since that time, several studies have used patient series to assess the feasibility and accuracy of navigation for pedicle screw placement in the subaxial cervical spine.

Kotani et al evaluated the placement of CT-based navigated pedicle screws in 17 patients with difficult cervical anatomy, including those with spondylotic myelopathy with segmental instability, metastatic spinal tumors, rheumatoid spine, and post-laminectomy kyphosis.[5] A total of 78 pedicle screws were placed using CT-guided navigation between C2 and C7, and compared to a control group of 669 screws placed using free-hand technique. The authors reported that the rate of pedicle wall perforation was significantly lower in the navigation group (1 of 78, 1.2%) compared to the freehand technique (45 of 669, 6.7%, $p < 0.01$). The authors concluded that CT-based navigation is a safe and reliable tool for cervical pedicle screw placement.[5]

In a 2005 study by Richter et al, the authors prospectively compared the implantation of cervical pedicle screws in 52 consecutive patients with or without navigation.[10] The authors compared 92 screws in 20 patients implanted using conventional technique with 167 screws in 32 patients using CT-based

navigation techniques. While no screws caused a neurovascular compromise, the authors found that 8.6% of the non-navigated screws violated the bony cortex compared to 3.0% of the navigated screws.[10] The authors concluded that navigation-based pedicle screw placement from C3 to C6 reduces the risk of screw misplacement, which may reduce the risk of neurovascular injury.[10]

In 2011, Ishikawa et al performed a retrospective review of 21 consecutive patients undergoing a total of 108 cervical pedicle screws with the use of intraoperative CT-based navigation using the O-arm system.[11] Of the 108 pedicle screws, 96 (88.9%) were classified as Grade 0 (no perforation), 9 (8.3%) as Grade 1 (perforations < 2 mm), and 3 (2.8%) as Grade 2 (perforations between ≥ 2 and < 4 mm). The authors concluded that while intraoperative CT with the O-arm system can facilitate accurate cervical pedicle screw placement, there was still a 2.8% rate of major pedicle violations, which may lead to catastrophic complications.[11]

A 2014 study by Uehara et al was a retrospective review of 129 consecutive patients treated with CT-based computer-navigated pedicle screw placement.[12] Screw accuracy was classified as Grade 1 (no perforation); Grade 2 (minor perforation), indicating perforation of less than 50% of the screw diameter; and Grade 3 (major perforation), indicating perforation of 50% or more of the screw diameter. The authors found that 463 of 579 (80%) of screws were classified as Grade 1, 77 of 579 (13.3%) were Grade 2, and 39 of 579 (6.7%) were Grade 3.[12] While 6.7% of all pedicle screws were classified as a major perforation, there were no clinically significant complications, such as vertebral artery injury, spinal cord injury, or nerve root injury. Of the Grade 3 perforations, 30.8% of screws were medially perforated and 69.2% of screws were laterally perforated. The rate of perforation was significantly higher at C3–C5 compared to C6–C7 ($p = 0.0024$). The authors concluded that while CT-based navigation might increase the accuracy of cervical pedicle screw placement, great care is still needed while inserting cervical pedicle screws, particularly at the level of C3–C5.[12]

While most of these studies use CT-based navigation techniques, some newer studies have evaluated the use of intraoperative 3D-fluoroscopy imaging. Holly et al performed the first feasibility study using 3D fluoroscopic guidance to place percutaneous cervical pedicle screws in a cadaver model. Using an isocentric C-arm, the authors placed a total of 42 percutaneous pedicle screws into the cervical spine. Postprocedure CT scans were used to determine screw position. The authors reported that a total of 41 of 42 (97.6%) screws were placed accurately.[13] The authors concluded that the use of 3D fluoroscopy enables highly accurate, percutaneous cervical pedicle screw placement.[13]

In 2008, Ito and colleagues reported on their initial 50 cases using 3D-fluoroscopy-assisted cervical screw insertion, including 176 pedicle screws, 58 lateral mass screws, and 5 odontoid screws into the C1–C7 vertebrae.[14] All screws were placed by 3D-fluoroscopy and computer navigation, and postoperative fine-cut CT scans were used to assess the accuracy of screw insertion.[14] Of the 176 pedicle screws placed between C2 and C7, 171 screws (97.2%) of screws had no pedicle perforation. Importantly, the authors reported that no pedicle screws had a perforation > 2 mm, which was defined as a clinically significant screw deviation. The authors concluded that intraoperative 3D-fluoroscopy offers a number of advantages over CT-based navigation, and may be used for the accurate placement of cervical pedicle screws.

In 2010, Ishikawa published a similar study assessing the feasibility and accuracy of cervical pedicle screw placement using 3D-fluoroscopy-based navigation (3D-FN) compared to the conventional freehand technique with a lateral fluoroscopic view.[4] A total of 150 screws were placed using the 3D-FN technique, and compared to 126 screws placed using the conventional technique of a lateral fluoroscopic view. While there was no significant difference in the rate of pedicle perforation (27.0% conventional vs. 18.7% navigated), the rate of pedicle perforations measuring > 1 mm was significantly reduced by navigation. There was a higher prevalence of malpositioned cervical pedicle screws (defined as Grade 2 or higher [> 2 mm perforation]) in the conventional group compared to the 3D-FN group (17.5 vs. 7.3%, $p < 0.05$).[4] The authors concluded that 3D-fluoroscopy-based navigation had clear advantages in terms of accuracy over conventional techniques. However, they state that severe malpositioning of cervical pedicle screws can occur even with the assistance of 3D-based fluoroscopic navigation.[4]

A 2007 meta-analysis by Kosmopoulos compared the accuracy of 1,089 cervical pedicle screws placed without the use of navigation compared to 114 placed with image guidance. The authors found a higher accuracy among navigated pedicle screws (99.4%, range: 98.8–100%) compared to the conventional technique (93.3%, range: 71–100%).[15] The authors concluded that navigation improved the accuracy of the placement of pedicle screws.[15]

In addition to improving accuracy, navigation-based pedicle screw placement may reduce radiation exposure to the surgeon and surgical team. Navigation reduces the required amount of repetitive intraoperative fluoroscopy. While the radiation risk to the patient is likely slightly increased, it is still in an acceptable range.[16] Reducing radiation is likely more important for the operating surgeon and operating room staff, who are exposed to a significant amount of daily radiation during routine spinal procedures.

10.4 Limitations

CT-based navigation has several limitations. Many patients present with CT scans that lack the precision required for CT-based navigation. This patient must then undergo repeat CT scan, which increases the radiation exposure to the patient and increases cost of care. For insertion of pedicle screws at multiple levels, each vertebra must be registered and matched individually. This procedure is time consuming. Intraoperative registration is not possible in certain situations, such as following prior laminectomies, as the registration frame cannot be attached. As mentioned previously, a major limitation of CT-based navigation is that intervertebral anatomic relationships with the patient in the prone position during surgery may not match the preoperative CT data obtained while the patient is in the supine position. This discrepancy may be overcome by obtaining intraoperative 3D CT-based navigation. Shimokawa et al compared the rate of cervical pedicle screw misplacement in patients undergoing CT-based navigation with either preoperative or intraoperative CT scans.[17] The authors found a higher rate of pedicle screw misplacement (more than half of screw outside the pedicle) using a preoperative CT-based navigation system (15 of 452 screws, 3.3%) compared to an intraoperative CT-based navigation system (2 of 310 screws, 0.6%). Despite these cortical perforations, the authors did not identify any neural or vascular complications associated with the use of CT-based pedicle screw placement in the cervical spine.[17] Intraoperative CT scans have an advantage, in that registration occurs automatically. 3D-fluoroscopy shares this same benefit, as registration can be performed automatically.

Another major limitation is cost. Intraoperative CT scanners and 3D-fluoroscopy machines are expensive and not available at all centers. There is an additional cost of the navigation computer and associated instruments. Lastly, intraoperative imaging may require specialized radiolucent head holders or tables not available at all centers.

There is a learning curve associated with the adoption of any new technology or technique. The learning curve for image-guided navigation has not been reported specifically for cervical pedicle screw placement. However, it has been reported for the use of image-guided navigation in other areas of spine surgery.[18,19] The major difficulties when using navigation-guided pedicle screw placement is the ability to direct instruments based on imaging visualized on a screen and the ability to replicate in-line maneuvers when placing instrumentation.[20]

Lastly, it is important to note that while navigation improves the accuracy of cervical pedicle screw placement, perforation remains an issue, and is most common in the cervical spine. Uehara et al retrospectively reviewed a total of 3,413 pedicle screws placed from C2 to L5 using a CT-based navigation system.[21] Postoperative CT scans were used to assess the accuracy of pedicle screw placement. The authors found that the highest rate of Grade 2 or 3 perforations (Grade 2 defined as 2–4 mm perforation of the pedicle, Grade 3 defined as > 4 mm perforation of the pedicle) occurred in the middle cervical spine (11.4% for C3–C5), followed by 10.4% for T1–T4, 8.8% for T5–T8, 7.0% for C6–C7, 5.0% for C2, 4.5% for T9–T12, and 3.8% for L1–L5.[21] The authors concluded that even with the added benefit of CT-based navigation, it is especially important to take care when inserting pedicle screws in the cervical spine given the high perforation rate.[21]

10.5 Discussion

Navigation-based cervical pedicle screw placement increases the accuracy and reliability of this technically challenging procedure. It has yet to be established that this increased accuracy translates into a decreased rate of arterial or neurological injuries. In addition, no study has demonstrated improved clinical or functional outcome scores with navigation-based pedicle screw placement compared to conventional techniques. Therefore, navigation-based pedicle screw placement at present should not be considered the gold-standard compared to conventional techniques. Given the increased operating room time, potential learning curve, and high cost of this technology, future high-quality studies are needed to demonstrate improved clinical and functional outcomes and a decreased risk of complications before adopting this technology as a gold standard. While not considered the standard of care, navigated cervical spine screw instrumentation may be indicated in certain complex anatomical situations, such as revision surgeries or malformations.

References

[1] Abumi K, Shono Y, Ito M, Taneichi H, Kotani Y, Kaneda K. Complications of pedicle screw fixation in reconstructive surgery of the cervical spine. Spine. 2000; 25(8):962–969

[2] Hojo Y, Ito M, Suda K, Oda I, Yoshimoto H, Abumi K. A multicenter study on accuracy and complications of freehand placement of cervical pedicle screws under lateral fluoroscopy in different pathological conditions: CT-based evaluation of more than 1,000 screws. Eur Spine J. 2014; 23(10):2166–2174

[3] Neo M, Sakamoto T, Fujibayashi S, Nakamura T. The clinical risk of vertebral artery injury from cervical pedicle screws inserted in degenerative vertebrae. Spine. 2005; 30(24):2800–2805

[4] Ishikawa Y, Kanemura T, Yoshida G, Ito Z, Muramoto A, Ohno S. Clinical accuracy of three-dimensional fluoroscopy-based computer-assisted cervical pedicle screw placement: a retrospective comparative study of conventional versus computer-assisted cervical pedicle screw placement. J Neurosurg Spine. 2010; 13(5):606–611

[5] Kotani Y, Abumi K, Ito M, Minami A. Improved accuracy of computer-assisted cervical pedicle screw insertion. J Neurosurg. 2003; 99(3) Suppl:257–263

[6] Kaneyama S, Sugawara T, Sumi M. Safe and accurate midcervical pedicle screw insertion procedure with the patient-specific screw guide template system. Spine. 2015; 40(6):E341–E348

[7] Tauchi R, Imagama S, Sakai Y, et al. The correlation between cervical range of motion and misplacement of cervical pedicle screws during cervical posterior spinal fixation surgery using a CT-based navigation system. Eur Spine J. 2013; 22(7):1504–1508

[8] Barsa P, Fröhlich R, Šercl M, Buchvald P, Suchomel P. The intraoperative portable CT scanner-based spinal navigation: a viable option for instrumentation in the region of cervico-thoracic junction. Eur Spine J. 2016; 25(6):1643–1650

[9] Ludwig SC, Kramer DL, Balderston RA, Vaccaro AR, Foley KF, Albert TJ. Placement of pedicle screws in the human cadaveric cervical spine: comparative accuracy of three techniques. Spine. 2000; 25(13):1655–1667

[10] Richter M, Cakir B, Schmidt R. Cervical pedicle screws: conventional versus computer-assisted placement of cannulated screws. Spine. 2005; 30(20):2280–2287

[11] Ishikawa Y, Kanemura T, Yoshida G, et al. Intraoperative, full-rotation, three-dimensional image (O-arm)-based navigation system for cervical pedicle screw insertion. J Neurosurg Spine. 2011; 15(5):472–478

[12] Uehara M, Takahashi J, Ikegami S, et al. Screw perforation features in 129 consecutive patients performed computer-guided cervical pedicle screw insertion. Eur Spine J. 2014; 23(10):2189–2195

[13] Holly LT, Foley KT. Percutaneous placement of posterior cervical screws using three-dimensional fluoroscopy. Spine. 2006; 31(5):536–540, discussion 541

[14] Ito Y, Sugimoto Y, Tomioka M, Hasegawa Y, Nakago K, Yagata Y. Clinical accuracy of 3D fluoroscopy-assisted cervical pedicle screw insertion. J Neurosurg Spine. 2008; 9(5):450–453

[15] Kosmopoulos V, Schizas C. Pedicle screw placement accuracy: a meta-analysis. Spine. 2007; 32(3):E111–E120

[16] Mendelsohn D, Strelzow J, Dea N, et al. Patient and surgeon radiation exposure during spinal instrumentation using intraoperative computed tomography-based navigation. Spine J. 2016; 16(3):343–354

[17] Shimokawa N, Takami T. Surgical safety of cervical pedicle screw placement with computer navigation system. Neurosurg Rev. 2017; 40(2):251–258

[18] Sasso RC, Garrido BJ. Computer-assisted spinal navigation versus serial radiography and operative time for posterior spinal fusion at L5-S1. J Spinal Disord Tech. 2007; 20(2):118–122

[19] Bai YS, Zhang Y, Chen ZQ, et al. Learning curve of computer-assisted navigation system in spine surgery. Chin Med J (Engl). 2010; 123(21):2989–2994

[20] Nottmeier EW. A review of image-guided spinal surgery. J Neurosurg Sci. 2012; 56(1):35–47

[21] Uehara M, Takahashi J, Ikegami S, Kuraishi S, Futatsugi T, Kato H. Screw perforation rates in 359 consecutive patients receiving computer-guided pedicle screw insertion along the cervical to lumbar spine. Eur Spine J. 2017; 26(11):2858–2864

11 Navigated Anterior Transoral Surgery for C1 and C2 Pathologies

Christine L. Hammer and James J. Evans

Abstract:

The transoral approach to the cervical spine is an essential technique that uniquely allows for direct anterior cervical spine decompression. It may be done as a standalone procedure or part of a staged anterior decompression and posterior fusion approach. A microscope is generally used, yet visualization may be improved with concurrent use of a transnasal endoscope. Accuracy may be further improved with either 2D or 3D navigation.

Keywords: transoral, transoral–transpalatal, navigation, anterior cervical

11.1 Introduction

Accessing the anterior aspects of the upper cervical spine in patients with ventral cervical spine pathology has historically presented a challenge to surgeons. Classic approaches include the transoral and transoral–transpalatal, as well as more expanded approaches including the transoral–transmandibular and the transoral-extended maxillotomy (open door) approaches (▶ Fig. 11.1).

Credit for popularizing these techniques may be given to many such as Sherman (1935), Fang and Ong for their work for infection (1962), Greenberg (1968), and many others including Crockard (1985) who designed the well-known Crockard retractor.[1,2] More recently, the endoscopic transnasal approaches have been popularized either as independent approaches or in combination with the transoral approach. This chapter will analyze the utility and limits of these approaches to the upper cervical spine when coupled with intraoperative navigation techniques.

Nearly a century of experience has increased the success of the transoral or transoral–transpalatal approaches for pathology of the upper cervical spine while simultaneously simplifying and standardizing the optimal preoperative and postoperative care. The challenges of operating in a small corridor have been partially addressed through the development and implementation of modern technology including microscopes, endoscopes, and malleable or angled instruments. Furthermore, these new technologies have helped limit the approach-related damage to normal anatomy not directly involved with the pathology. This is particularly true of the endoscopic transoral and transnasal approaches. Additionally, as with other surgical disciplines, the use of two-dimensional (2D) or three-dimensional (3D) intraoperative image-guided navigation has dramatically increased surgical precision and improved outcomes in the anterior approach to ventral pathologies of the cervical spine.[1]

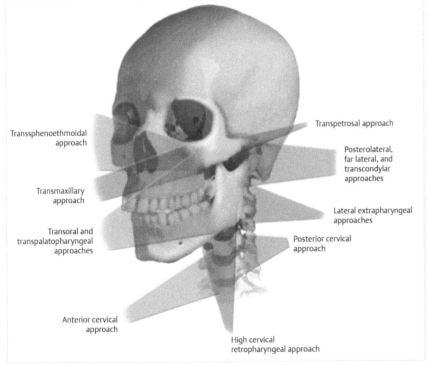

Fig. 11.1 Surgical approaches to the craniocervical junction.

Transsphenoethmoidal approach

Transmaxillary approach

Transoral and transpalatopharyngeal approaches

Anterior cervical approach

High cervical retropharyngeal approach

Transpetrosal approach

Posterolateral, far lateral, and transcondylar approaches

Lateral extrapharyngeal approaches

Posterior cervical approach

11.2 Indications

Indications for the transoral approach to the anterior cervical spine include, but are not limited to, accessing the following pathologies which may involve the craniovertebral junction, also known as the craniocervical junction (CCJ):

- Pathology of the bone:
  - Traumatic bone fracture.
  - Removal of foreign objects (e.g., ballistics).
  - Basilar impression/invagination or upward migration of the occipital condyles.
  - Pannus related to rheumatoid arthritis. (This is more historic given the frequency of posterior instrumented arthrodesis in these patients.)
- Extradural mass:
  - Abscess.
  - Chordoma.
  - Metastasis (e.g., renal).
  - Primary bone or central nervus system (CNS) tumor.
- Intradural extramedullary mass (e.g., schwannoma, meningioma, neurofibroma).

11.3 Anatomy

The CCJ includes the inferior clivus at the junction of the foramen magnum, the atlas and axis, as well as the associated ligaments such as the anterior atlanto-occipital ligament (continuation of the anterior longitudinal ligament [ALL]), the apical and alar ligaments, and tectorial membrane (▶ Fig. 11.2). The pharyngeal wall consists of several layers which have been studied and described by Wang et.al.[3]

The posterior pharyngeal wall was found to range in thickness from 2.9 to 4.3 mm at the C1 tubercle and 5.2 to 7.1 mm at the C1 lateral mass, and 4.3 to 6.5 mm at the central portion of the C2 vertebral body (▶ Table 11.1). Through these dissections, five layers were identified and described: mucosa, muscularis mucosae, prevertebral fascia, prevertebral muscles (longus capitis and longus cervices), and the anterior longitudinal ligament which drapes the dens anteriorly.[3]

Several major veins and arteries (i.e., pharyngeal branches of carotid, palatine, and pharyngeal arteries and veins) were noted to be in the space between the muscularis mucosae and the prevertebral fascia (retropharyngeal space). The internal carotid artery (ICA) is most susceptible to injury at the level of C1 because it resides anterolaterally to the C1 arch before it enters the skull base. The C2 segment lies more anteromedially than the C1 segment.

When discussing the safe exposure zone in the transoral approach, it is important to consider that an expected width ranges 35.5 to 43.7 mm and expected length ranges 44.3 to 62.0 mm. Additional exposure from soft palate splitting may provide nearly 1.5 cm more length[3,4] (▶ Fig. 11.3).

With microscopic visualization, it is recommended that the entrance to the oral cavity must be at least 2.5 to 3.0 cm between incisors in order to have adequate visualization and working room. This may be circumvented by the use of endoscopic transoral visualization and angled instruments.[4]

11.4 Navigation

Intraoperative computed tomography (CT) image-guided navigation for the treatment of anterior cervical pathologies has been well studied and shown to improve accuracy and decrease morbidity. It can aid the surgeon in creating a safe exposure with minimal dissection (i.e., minimal access) as well as preventing injuries to neural and vascular structures. The use of image-guided navigation also limits the use of fluoroscopy, thereby decreasing radiation exposure to the patient and operating room staff and it allows a similar or greater degree of accuracy which is critical when working in this high-risk

Table 11.1 Average posterior pharyngeal wall thickness

Posterior pharyngeal wall thickness at the C1 tubercle	2.9–4.3 mm
Posterior pharyngeal wall thickness at the C1 lateral mass (at the central portion of the C2 vertebral body)	4.3–6.5 mm

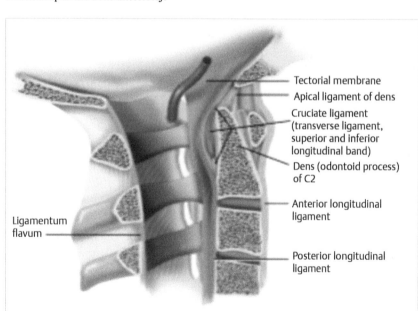

Tectorial membrane

Apical ligament of dens

Cruciate ligament (transverse ligament, superior and inferior longitudinal band)

Dens (odontoid process) of C2

Anterior longitudinal ligament

Posterior longitudinal ligament

Ligamentum flavum

Fig. 11.2 Ligaments encountered at the craniocervical junction during the transoral approach.

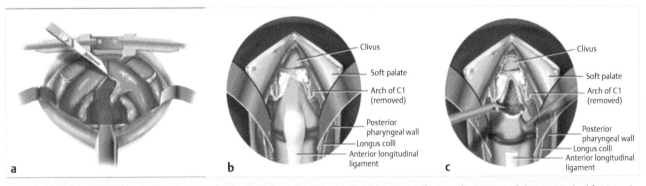

Fig. 11.3 **(a)** Exposure of the oral cavity and pharynx using Dingman or Crockard oral retractors. **(b)** Lateral retraction of the prevertebral fascia and longus colli muscles revealing the clivus, the C1 arch, and the odontoid peg. **(c)** Removal of the C1 anterior arch, clivus, and odontoid peg using Kerrison rongeurs and a high-speed drill.

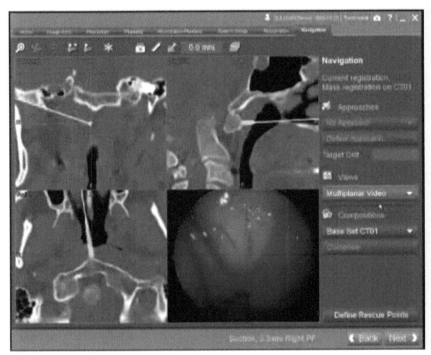

Fig. 11.4 2D navigation software showing coronal, sagittal, and axial views with the concurrent transnasal endoscope image in the bottom right.

location. Indications for use and, furthermore, 2D versus 3D may include complex and disrupted anatomy.

The use of navigation, or image guidance, for anterior approaches to the upper cervical spine has been increasingly studied with continued refinement of the registration process, given that the transoral approaches to the anterior cervical spine have been complicated by the lack of anatomically consistent or characteristic landmarks for obtaining registration.[5,6,7] There are several systems that utilize 2D or 3D image guidance for intraoperative assistance. The 2D navigation systems are similar to those used for cranial cases which are registered through point system, fiducials, or another form of tracker designed for placement on the soft tissue such as a face mask. An example of this is the commonly used CranialMask Tracker (Stryker) which is paired with LED-based instrumentation and the compatible software system. This software, like other systems, provide image fusion between image modalities including CT and magnetic resonance imaging (MRI; ▶ Fig. 11.4).

The 3D options require the use of a reference frame and trackers which may be attached to the headrest, bone, or skin.

These are often referred to as "real-time" navigation and include the Airo Mobile Intraoperative CT-Based Spinal Navigation (Brainlab, Westchester, IL) system, the Stealth Station Spine Surgery Imaging and Surgical Navigation with O-arm (Medtronic Inc, Minneapolis, MN), Stryker Spinal Navigation with SpineMask and SpineMap Software (Stryker, Kalamazoo, MI), and Ziehm Vision FD Vario 3D with NaviPort (Ziehm Imaging, Orlando, FL).[8]

Both 2D and 3D image guidance system and intraoperative CT scanning systems have anatomical reference clamps, pins, or surface attachments that require placement at various points before or after exposure. The most significant challenge with using 3D image guidance navigation is ensuring that the dynamic reference frame remains fixed during the case.[9] In cases of the anterior cervical spine approaches including transoral, it is difficult to find a bony attachment and novel approaches have been discussed including attachment to the forehead.[9] In most cases, the 2D systems are adequate for achieving the goals of both accuracy and minimal exposure.

11.5 Preoperative Considerations

The transoral approach to the anterior cervical spine must be considered with the following limitations in mind: adequacy of visualization beyond midline, limitations of oral retraction, velopharyngeal incompetence postoperatively, the indications for a tracheostomy and gastric tube, as well as how to address healing problems.

The transoral approach is considered a class II (clean contaminated) surgical wound with increased healing time given the rich blood supply of this region.[10] However, studies have shown that preoperative oropharyngeal inflammation are more likely to have a postoperative infection.[10] Treatment may be initiated with a few days of oral cavity cleaning including chlorhexidine rinses and prophylactic antibiotic use, smoking cessation, and optimizing nutrition status through consultation with a nutritionist who may recommend vitamins or supplements based on laboratory results.[10] Patients should be evaluated for natural jaw excursion with the minimum recommended opening of 2.5 cm between the incisors when microscopic visualization is used.[11] Additionally, patients should be evaluated for congenital flexion deformities or for limited range of motion since extension of the neck aids in ease of the exposure.

The patient's nutrition status and neurological exam may guide preoperative planning for a gastric tube and a preoperative tracheostomy.[10] Consider tracheotomy with vagal, hypoglossal, and/or glossopharyngeal nerve dysfunction.[12] A percutaneous endoscopic gastrostomy (PEG) and tracheostomy may be planned in cases of extended exposure, given the increased risk of infection and velopharyngeal incompetence or nasal regurgitation.[13] Preoperative imaging includes the one that provides appropriate diagnosis including CT and MRI.

11.6 Operative Approach

11.6.1 Exposure

The patient is intubated via an orotracheal or nasotracheal intubation or according to preoperative plans for a tracheostomy.[14] Five percent cortisone cream is recommended for coating the lips and tongue to minimize swelling with subsequent phisohex solution rinse for oral preparation.[11] The head is placed in a three-pin Mayfield head holder or on a circular head rest, or on a halo-headrest, with the patient positioned similar to an anterior cervical procedure. Retractors, such as the Dingman or Crockard oral retractors, or the use of sutures open the operative corridor.[4] A red rubber catheter sutured to the uvula can be used for increased retraction of the uvula. Alternatively, the uvula may be removed and red rubber catheters may be inserted into the bilateral nares to retract the soft palate.

A common theme among the experiences with this approach is the importance of respecting soft-tissue planes.[3] A midline incision should be made with dissection laterally. The ALL may be dissected in a subperiosteal fashion with electrocautery. Preserving the tissue planes for at least a two-layer closure is important for transoral surgery.

11.6.2 Closure

Long needle holders with 3.0 Vicryl are recommended for both the mucosal and muscle layers.[1,11,12,15] When working transnasal, the closure is less of an issue since the surgical corridor is mainly above the palatal plane. In intradural cases with high potential of a CSF leak, a lumbar drain should be considered in addition to attempted reconstruction through grafting such as fascia lata or fat. Antibiotics with CNS penetration should be provided as well for up to 1 week postoperatively.[4,11]

11.6.3 Endoscope

The use of the endoscope in both the transnasal and transoral approach provides improved visualization without further dissection or exposure, such as palate splitting or extended maxillotomy procedures.[4,7,16] This avoids injury to normal anatomical structures uninvolved with the pathology. The benefits to the patient include decreased airway and swallowing morbidity, decreased postoperative pain, better sinonasal function, and reduced need for tracheostomies or feeding tubes.[4] It may be wise to consider the endoscope use in the transoral approaches in patients with limited mouth opening, minimal occipital cervical fusion, temporomandibular joint arthritis, or trismus.[4] Angled scopes improve craniocaudal and lateral visualization which can facilitate improved resections.[17] The transnasal approach is a favored approach, given the less invasive access with limited to no retraction. A combined approach of transnasal and transoral is recommended for maximizing the working room without increasing the invasiveness of the approach (i.e., avoiding splitting the palate; ▶ Fig. 11.5).

Additional benefits include the ability to use malleable instruments which were designed for maximizing surgeons' ability to maneuver in small corridors and reach around corners where angled endoscopes can visualize.

11.6.4 Postoperative Considerations

An obvious issue to address both in preoperative consultation and in the postoperative setting is that of the nutrition plan and status. As discussed, a tracheostomy and preoperative PEG may be indicated in cases of existing cranial nerve deficits or plans for extended approaches. For less complex pathologies and approaches, one may restart an oral diet of modified consistency on postoperative day one.[3,10]

11.7 Pearls and Pitfalls

Complications associated with the transoral and transoral–transpalatal approach include velopharyngeal incompetence, hypernasal speech and nasal reflux, dental injury, tongue necrosis, upper airway obstruction, wound dehiscence, odynophagia, meningitis from cerebrospinal fluid leaks, and temporomandibular joint syndrome.[4]

Limiting the width of the exposure to approximately 3.0 cm prevents inadvertent injury to the eustachian tubes, vertebral arteries, and hypoglossal nerves and the carotid artery as it passes in front of the C1 arch laterally.[4] Studies comparing endoscope use in the transoral and/or transnasal approach in combination with the use of image guidance suggested that one may obtain the least invasive exposure while providing the most precision.[7] The combined approach, in cases of this upper cervical pathology, addresses the limits of the transnasal

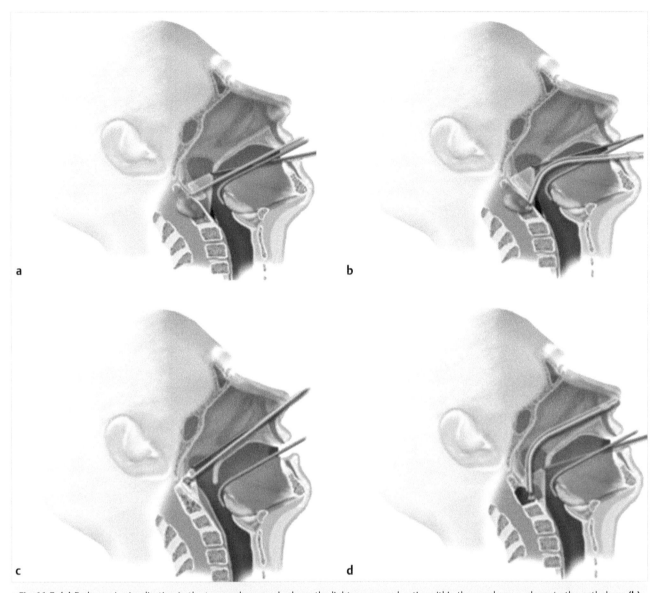

Fig. 11.5 **(a)** Endoscopic visualization in the transoral approach places the light source and optics within the oropharynx, closer to the pathology. **(b)** Angled endoscopes and drills broaden the craniocaudal and lateral extent of resection within the retropharyngeal incision. **(c)** Endoscopic visualization in the transnasal and transoral approach. **(d)** Angled transnasal drill with a transoral endoscope.

approach which is the angle and length of the hard palate (▶ Fig. 11.6). Examples would be in the cases of a clival–cervical chordoma or basilar invagination (▶ Fig. 11.7, ▶ Fig. 11.8). In these latter examples, the normal anatomy is not present, therefore proving the importance of navigation for a safe and effective surgery, which will likely improve the patient's outcome.

11.8 Case Discussion

The patient is a 45-year-old female with history of Ehlers-Danlos. She presented with a 1-year history of repeated falls and gait instability. On examination, she was hyperreflexic in both the upper and lower extremities. The preoperative MRI showed basilar invagination with cord compression (▶ Fig. 11.9). The preoperative CT scan showed apparent overgrowth of the clivus with a shortened dens which was likely a congenital anomaly (▶ Fig. 11.9). She underwent a two-stage procedure on the same day. First, she had a transoral, 3D-navigated surgery to decompress her spinal cord (▶ Fig. 11.10). Second, she had a posterior occipital-to-cervical fusion. The patient recovered well neurologically with improvement in gait and balance. She was started on oral diet on postoperative day one.[3,5,6,7,15,16,17,18,19,20,21,22]

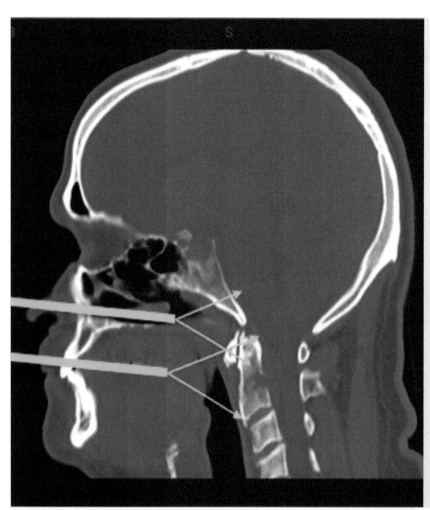

Fig. 11.6 The limits of the transnasal and transoral approach.

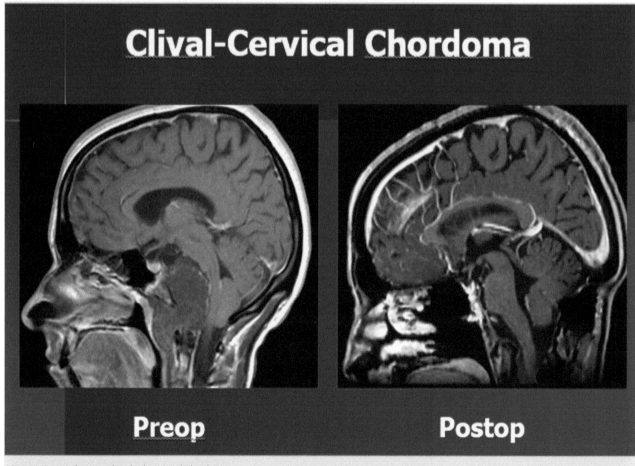

Fig. 11.7 MRI showing the clival–cervical chordoma.

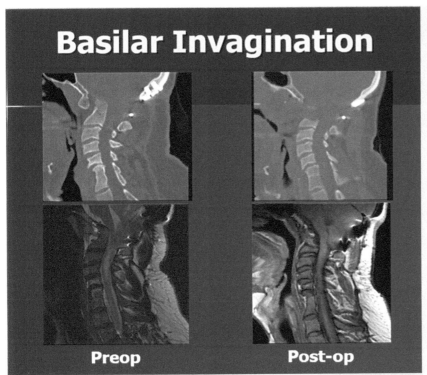

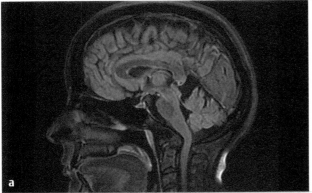

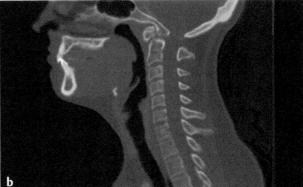

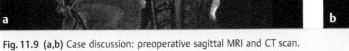

Fig. 11.8 CT and MRI imaging of a case of basilar invagination.

Fig. 11.9 (a,b) Case discussion: preoperative sagittal MRI and CT scan.

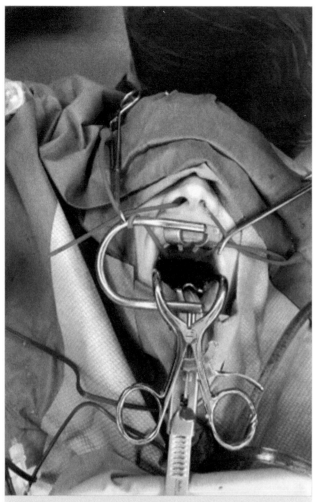

Fig. 11.10 Intraoperative placement of retractors and bilateral intranasal red rubber catheters for retraction used in this transoral navigated case.

References

[1] Crockard HA. The transoral approach to the base of the brain and upper cervical cord. Ann R Coll Surg Engl. 1985; 67(5):321–325

[2] Crockard HA, Bradford R. Transoral transclival removal of a schwannoma anterior to the craniocervical junction. Case report. J Neurosurg. 1985; 62(2):293–295

[3] Wang Z, Xia H, Wu Z, Ai F, Xu J, Yin Q. Detailed anatomy for the transoral approach to the craniovertebral junction: an exposure and safety study. J Neurol Surg B Skull Base. 2014; 75(2):133–139

[4] Singh H, Harrop J, Schiffmacher P, Rosen M, Evans J. Ventral surgical approaches to craniovertebral junction chordomas. Neurosurgery. 2010; 66 (3) Suppl:96–103

[5] Miyahara J, Hirao Y, Matsubayashi Y, Chikuda H. Computer tomography navigation for the transoral anterior release of a complex craniovertebral junction deformity: a report of two cases. Int J Surg Case Rep. 2016; 24:142–145

[6] Veres R, Bagó A, Fedorcsák I. Early experiences with image-guided transoral surgery for the pathologies of the upper cervical spine. Spine. 2001; 26(12):1385–1388

[7] Pillai P, Baig MN, Karas CS, Ammirati M. Endoscopic image-guided transoral approach to the craniovertebral junction: an anatomic study comparing surgical exposure and surgical freedom obtained with the endoscope and the operating microscope. Neurosurgery. 2009; 64(5) Suppl 2:437–442, discussion 442–444

[8] Overley SC, Cho SK, Mehta AI, Arnold PM. Navigation and robotics in spinal surgery: where are we now? Neurosurgery. 2017; 80 3S:S86–S99

[9] Jang SH, Cho JY, Choi WC, Lee HY, Lee SH, Hong JT. Novel method for setting up 3D navigation system with skin-fixed dynamic reference frame in anterior cervical surgery. Comput Aided Surg. 2015; 20(1):24–28

[10] Yin Q, Xia H, Wu Z, et al. Surgical site infections following the transoral approach: a review of 172 consecutive cases. Clin Spine Surg. 2016; 29(10):E502–E508

[11] Liu JK, Couldwell WT, Apfelbaum RI. Transoral approach and extended modifications for lesions of the ventral foramen magnum and craniovertebral junction. Skull Base. 2008; 18(3):151–166

[12] Jones DC, Hayter JP, Vaughan ED, Findlay GF. Oropharyngeal morbidity following transoral approaches to the upper cervical spine. Int J Oral Maxillofac Surg. 1998; 27(4):295–298

[13] Choi D, Crockard HA. Evolution of transoral surgery: three decades of change in patients, pathologies, and indications. Neurosurgery. 2013; 73(2):296–303, discussion 303–304

[14] Hsu W, Wolinsky JP, Gokaslan ZL, Sciubba DM. Transoral approaches to the cervical spine. Neurosurgery. 2010; 66(3) Suppl:119–125

[15] El-Sayed IH, Wu JC, Ames CP, Balamurali G, Mummaneni PV. Combined transnasal and transoral endoscopic approaches to the craniovertebral junction. J Craniovertebr Junction Spine. 2010; 1(1):44–48

[16] Pillai P, Sammet S, Ammirati M. Image-guided, endoscopic-assisted drilling and exposure of the whole length of the internal auditory canal and its fundus with preservation of the integrity of the labyrinth using a retrosigmoid approach: a laboratory investigation. Neurosurgery. 2009; 65(6) Suppl:53–59, discussion 59

[17] Lee A, Sommer D, Reddy K, Murty N, Gunnarsson T. Endoscopic transnasal approach to the craniocervical junction. Skull Base. 2010; 20(3):199–205

[18] Chaudhry NS, Ozpinar A, Bi WL, Chavakula V, Chi JH, Dunn IF. Basilar invagination: case report and literature review. World Neurosurg. 2015; 83(6):1180.e7–1180.e11

[19] Guppy KH, Chakrabarti I, Banerjee A. The use of intraoperative navigation for complex upper cervical spine surgery. Neurosurg Focus. 2014; 36(3):E5

[20] Jackson GJ, Sedney CL, Fancy T, Rosen CL. Intraoperative neuronavigation for transoral surgical approach: use of frameless stereotaxy with 3D rotational C-arm for image acquisition. W V Med J. 2015; 111(3):30–32, 34

[21] Jeszenszky D, Fekete TF, Melcher R, Harms J. C2 prosthesis: anterior upper cervical fixation device to reconstruct the second cervical vertebra. Eur Spine J. 2007; 16(10):1695–1700

[22] Van Abel KM, Mallory GW, Kasperbauer JL, et al. Transnasal odontoid resection: is there an anatomic explanation for differing swallowing outcomes? Neurosurg Focus. 2014; 37(4):E16

12 Navigated Posterior Correction of Pediatric Scoliosis

Justin C. Paul, Arya Varthi, and Raj J. Gala

Abstract:

A significant number of pediatric scoliosis patients undergo an operation that carries substantial risk. Avoiding complications is critical and some of the most devastating complications can arise from malpositioned hardware. Pedicle screw instrumentation of the spine is the most common instrumentation technique, and proper placement of each anchor point can be assisted by 3D navigation. In the best cases, these techniques can improve fidelity and reduce radiation. In the future, there is potential for improved efficiency and costs.

Keywords: pediatric, scoliosis, navigation, pedicle, screw, radiation, 3D

12.1 Introduction

Over 600,000 children in the United States have pediatric scoliosis, with the vast majority diagnosed with adolescent idiopathic scoliosis (AIS).[1] While many of these patients are managed with nonoperative care, a significant number undergo an operation, which is often a major undertaking that carries substantial risk. When the decision is made to operate, it is often not for current symptoms, as most patients are asymptomatic.[2] Thus, avoiding complications, both short-term and long-term, is one of the most important aspects of surgical care of this pathology.

12.2 Surgical Approach to Pediatric Scoliosis

Surgical treatment of AIS is generally recommended when curvature is greater than 45° and progressing or when the terminal curvature exceeds 50 degrees.[3] The principal aims of surgery are primarily to halt curve progression with spinal fusion and secondarily correct existing curvature with rod-and-screw constructs. The surgical approach to spinal fusion can be through open anterior, posterior, or combined approaches. There are also posterior percutaneous or "minimally invasive" approaches to AIS correction.[4,5,6]

While there are a variety of options, operative treatment of pediatric scoliosis is most often performed through a posterior approach.[2] Through the posterior approach, deformity correction can be achieved through rod contouring and derotation maneuvers, as well as through various osteotomies.[7,8,9] Some of the more involved osteotomies, such as pedicle subtraction osteotomies and vertebral column resections carry significantly higher risk of complications.[9,10] In addition, the current surgical trends for pediatric scoliosis have shifted away from hook-and-wire fixation, toward pedicle screw instrumentation.[11,12,13] In the pediatric spine, pedicle screw placement has been shown to be safe in the vast majority of cases, but there remains a risk for malpositioned screws that may result in neurologic injury.[14] The deformities seen in congenital scoliosis and neuromuscular scoliosis can be even more challenging as the rotation of the vertebral bodies can make pedicle screw placement difficult and sometimes impossible.

12.3 Pedicle Screw Instrumentation

Posterior instrumentation in AIS includes screws inserted into pedicles of the vertebra that are connected by a rod to fix the spine while fusion occurs.[15] The placement of these pedicle screws can be guided by either anatomical landmarks or computer-guided navigation.[16] Inappropriate pedicle screw placement may result in intraoperative pedicle fractures, wound infection, and encroachment on the spinal canal causing neurological complications.[17] Studies of non-navigated, freehand screw placement have established baseline levels of inappropriate screw placement.[18,19,20,21]

Pedicle screws can be placed with "freehand" technique, meaning with the use of bony landmarks and palpation of the bony canal through the pedicle. But imaging can be used to assist the instrumentation process with several technological advances. The most recent advancement is the use of the intraoperative CT for navigation of pedicle screw placement. While navigation can assist with osteotomies, including hemivertebral resections for cases of congenital scoliosis,[22] the most natural use of navigation is to increase the accuracy of pedicle screw placement.[23,24] Moreover, navigation can allow for placement of pedicle screws in situations previously deemed unsafe, such as severe rotational deformity or narrow pedicles.[25,26,27,28,29] Additionally, in cases of revision surgery for pediatric scoliosis, the normal landmarks for freehand pedicle screw placement may be distorted. Navigation can be useful in these situations, as well as if an osteotomy through the prior fusion mass is needed.[30] Lastly navigation may also have a role in minimally invasive techniques for pediatric scoliosis.[31]

12.4 Freehand Technique

Freehand technique has been used widely in orthopedics to place implants. Before more widespread use of intraoperative fluoroscopy, percutaneous pinning of the hip was performed freehand with external landmarks and tactile feedback. Radiographs were performed to confirm proper positioning after placement of implants. However, in the age where imaging is readily available intraoperatively, most surgeons use a combination of visual landmarks, tactile feedback, and fluoroscopic imaging to place screws. Freehand placement of pedicle screws can be fast and safe, but it is important to evaluate the results of this technique. Many surgeons do not get postoperative CT and do not look critically at screw placement other than plain films, but some centers have tried to answer this question.

A seminal study was conducted to critically evaluate freehand screws using a postoperative CT. In 112 screws that were assessed, 12.5% screws were misplaced and two screws were on the aorta.[32] Another report of over a thousand freehand screws placed in 60 pediatric deformity patients evaluated with postoperative CT showed about 10% had significant medial or lateral pedicle wall violations.[33] The T4–T9 screws placed in the concavity were seen to be the highest risk after evaluating freehand thoracic screws.[34] Overall it appears that about 1 in 10 freehand screws is in a suboptimal location, but they may not have negative clinical effects. Medial and lateral breach is often well tolerated and even anterior penetration can have no effect in many cases as aortic and esophageal injury is exceedingly rare.

12.5 Freehand Technique with Image Guidance

Two-dimensional (2D) imaging can be performed readily at most hospitals. When freehand technique is used, plain radiography can demonstrate the cascade of the screws in two planes. This can be time consuming as films need to be printed and repeated if images are inadequate. These films do not assess the axial plane, where most errors are usually detected.

Another technique involves the mobile C-arm. The image intensifier can be draped into the surgical field and used flexibly to image in any plane but only takes one image at a time. Two C-arms can be used to take simultaneous biplanar images to save time. Still, axial plan information is difficult to interpret and surgery must be performed wearing lead. The patient and staff are all at risk for radiation exposure.

Limitations in these 2D techniques led to the development of intraoperative CT scans (e.g., O-arm), which can be used with or without navigation. Without navigation, the CT can be performed after implant placement to critically assess pedicle screw location after freehand technique, using the axial plane, which is more ideal. Using the CT with navigation allows real-time confirmation of the surgeon's visual and tactile information showing the containment in the pedicle and the length and diameter of the screw. This maximizes the size of the screw that can be placed safely. The drawbacks include the expense of the machinery and the radiation exposure to the patient.

12.6 Navigation Technique

Navigation is the synthesis of physical landmarks on the surgical field with previously obtained or intraoperatively obtained imaging to form a visual guide for the surgeon when the target is deep to the surgical exposure. In spine surgery, navigation techniques elucidate pedicle morphology since the pedicle is usually not directly palpable or viewable during surgery unless a decompression or osteotomy is performed. In most modern systems, a posterior exposure is performed normally. Then a CT scan is performed with an O-arm (▶ Fig. 12.1) after a 3D array is attached to the spinous process (▶ Fig. 12.2) usually using the most cephalad spinous process exposed. When draping is complete (▶ Fig. 12.3a), the entire team is evacuated from the room and the CT is run (▶ Fig. 12.3b, c) and is uploaded to the navigation station. The surgeon registers the probe after the CT scan (▶ Fig. 12.4). Previous navigation systems used registration of anatomic landmarks after this step, but more recent CT-based systems have obviated this time-consuming step. These newer systems register the probe immediately and the probe becomes "live," meaning it can be seen on the monitor superimposed on the anatomic structures in the axial plane with the invisible structures beneath the probe in line with the axis of the probe (▶ Fig. 12.5a).

The image translation to the flat panel display screen shows the tip of the probe placed at a proposed starting point or bony landmark and the projected trajectory of any length-and-diameter screw before it is placed. These can be color coded for better visualization (▶ Fig. 12.5b). One can then move the hand in space in order to optimize angulation in any plane. The awl, probe, tap, and screw can also be done under navigation or by freehand depending on surgeon preference.

Since the ideal way to assess the fidelity of screw placement is to use postoperative low-dose CT examination to visualize the screws in the pedicle, these systems can be compared to freehand techniques.[28,35] Compared to freehand screw placement, navigated techniques have been associated in these studies with more optimally placed screws, fewer unacceptably placed screws, and fewer screw removals.[28] Moreover, 2D navigation performs favorably compared with non-navigated techniques and 3D navigation performs favorably compared with 2D navigation.[26,36,37,38] In combination with the navigation, a robotic arm can be attached to the bed and the trajectories confirmed by the surgeon can be instrumented by the robot. Robot-assisted implantation of pedicle screws has not yet been shown to outperform other navigation techniques.[39,40] Notably, navigation setup times and cost increase with the complexity of navigation.

12.7 Radiation

Pediatric spine surgery is associated with radiation exposure to the surgeon, OR staff, as well as the patient. Fluoroscopy is traditionally used for procedures during localization and instrumentation. Notably, within orthopedics, a spine surgeon experiences 50 times the lifetime radiation exposure compared to a hip surgeon.[41] Riis et al demonstrated that intraoperative CT-guided navigation does not result in significantly different effective radiation dose to the patient while it does decease radiation exposure to providers.[42] For example, if a surgeon uses 4 to 6 images per screw and places 12 screws in a thoracic spine fusion, the C-arm uses 40 to 70 images, whereas an O-arm uses 2.86 mSv (approximately 20–40 C-arm images). Both techniques subject the patient to a large amount of radiation, but radiation to surgical team may be mitigated with the O-arm.

One study measured neck, torso, and dominant hand radiation to surgeon with fluoroscopy-assisted screw placement in cadavers showing much higher levels than other nonspine procedures.[43] A group comparing cadavers irradiated with C-arm vs. a navigation tool called the Stealth-Station Iso-C reported that the surgeon was exposed 13 times more when using the C-arm.[44]

In regard to patient exposure, several studies have shown increased radiation to the patient when using navigation. Richerand et al retrospectively compared radiation dosages to children with spinal deformities who underwent either CT-guided navigated surgery or C-arm fluoroscopy-guided

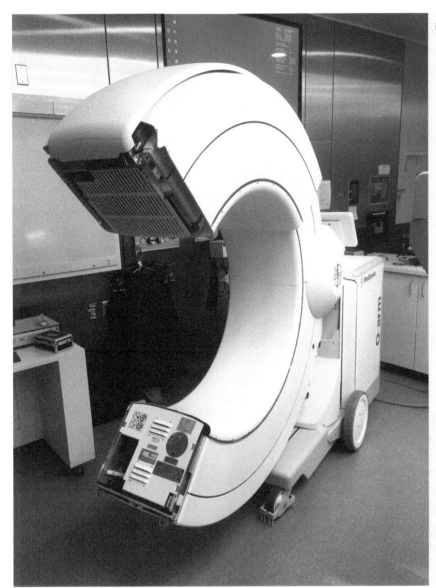

Fig. 12.1 O-arm for intraoperative CT.

surgery.[45] They found the average effective dose was 1.48 ± 1.66 mSv for the CT patients and 0.34 ± 0.36 mSv for the C-arm patients. In addition, they found that the most obese patients had the highest effective doses of radiation when undergoing CT navigation. Similarly a 2018 study showed that CT navigation in AIS resulted in a mean increase of 680 mGy-cm radiation dose, as compared to traditional intraoperative fluoroscopy.[46] In order to try and reduce the radiation dose when using the O-arm in pediatric spine surgery, a pediatric protocol was developed that cuts the radiation to one-tenth of the default protocol.[47] When this low-dose protocol for navigation was compared to traditional C-arm fluoroscopy in AIS, it was found that the O-arm group patients received a total effective dose approximately four times higher than the C-arm patients.[48]

A major concern in navigated pedicle screw placement is the need to limit patient and provider exposure to radiation. While 3D and 2D navigation both expose the patient and surgeon to significant doses of radiation, there exists evidence that the 3D O-arm system might reduce radiation exposure to surgeons relative to 2D C-arm fluoroscopy.[40,42,48,49]

12.8 Screw Accuracy

Pediatric scoliosis surgery can be challenging, secondary to angular and rotational deformity in vertebral anatomy and due to small pedicle size (▶ Fig. 12.6a, b). Consequently, the accuracy of pedicle screw placement in pediatric scoliosis surgery is lower than in spine procedures related to degenerative disease or trauma.[50] Screw malalignment can lead to nerve root or spinal cord injury or spinal column instability.[51] Without navigation, the accuracy of pedicle screw placement in pediatric scoliosis has been reported to be between 77 and 99%.[34,52,53] The accuracy is even lower at 73% in patients with neuromuscular scoliosis.[54] Recent studies using navigation have demonstrated 98.9 and 99.3% screw tract accuracy in AIS and congenital scoliosis, respectively.[25,55]

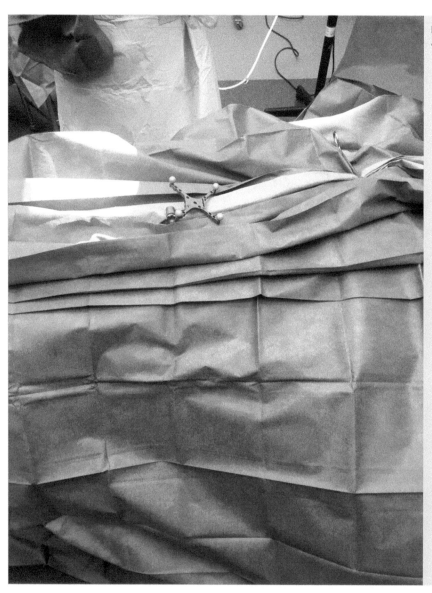

Fig. 12.2 3D array attached to spinous process and surgical field covered by sterile drapes.

In AIS cases, navigation has been shown to increase accuracy of pedicle screw placement. In a 2012 retrospective study of AIS cases, 300 CT-guided navigated thoracic pedicle screws were compared to 185 non-navigated screws.[28] Seventy-four percent of the CT-guided screws were optimally placed, compared to 42% of the non-navigated screws. Furthermore, 9% of non-navigated screws were considered potentially unsafe, compared to 3% of navigated screws. The study noted that without navigation, the odds of a significant medial breach were 7.6 times higher, and the odds of screw removal were 8.3 times higher. Vissarionov et al used an ambispective study design to compare 32 navigated cases of AIS to 30 freehand cases.[55] They found that navigated screws overall had a 1.6% rate of pedicle integrity breach, compared to 5.1% in freehand placement. In a separate study, with instrumentation of extremely small pedicles (≤ 2 mm diameter), navigation was shown to have a significantly higher accuracy rate (84.3%) than the freehand technique (62.7%).[26]

Other types of pediatric scoliosis, non-AIS, have also seen benefit in screw placement with using navigation. In a study of

the apical region of dystrophic scoliosis in patients with neurofibromatosis type I, 92 pedicle screws placed using navigation were compared to 121 screws placed using freehand technique.[29] Pedicle violation was graded from 0 (no perforation) to 3 (> 4 mm of penetration). Navigated screws showed statistically higher rates of grade 0 and 1 screws (79% compared to 67% with freehand technique). Navigation also resulted in significantly less medial perforations, and a significant increase in screw density in the apical region. In a case series of children with congenital scoliosis, 1 screw out of 142 that were placed with navigation required repositioning, which amounted to a 99.3% screw accuracy rate.[25] Similarly, when navigation was used for pedicle screw placement in children 10 years or younger with a variety of diagnoses, 3 screws out of 137 required revision (97.8% accuracy).[27]

Although navigation techniques now have a proven record of accuracy, they have several drawbacks. These devices require a direct line of sight between guided instruments and the tracking camera, camera quality, and surgeon skill to function

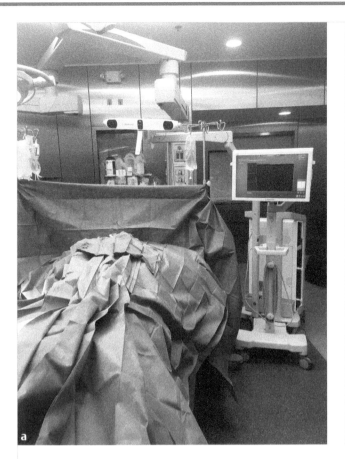

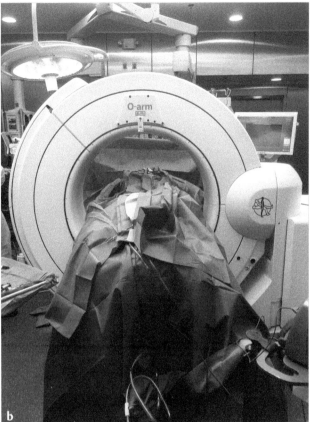

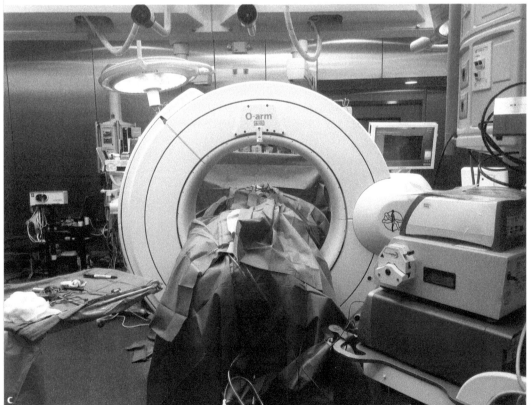

Fig. 12.3 (a) Complete draping of the patient and 3D array. (b) Intraoperative CT scan begins. (c) CT scan is complete and staff re-enter room.

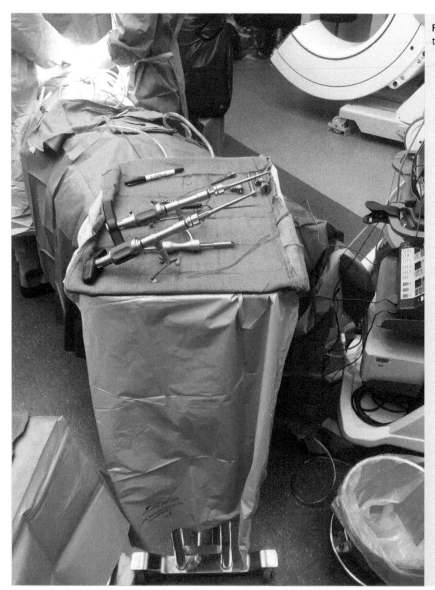

Fig. 12.4 Probe and other tools can be registered to the navigation system.

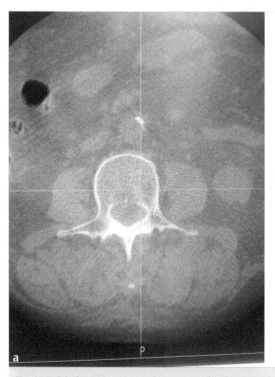
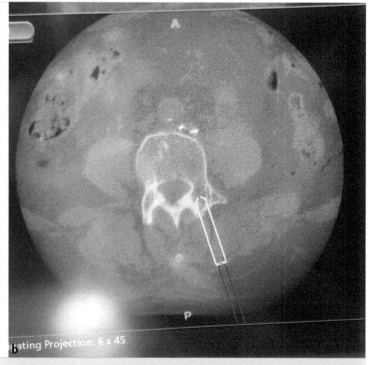

Fig. 12.5 **(a)** The CT is seen on the monitor. **(b)** The surgical tools can be seen on the monitor and observed with live movement as they relate to structures deep to the surgical field.

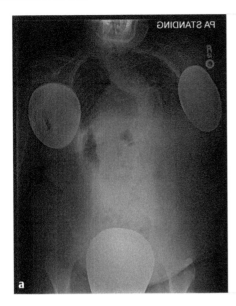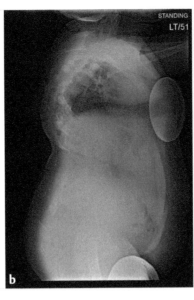

Fig. 12.6 (a,b) Posteroanterior and lateral views of a complex scoliosis with severe rotational deformity.

appropriately.[56] Robot-assisted surgery is being explored to solve some of the shortcomings of navigation methods. One robotic device, the SpineAssist/Renaissance robot (MAZOR Robotics Inc, Orlando, FL), can be attached directly to a spinous process or an external frame.[57] Cadaveric studies demonstrate an average of less than 1 mm of deviation between final implant and preoperative templating.[58] Multiple clinical studies demonstrate 95 to 99% accuracy of pedicle instrumentation using the SpineAssist robot.[40,59,60] Further, Macke et al demonstrated 2.4% screw malpositioning and 0% medial pedicle wall breach with CT-guided and robot-assisted pediatric deformity correction.[61]

In addition, MRI and CT coregistration is being explored to increase image resolution and further reduce radiation exposure. In this scenario, a low-radiation intraoperative scan could be matched to images obtained with a preoperative MRI. Further, navigation based solely on MRI may be a possibility that would allow visualization of both bony and neural elements without any radiation exposure to patient or providers.[56]

12.9 The Cost of Screw Accuracy

In a new era of patient safety where government, payers, and patients are measuring outcomes such as intraoperative neurologic events and unanticipated return to the OR, misplaced screws may be considered a "near-miss" event, which is of concern to patient safety administrators. Still, the question remains whether intraoperative CT prevents an immediate danger of a misplaced screw but increases the risk of long-term danger such as a malignancy from radiation. Some studies have shown increased rates of radiation to the patient without dramatic improvement in the screw accuracy.[42,45,46,47,48,62] The length of surgery is likely slightly increased when navigation is used.[55,63] Finally, the concern of cost looms large in the current era of economic medicine.[64,65]

12.10 Conclusion

Navigated techniques in AIS surgery can optimize screw placement and should be of significant interest to surgeons. Modern systems can help determine pedicle screw position and maximize screw size and length for more powerful correction of deformity. 3D navigation may be of particular benefit in cases where pedicles are very small or difficult to visualize. Furthermore, robot-assisted pedicle screw placement holds significant promise to reduce surgical errors to a minimum.

References

[1] Weinstein SL, Dolan LA. The evidence base for the prognosis and treatment of adolescent idiopathic scoliosis: the 2015 Orthopaedic Research and Education Foundation Clinical Research Award. J Bone Joint Surg Am. 2015; 97(22): 1899–1903

[2] Weinstein SL, Dolan LA, Cheng JC, Danielsson A, Morcuende JA. Adolescent idiopathic scoliosis. Lancet. 2008; 371(9623):1527–1537

[3] Asher MA, Burton DC. Adolescent idiopathic scoliosis: natural history and long term treatment effects. Scoliosis. 2006; 1(1):2

[4] Sarwahi V, Wollowick AL, Sugarman EP, Horn JJ, Gambassi M, Amaral TD. Minimally invasive scoliosis surgery: an innovative technique in patients with adolescent idiopathic scoliosis. Scoliosis. 2011; 6:16

[5] Anand N, Rosemann R, Khalsa B, Baron EM. Mid-term to long-term clinical and functional outcomes of minimally invasive correction and fusion for adults with scoliosis. Neurosurg Focus. 2010; 28(3):E6

[6] Sarwahi V, Horn JJ, Kulkarni PM, et al. Minimally invasive surgery in patients with adolescent idiopathic scoliosis: is it better than the standard approach? A 2-year follow-up study. Clin Spine Surg. 2016; 29(8):331–340

[7] Geck MJ, Rinella A, Hawthorne D, et al. Anterior dual rod versus posterior pedicle fixation surgery for the surgical treatment in Lenke 5C adolescent idiopathic scoliosis: a multicenter, matched case analysis of 42 patients. Spine Deform. 2013; 1(3):217–222

[8] Neal KM, Siegall E. Strategies for surgical management of large, stiff spinal deformities in children. J Am Acad Orthop Surg. 2017; 25(4):e70–e78

[9] Lewis SJ, Zamorano JJ, Goldstein CL. Treatment of severe pediatric spinal deformities. J Pediatr Orthop. 2014; 34 Suppl 1:S1–S5

[10] Saifi C, Laratta JL, Petridis P, Shillingford JN, Lehman RA, Lenke LG. Vertebral column resection for rigid spinal deformity. Global Spine J. 2017; 7(3):280–290

[11] Kim YJ, Lenke LG, Cho SK, Bridwell KH, Sides B, Blanke K. Comparative analysis of pedicle screw versus hook instrumentation in posterior spinal fusion of adolescent idiopathic scoliosis. Spine. 2004; 29(18):2040–2048

[12] Yilmaz G, Borkhuu B, Dhawale AA, et al. Comparative analysis of hook, hybrid, and pedicle screw instrumentation in the posterior treatment of adolescent idiopathic scoliosis. J Pediatr Orthop. 2012; 32(5):490–499

[13] Cuartas E, Rasouli A, O'Brien M, Shufflebarger HL. Use of all-pedicle-screw constructs in the treatment of adolescent idiopathic scoliosis. J Am Acad Orthop Surg. 2009; 17(9):550–561

[14] Ledonio CG, Polly DW, Jr, Vitale MG, Wang Q, Richards BS. Pediatric pedicle screws: comparative effectiveness and safety: a systematic literature review from the Scoliosis Research Society and the Pediatric Orthopaedic Society of North America task force. J Bone Joint Surg Am. 2011; 93(13):1227–1234

[15] Suk SI. Pedicle screw instrumentation for adolescent idiopathic scoliosis: the insertion technique, the fusion levels and direct vertebral rotation. Clin Orthop Surg. 2011; 3(2):89–100

[16] Aubin CE, Labelle H, Ciolofan OC. Variability of spinal instrumentation configurations in adolescent idiopathic scoliosis. Eur Spine J. 2007; 16(1):57–64

[17] Di Silvestre M, Parisini P, Lolli F, Bakaloudis G. Complications of thoracic pedicle screws in scoliosis treatment. Spine. 2007; 32(15):1655–1661

[18] Vaccaro AR, Rizzolo SJ, Allardyce TJ, et al. Placement of pedicle screws in the thoracic spine. Part I: Morphometric analysis of the thoracic vertebrae. J Bone Joint Surg Am. 1995; 77(8):1193–1199

[19] Vaccaro AR, Rizzolo SJ, Balderston RA, et al. Placement of pedicle screws in the thoracic spine. Part II: An anatomical and radiographic assessment. J Bone Joint Surg Am. 1995; 77(8):1200–1206

[20] Farber GL, Place HM, Mazur RA, Jones DE, Damiano TR. Accuracy of pedicle screw placement in lumbar fusions by plain radiographs and computed tomography. Spine. 1995; 20(13):1494–1499

[21] Gertzbein SD, Robbins SE. Accuracy of pedicular screw placement in vivo. Spine. 1990; 15(1):11–14

[22] Takahashi J, Ebara S, Hashidate H, et al. Computer-assisted hemivertebra resection for congenital spinal deformity. J Orthop Sci. 2011; 16(5):503–509

[23] Chan A, Parent E, Narvacan K, San C, Lou E. Intraoperative image guidance compared with free-hand methods in adolescent idiopathic scoliosis posterior spinal surgery: a systematic review on screw-related complications and breach rates. Spine J. 2017; 17(9):1215–1229

[24] Larson AN, Santos ER, Polly DW, Jr, et al. Pediatric pedicle screw placement using intraoperative computed tomography and 3-dimensional image-guided navigation. Spine. 2012; 37(3):E188–E194

[25] Larson AN, Polly DW, Jr, Guidera KJ, et al. The accuracy of navigation and 3D image-guided placement for the placement of pedicle screws in congenital spine deformity. J Pediatr Orthop. 2012; 32(6):e23–e29

[26] Liu Z, Jin M, Qiu Y, Yan H, Han X, Zhu Z. The superiority of intraoperative O-arm navigation-assisted surgery in instrumenting extremely small thoracic pedicles of adolescent idiopathic scoliosis: a case-control study. Medicine (Baltimore). 2016; 95(18):e3581

[27] Luo TD, Polly DW, Jr, Ledonio CG, Wetjen NM, Larson AN. Accuracy of pedicle screw placement in children 10 years or younger using navigation and intraoperative CT. Clin Spine Surg. 2016; 29(3):E135–E138

[28] Ughwanogho E, Patel NM, Baldwin KD, Sampson NR, Flynn JM. Computed tomography-guided navigation of thoracic pedicle screws for adolescent idiopathic scoliosis results in more accurate placement and less screw removal. Spine. 2012; 37(8):E473–E478

[29] Jin M, Liu Z, Liu X, et al. Does intraoperative navigation improve the accuracy of pedicle screw placement in the apical region of dystrophic scoliosis secondary to neurofibromatosis type I: comparison between O-arm navigation and free-hand technique. Eur Spine J. 2016; 25(6):1729–1737

[30] Vital JM, Boissière L, Bourghli A, Castelain JE, Challier V, Obeid I. Osteotomies through a fusion mass in the lumbar spine. Eur Spine J. 2015; 24 Suppl 1: S107–S111

[31] Zhu W, Sun W, Xu L, et al. Minimally invasive scoliosis surgery assisted by O-arm navigation for Lenke Type 5C adolescent idiopathic scoliosis: a comparison with standard open approach spinal instrumentation. J Neurosurg Pediatr. 2017; 19(4):472–478

[32] Smorgick Y, Millgram MA, Anekstein Y, Floman Y, Mirovsky Y. Accuracy and safety of thoracic pedicle screw placement in spinal deformities. J Spinal Disord Tech. 2005; 18(6):522–526

[33] Lehman RA, Jr, Lenke LG, Keeler KA, Kim YJ, Cheh G. Computed tomography evaluation of pedicle screws placed in the pediatric deformed spine over an 8-year period. Spine. 2007; 32(24):2679–2684

[34] Sarlak AY, Tosun B, Atmaca H, Sarisoy HT, Buluç L. Evaluation of thoracic pedicle screw placement in adolescent idiopathic scoliosis. Eur Spine J. 2009; 18(12):1892–1897

[35] Berlemann U, Heini P, Müller U, Stoupis C, Schwarzenbach O. Reliability of pedicle screw assessment utilizing plain radiographs versus CT reconstruction. Eur Spine J. 1997; 6(6):406–410

[36] Sembrano JN, Polly DW, Jr, Ledonio CG, Santos ER. Intraoperative 3-dimensional imaging (O-arm) for assessment of pedicle screw position: does it prevent unacceptable screw placement? Int J Spine Surg. 2012; 6: 49–54

[37] Kim TT, Johnson JP, Pashman R, Drazin D. Minimally invasive spinal surgery with intraoperative image-guided navigation. BioMed Res Int. 2016; 2016: 5716235

[38] Tabaraee E, Gibson AG, Karahalios DG, Potts EA, Mobasser JP, Burch S. Intraoperative cone beam-computed tomography with navigation (O-ARM) versus conventional fluoroscopy (C-ARM): a cadaveric study comparing accuracy, efficiency, and safety for spinal instrumentation. Spine. 2013; 38(22):1953–1958

[39] Marcus HJ, Cundy TP, Nandi D, Yang GZ, Darzi A. Robot-assisted and fluoroscopy-guided pedicle screw placement: a systematic review. Eur Spine J. 2014; 23(2):291–297

[40] Ringel F, Stüer C, Reinke A, et al. Accuracy of robot-assisted placement of lumbar and sacral pedicle screws: a prospective randomized comparison to conventional freehand screw implantation. Spine. 2012; 37(8):E496–E501

[41] Theocharopoulos N, Perisinakis K, Damilakis J, Papadokostakis G, Hadjipavlou A, Gourtsoyiannis N. Occupational exposure from common fluoroscopic projections used in orthopaedic surgery. J Bone Joint Surg Am. 2003; 85-A(9):1698–1703

[42] Riis J, Lehman RR, Perera RA, et al. A retrospective comparison of intraoperative CT and fluoroscopy evaluating radiation exposure in posterior spinal fusions for scoliosis. Patient Saf Surg. 2017; 11:32

[43] Rampersaud YR, Foley KT, Shen AC, Williams S, Solomito M. Radiation exposure to the spine surgeon during fluoroscopically assisted pedicle screw insertion. Spine. 2000; 25(20):2637–2645

[44] Smith HE, Welsch MD, Sasso RC, Vaccaro AR. Comparison of radiation exposure in lumbar pedicle screw placement with fluoroscopy vs computer-assisted image guidance with intraoperative three-dimensional imaging. J Spinal Cord Med. 2008; 31(5):532–537

[45] Dabaghi Richerand A, Christodoulou E, Li Y, Caird MS, Jong N, Farley FA. Comparison of effective dose of radiation during pedicle screw placement using intraoperative computed tomography navigation versus fluoroscopy in children with spinal deformities. J Pediatr Orthop. 2016; 36(5):530–533

[46] Urbanski W, Jurasz W, Wolanczyk M, et al. Increased radiation but no benefits in pedicle screw accuracy with navigation versus a freehand technique in scoliosis surgery. Clin Orthop Relat Res. 2018; 476(5):1020–1027

[47] Su AW, Luo TD, McIntosh AL, et al. Switching to a pediatric dose O-arm protocol in spine surgery significantly reduced patient radiation exposure. J Pediatr Orthop. 2016; 36(6):621–626

[48] Su AW, McIntosh AL, Schueler BA, et al. How does patient radiation exposure compare with low-dose O-arm versus fluoroscopy for pedicle screw placement in idiopathic scoliosis? J Pediatr Orthop. 2017; 37(3):171–177

[49] Abt NB, De la Garza-Ramos R, Olorundare IO, et al. Thirty day postoperative outcomes following anterior lumbar interbody fusion using the National Surgical Quality Improvement Program database. Clin Neurol Neurosurg. 2016; 143:126–131

[50] Zhu F, Sun X, Qiao J, Ding Y, Zhang B, Qiu Y. Misplacement pattern of pedicle screws in pediatric patients with spinal deformity: a computed tomography study. J Spinal Disord Tech. 2014; 27(8):431–435

[51] Mac-Thiong JM, Parent S, Poitras B, Joncas J, Hubert L. Neurological outcome and management of pedicle screws misplaced totally within the spinal canal. Spine. 2013; 38(3):229–237

[52] Brown CA, Lenke LG, Bridwell KH, Geideman WM, Hasan SA, Blanke K. Complications of pediatric thoracolumbar and lumbar pedicle screws. Spine. 1998; 23(14):1566–1571

[53] Rajasekaran S, Vidyadhara S, Ramesh P, Shetty AP. Randomized clinical study to compare the accuracy of navigated and non-navigated thoracic pedicle screws in deformity correction surgeries. Spine. 2007; 32(2):E56–E64

[54] Modi HN, Suh SW, Fernandez H, Yang JH, Song HR. Accuracy and safety of pedicle screw placement in neuromuscular scoliosis with free-hand technique. Eur Spine J. 2008; 17(12):1686–1696

[55] Vissarionov S, Schroeder JE, Novikov SN, Kokyshin D, Belanchikov S, Kaplan L. The utility of 3-dimensional-navigation in the surgical treatment of children with idiopathic scoliosis. Spine Deform. 2014; 2(4):270–275

[56] Overley SC, Cho SK, Mehta AI, Arnold PM. Navigation and robotics in spinal surgery: where are we now? Neurosurgery. 2017; 80 3S:S86–S99

[57] Shoham M, Burman M, Joskowicz L, Batkilin E, Kunicher Y. Bone-mounted miniature robot for surgical procedures: concept and clinical applications. Ieee T Robotic Autom.. 2003; 19(5):893–901

[58] Togawa D, Kayanja MM, Reinhardt MK, et al. Bone-mounted miniature robotic guidance for pedicle screw and translaminar facet screw placement: part 2—Evaluation of system accuracy. Neurosurgery. 2007; 60(2) Suppl 1: ONS129–ONS139, discussion ONS139

[59] Kantelhardt SR, Martinez R, Baerwinkel S, Burger R, Giese A, Rohde V. Perioperative course and accuracy of screw positioning in conventional, open

robotic-guided and percutaneous robotic-guided, pedicle screw placement. Eur Spine J. 2011; 20(6):860–868

[60] Schizas C, Thein E, Kwiatkowski B, Kulik G. Pedicle screw insertion: robotic assistance versus conventional C-arm fluoroscopy. Acta Orthop Belg. 2012; 78(2):240–245

[61] Macke JJ, Woo R, Varich L. Accuracy of robot-assisted pedicle screw placement for adolescent idiopathic scoliosis in the pediatric population. J Robot Surg. 2016; 10(2):145–150

[62] Kobayashi K, Ando K, Ito K, et al. Intraoperative radiation exposure in spinal scoliosis surgery for pediatric patients using the O-arm® imaging system. Eur J Orthop Surg Traumatol. 2018; 28(4):579–583

[63] Meng XT, Guan XF, Zhang HL, He SS. Computer navigation versus fluoro-scopy-guided navigation for thoracic pedicle screw placement: a meta-analy-sis. Neurosurg Rev. 2016; 39(3):385–391

[64] Qureshi S, Lu Y, McAnany S, Baird E. Three-dimensional intraoperative imag-ing modalities in orthopaedic surgery: a narrative review. J Am Acad Orthop Surg. 2014; 22(12):800–809

[65] Dea N, Fisher CG, Batke J, et al. Economic evaluation comparing intraoperative cone beam CT-based navigation and conventional fluoroscopy for the place-ment of spinal pedicle screws: a patient-level data cost-effectiveness analysis. Spine J. 2016; 16(1):23–31

13 Navigated Posterior Instrumentation of the Arthrodesed Spine

Erika A. Dillard, James S. Harrop, and I. David Kaye

Abstract

Since the first published case in 1995 describing the use of image-guided computer-assisted navigation (CAN) for placement of lumbar posterior instrumentation, several technological modifications in surgical navigation systems have transformed the way spine surgery is performed. Image guidance has been particularly useful in cases where "normal" bony anatomy is obscured, secondary to congenital, degenerative, or iatrogenic factors (e.g., previous fusion). Anatomical abnormalities increase the risk of inaccurately implanted hardware, which may increase the risk of neurological deficits from spinal cord or nerve root injury, cerebrospinal fluid leak from dural openings, and blood loss from vascular injury. Therefore, intraoperative navigation has become an additional tool for placement of posterior instrumentation in complex cases such as in the arthrodesed or ankylosed spine.

The most widely used instrumentation for posterior arthrodesis in the thoracolumbar spine is the pedicle screw construct. Some studies have demonstrated increased accuracy in the placement of navigated pedicle screws in the naïve spine; however, only a few studies have addressed its benefit in revision cases. In this chapter, we will briefly discuss failed back surgery and the indication for revision surgery. We will review the studies evaluating the accuracy of navigated instrumentation relative to conventional revision strategies, describe methods used for determining accuracy, and provide several illustrative examples of navigated posterior instrumentation in the arthrodesed spine.

Keywords: accuracy, arthrodesis, breach, computer-assisted, deformity, fusion mass, image-guidance, navigation, pedicle screw, revision

13.1 Revision Spine Surgery

13.1.1 Prevalence and Etiology

There has been a recent increase in spinal surgery with over one million spine procedures occurring annually.[1] Of these patients, up to 40% will not meet their postoperative expectations of improvement and may suffer from persistent or recurrent back and/or radicular pain that is resistant to conservative measures.[2] In addition, approximately 15% of patients that fail to improve will require revision surgery, with the majority attributable to postdiskectomy and postlaminectomy syndrome.[3] Pateder et al showed that in adult scoliosis patients with pseudarthrosis following multiple revisions, successful fusion was achieved in 90% of patients and was dependent on restoration of sagittal alignment,[4] yet overall, the evidence for improvement with surgical revision is variable.[2,5,6] Failure to improve from the initial surgery may be multifactorial. Underlying causes include preoperative factors such as poor patient selection and unrealistic postoperative expectations, intraoperative factors such as overly aggressive surgical decompression leading to spinal instability, and/or postoperative factors such as development of Flat Back Syndrome and pseudarthrosis.[2,7]

13.1.2 Management

Success rates of revision surgery may decrease with each reoperation of spinal fusion with 50% success in the first reoperation, 30% in the second, and 15% in the third.[2,5] Therefore, optimal medical management should first be considered, including efficient pain control and physical therapy; however, deteriorating neurological function or overt hardware malfunction causing instability may necessitate treatment. Patient evaluation should be performed to determine candidacy for less-invasive measures such as epidural injections or a spinal cord stimulator trial. If these strategies are not sufficient or fail, revision surgery should be considered as a treatment option.

13.2 Posterior Arthrodesis: The Pedicle Screw

13.2.1 Pedicle Screw

The majority of spine revisions, particularly in the thoracolumbar spine, are performed by a posterior or posterolateral approach and the most commonly utilized form of instrumentation is the pedicle screw. The pedicle screw instrumentation and constructs has the advantage of improved biomechanical stability due to its resistance to fatigue and increased pull-out strength. Because the pedicle screw is designed to span all three columns of the vertebrae, it provides overall support not offered by other fusion constructs (e.g., Harrington rods, wiring).[8,9] Traditionally, pedicle screw insertion is performed freehand, guided by a meticulous knowledge of bony anatomy and appreciation for key landmarks exposed during surgery, such as the pars articularis, mammillary body, and the transverse process (e.g., Roy-Camille method). This method can carry a breach rate of 55% associated with a 1 to 8% risk of injury to surrounding structures such as nerve roots, adjacent viscera, and vasculature.[10,11] This risk is amplified in revision cases where bony elements have been completely removed or modified and replaced with a fusion mass over time, making anatomical landmarks indiscernible.[10] In addition, surrounding scar tissue makes dura and nerve roots harder to delineate which escalates the risk of cerebrospinal fluid leak and of damage to underlying nerve roots.[8,12]

13.2.2 Determining Pedicle Screw Breach Rate

Breaches may reflect a violation of instrumentation out of the bony confines. Most studies that evaluate the accuracy or breach rate of pedicle screws in the spine do so with the aid of grading systems that classify breaches based on several features observed on postoperative imaging. These features include the extent of screw perforation outside of the pedicle (mm), directionality of the screw breach (medial vs. lateral), as well as degree and type of associated neurological deficits, if present (▶ Fig. 13.1). Below are several grading systems for pedicle breaches used to determine accuracy of techniques for screw placement (▶ Table 13.1). Variations do exist among the breach grading systems. These differences should be appreciated as they may affect the ability to compare accuracy rates of screw placement methods across studies.

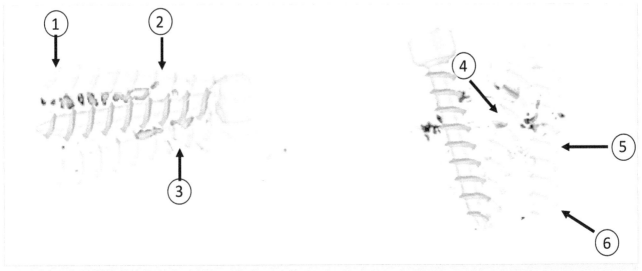

Fig. 13.1 **Pedicle screw breaches.** Through the superior end plate into the intervertebral space (1); superior pedicle breach (2); inferior pedicle breach (3) with higher risk of affecting the exiting nerve root; medial breach (4) with higher risk of spinal cord injury if in the cervicothoracic spine or thecal sac in the lumbar spine; lateral breach (5); anterior breach (6) with higher risk of damage to adjacent viscera or vasculature.

Table 13.1 Grading systems for pedicle screw breaches[18,19,20,21]

a. Laine et al (2000)	
Direction	**Perforation (mm)**
Lateral	<2
Inferior	2–4
Medial	4–6
Superior	>6

b. Mirza 3-Tier classification (2003)	
Grade	**Perforation (mm)**
1, Encroachment	None (cortex not visualized)
2, Minor	<3
3, Moderate	3–6
4, Severe	>6

c. Hsieh et al (2014)		
Grade	**Perforation (mm)**	**Description**
Good	<1	Optimal
Fair	1–3	Suboptimal
Poor	>3	Unsound[a]

d. Aoude et al (2018)					
Direction	**Perforation (mm)**				**Neuro-deficit**
	<2	2–4	4–6	>6	
Medial	1	2	3	4	None 0
Inferior	0	1	2	2	Sensory loss 1
Lateral	0	1	2	2	Weakness 4
Superior	0	0	1	1	New radicular pain 4
Anterior	0	0	1	1	

SCORE (0–8)[b]

[a] Revision recommended. [b] For score >6, revision recommended.

Table 13.2 Advantages and disadvantages of CT-guided computer-assisted navigation

Advantages	Disadvantages
Multiplanar images	Learning curve
Automated registration	Longer operative times
Reduced radiation exposure	Inaccuracies from altered DRA position
Real time trajectory planning	Image interference from hardware artifact
Decreased tissue disruption	Costs
Increased accuracy/Decreased breach rate	
Increased screw-to-pedicle ratio	

13.3 Navigation

13.3.1 Pros and Cons of CT-Guided Computer-Assisted Navigation

Image-guided techniques for placement of posterior instrumentation in the spine ranges from plain serial radiography, C-arm fluoroscopy, to 2D Fluoro/3D CT-guided computer-assisted navigation (CAN). Furthermore, 3D navigation systems may use either preoperatively or intraoperatively acquired imaging for registration. Specifically, CT-guided CAN offers several advantages in the placement of posterior instrumentation (▶ Table 13.2). As mentioned, this technique allows the acquisition of multiplanar images that readily interface with the externally referenced navigation system. This eliminates the time-consuming and error-prone step of manual registration as the images are automatically registered and formatted on the workstation for use during navigation. Preoperative gantry settings can be adjusted to provide as low as reasonably achievable (ALARA) image acquisition resulting in lower doses of radiation exposure.[17] Planning of screw trajectory can be done in real time, which also allows for instantaneous adjustments of implants during the procedure. Further, the ability to acquire images intraoperatively while the patient is in final position using mobile CT technology reduces error introduced by positional changes that occur when images are acquired preoperatively with the patient positioned supine.[18] Use of CT-guided CAN may result in a significantly larger screw to pedicle ratio that enhances pull-out strength of implanted constructs and, indirectly, decreases the risk of future revision.[8] These advantages are not just limited to the thoracolumbar spine but have been proven in the placement of pedicle screws in the cervical spine as well.[19]

Despite the advantages, several shortcomings have been suggested. These include longer operative times amplified by the learning curve necessary for surgeons and staff to become familiar with the navigation procedure, more exposure to radiation, and overall increased costs associated with purchase and upkeep of a navigation system. In addition, despite the numerous studies that have shown decreased breach rates with image guidance, these results have not translated into significantly improved clinical outcomes. Technical aspects of navigation

have been implicated in hindering the accurate placement of pedicle screws as well. These include accidental shifts in position of the DRA after registration due to presence of abutting scar tissue or jolting from hand movements during space-occupying steps such as tapping or screw placement.[20] Also, in patients with previous fusion implants, metal artifact can impede visualization of bony anatomy on imaging.[21] Yet, as the technology continues to evolve, evidence of these proposed shortcomings are becoming increasingly invalidated.[17,20,22,23,24,25,26,27,28,29]

13.3.2 Accuracy of Image-Guided Navigated Pedicle Screws in the Arthrodesed Spine

Pedicle screw insertion accuracy and breach rate using 3D CT-guided CAN has been studied more extensively in patients undergoing spine surgery for the first time.[30,31,32] Less available are studies evaluating navigated screw placement in revision cases, specifically through an established fusion mass in comparison to more conventional methods. These studies utilize various models (cadaver vs. surgical patients), breach classification systems, and navigation technology (2D vs. 3D; IsoC vs. O-arm) as seen in ▶ Table 13.3.

For instance, using a cadaver model in which posterior spinal elements are obscured by cement to simulate a posterior fusion mass, Austin et al evaluated pedicle perforation distance (mm) into either the spinal canal or neural foramen based on direct visualization of each specimen. An accuracy rate of 100% was observed for pedicle screws placed from T6 to S1 (n=24 screws) with a 0% breach rate using CT-guided CAN. On the other hand, freehand placement of pedicle screws resulted in a 21.43% breach rate in the fusion mass models versus 14.29% in models with normal anatomy. This supports the hypothesis that the presence of a fusion mass inherently increases the risk of inaccurate placement of hardware despite the method of placement. However, with navigation, accuracy does not just match but exceeds that of screws placed freehand with nonobscured anatomy.[33]

Most data on the accuracy of image-guided CAN for screw placement in surgical patients has been done so, retrospectively. An example includes a single-center chart review of 231 thoracolumbar-navigated pedicle screws using preoperative-acquired CT imaging. Approximately 50% of these cases were revision surgeries, resulting in evaluation of 122 screws placed into previous fusion masses. Based on axial cuts of postoperative CT imaging, an overall breach rate of 4.1% was observed in previously fused levels compared to 5.5% in nonfused levels. These rates were not significantly different from the overall breach rate of 4.8%.[34] Breach rates were determined using the method described previously by Laine et al[13] (▶ Table 13.1a).

Another retrospective analysis revealed a 0% breach rate based on analysis of 45 screws in 30 patients who underwent revision surgery using O-arm CT-guided navigation. The surgical indication involved the redirection of misplaced screws in patients with pseudarthrosis, adjacent segment degeneration, sagittal imbalance, or unresolved neurological symptoms caused by the malpositioned screw. Screws excluded from the study were those placed using an intentional "in-out-in"

Table 13.3 Summary of studies evaluating image-guided computer-assisted navigation for placement of pedicle screws in the arthrodesed spine

Author (year)	Study type	Model used	Groups (n = screws)	AR/BR	Method for breach evaluation	CAN type	Additional outcome measures (if applicable)
Austin et al (2002)[33]	In vitro experimental study	Cadaver spine model	Freehand, fusion mass (14) Freehand, normal anatomy (14) Fluoro, fusion mass (12) Fluoro, normal anatomy (36) CAN, fusion mass (24)	BR: 21.43% BR: 14.29% BR: 8.33% BR: 8.33% BR: 0%	Direct visual inspection	Optical Tracking System (Radionics)	
Lim et al (2005)[34]	Retrospective Single Center Chart Review	Surgical patients	CAN revision with fusion mass (122) CAN revision without fusion mass (109)	BR: 4.1% BR: 5.5% Overall BR: 4.8%	Laine	Preoperative CT/ StealthStation	No NV injury Scoliosis BR: 13% Non-Scoliosis BR: 2%
Rampersaud et al (2007)[35]	Prospective Observational Cohort	Surgical patients	Fluoro primary surgery (102) CAN revision surgery (102)	AR: 84.3% AR: 81.4%	Mirza	Intraoperative C-arm/ FluoroNav	No NV injury
Nottmeier et al (2009)[10]	Retrospective Single Center Chart Review	Surgical patients	CAN primary surgery (669) CAN revision surgery (total) (282) CAN revision surgery, fusion mass (154)	BR: 7.7% BR:6.7% BR: 7.8 Overall BR: 7.5%	Mirza	Intraoperative C-arm/ Brainlab or O-arm/ StealthStation	0.9% NV injury Screw diameter >7.5 mm achieved in 71%
Luther et al (2015)[8]	Retrospective Single Center Cohort Series	Surgical patients	Lateral Fluoro[a] (708) CAN[b] (726)	AR: 88% AR: 82%	Mirza	Intraoperative C-arm/Brainlab	No NV injury Larger Screw: pedicle diameter (0.71 vs. 0.63)
Hsieh et al (2014)[15]	Retrospective Single Center Chart review	Surgical patients	CAN primary surgery (313) CAN revision surgery (429)	AR: 98.7% AR 98.6%	Hsieh	O-arm/ StealthStation	S1screw AR: Revision 80.6% Primary 100%
Yoon (2016)[12]	Retrospective Single Center Chart review	Surgical patients	CAN screw revisions (45)	BR 0%	Mirza	O-arm/ StealthStation	No NV injury

[a]44% with complex anatomy. [b] 76% with complex anatomy. Abbreviations: NV, neurovascular; AR, accuracy rate; BR, breach rate.

technique to enhance fixation in smaller pedicles and bicortical screws placed through the S1 promontory.[12] The breach rate was calculated based on axial postoperative CT images using the Mirza method[14] (▶ Table 13.1b).

Hsieh et al performed another retrospective single-center study that sought to determine the breach rate using O-arm-guided CAN in 313 screws placed during primary surgeries compared to 429 screws placed during revision cases with distorted anatomy. Screws were placed between C7 to the pelvis. The breach rate was determined based on a novel method described by the authors (▶ Table 13.1c). Accuracy rates overall were comparable regardless of anatomical distortion (98.7% in primary cases vs. 98.6% in revisions). S1 screws had a lower rate of accuracy in revision cases (80.6%) versus in primary surgeries (100%). A tendency for poorer placement of pelvic screws in revision cases was noted as well. This was likely a result of pelvic screws being mated to the inferior construct which ultimately influenced the ability to accomplish a specific trajectory. Only one screw required revision in the primary surgery group due to a breach causing postoperative pain but no screws required redirection in the revision cohort.[15]

Rampersaud et al published the only prospective study analyzing the use of image-guided navigation for placement of pedicle screws for revision.[35] This study utilized an observational matched cohort design for the evaluation of 24 patients with a history of previous thoracolumbar fusions using nonpedicle screw fixation (rod-hook, facet screws). These patients ultimately developed symptomatic adjacent segment degeneration requiring revision. Matched controls included patients undergoing initial instrumented fusion without obscured anatomy. Unlike the previous studies, image guidance was performed by intraoperative 2D computer-assisted fluoroscopy technique (FluoroNav-Medtronic Surgical Navigation technology, Louisville, CO). Of 102 pedicle screws placed through a mature posterolateral fusion mass, 81.4% were accurately placed in comparison to 84.3% in patients without previous surgery, which was not significantly different. The majority of breaches were a result of oversized screws, all clinically insignificant. Breaches were graded by a method similar to the Mirza classification but with Grade I signifying no breach and Grade IV representing a breach >4 mm.[35]

Weaknesses in the majority of studies described include their retrospective design with lack of randomization. Most are single-institution studies; therefore, results may not be applicable to the general patient population. Another limitation of these studies is the lack of a control cohort of patients with previous fusions using other conventional methods for pedicle screw placement such as the freehand technique or lateral fluoroscopy. The prospective trial discussed resulted in a significantly lower accuracy rate than was observed in the retrospective studies. This may be, in part, due to the 2D image-guided technique used in contrast to the CT-guided 3D systems most frequently used in other studies and in modern practice. Specific preoperative spinal pathologies such as scoliosis may amplify the risk of breach in revision cases. Additionally, variations in how breaches are defined can distort the overall determination of breach rate as some studies do not consider breaches of < 2 mm as inaccurate while others do. Lastly, despite these breach rates, the rate of neurovascular injury and of postoperative screw revision is low, so more studies are needed with a larger sample size and longer follow-up to truly detect differences in outcomes. In summary, the reported breach rate for navigated pedicle screws in the arthrodesed spine using image-guided CAN ranges from 0 to 18.6%. Altogether, the evidence implies that navigation, specifically CT guided, can achieve an accuracy comparable to that of primary cases with nondistorted anatomy but significantly higher than using conventional techniques.

13.3.3 Example Case: Revision Surgery in Flat Back Syndrome and Degenerative Kyphoscoliosis

A 70-year-old woman with comorbidities of atrial fibrillation, diabetes mellitus, multiple abdominal hernia repairs complicated by wound dehiscence, and two previous lumbar fusions 9 years prior presents with worsening back pain, decreased mobility, and severe leg radicular pain. Her initial symptoms improved for 2 years postfusion but then recurred. Nonoperative measures were attempted including pain control and physical therapy, and subsequently a thoracic spinal cord stimulator was placed that provided ~ 60% improvement in her back pain initially. Unfortunately, over time she experienced a decrease in stimulator efficacy to the point it provided no further pain relief and therefore it was removed. She continued nonoperative measures including multiple epidural steroid injections and physical therapy without relief. She reports worsening pain now radiating down both legs posteriorly, causing pain limited weakness for which she now requires a wheelchair. Her symptoms are accompanied by a significant loss in her quality of life.

An MRI and CT of the lumbar spine as well as EOS standing X-rays were completed. These revealed a progressive kyphotic thoracic deformity with multilevel degenerative foraminal and central stenosis, sagittal imbalance, and flat back deformity. Therefore, due to failure of nonoperative measures with progressive deterioration and based on the preoperative evaluation, she underwent removal of posterior instrumentation with replacement of pedicle screws and extension of fusion construct from T5 to S1 including iliac pelvic fixation. In addition, multilevel Smith-Pete osteotomies, revision L1–L4 laminectomies, an L1–L2 transforaminal lumbar interbody fusion, and

an L3 PSO were done using CT-guided computer-assisted navigation.

A postoperative CT scan revealed three breaches, 2 to 4 mm lateral breaches at T11 and T12, and a < 2-mm medial breach at L2. Each breach represented a score of 1 according to the Aoude scoring system.[16] In addition, all breaches were clinically insignificant; therefore, no screws required revision. Postoperative standing AP and lateral radiographs showed improvement in coronal and sagittal imbalance (▶ Fig. 13.2). At her 2-week follow-up appointment, the patient reported no back pain and 60% relief of her bilateral leg pain.

13.4 Use of Navigation in Complex Revisions

13.4.1 Osteotomies

Navigation can be valuable in the treatment of more complicated revision procedures such as with complex spinal deformities. Surgical management involves instrumentation in combination with corrective techniques such as the pedicle subtraction osteotomy (PSO) or vertebral column resection (VCR) for restoration of alignment. As with simple revisions, a thorough preoperative assessment is vital as well as a detailed analysis of preoperative imaging.[36] An example that emphasizes the feasibility and benefit of navigated correction and fusion in this scenario is described.

Case 1: A 54–year-old female presented following multiple thoracolumbar procedures for scoliosis. Preoperative standing scoliosis plain radiographs illustrated the previous T12–L4 posterior instrumentation with loss of the lumbar lordosis and significant positive sagittal vertical axis (SVA). Preoperative CT demonstrated a prominent fusion mass at the stated levels. Using intraoperative navigation, extension of fusion construct, an L4 PSO, and L5–S1 Ponte osteotomies were performed resulting in a 45-degree correction of lumbar lordosis[37] (▶ Fig. 13.3). The complex deformities and obliteration of normal anatomical landmarks can make revision surgery difficult. With navigation, there can be improved accuracy and potentially decreased risk of neurovascular injury.

13.4.2 Cervical Spine

Traditionally, lateral mass screw fixation has been the preferred method for posterior instrumented arthrodesis in the cervical spine. However, in cases where the lateral mass is unstable or destroyed due to fracture, infection, or previous surgery, or when hypoplastic lateral masses exist, the cervical pedicle screw (CPS) is a potential option. CPS placement is more challenging as pedicles in the cervicothoracic spine are much smaller than in the lower thoracic or lumbar spine. Following previous cervical arthrodesis, pedicle screw placement can be complicated due to limited flexibility of the cervical spine during positioning, which makes it difficult to achieve the appropriate angles for placement of screws.[38] This is amplified by the presence of kyphotic and/or scoliotic deformities at the cervicothoracic junction, which alters the normal orientation of the pedicles.

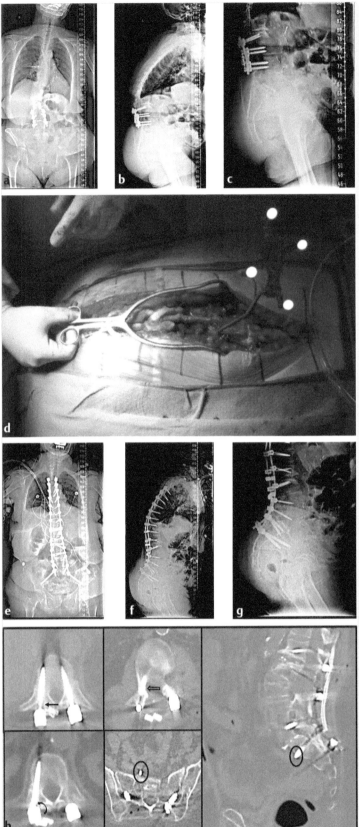

Fig. 13.2 Example case of revision surgery in flat back syndrome and degenerative kyphoscoliosis. Preoperative AP (**a**) and lateral (**b,c**) standing X-rays revealing combined imbalance. Intraoperative views of midline incision with placement of DRA attached to existing pedicle screws by a temporary rod (**d**). Postoperative AP (**e**) and lateral (**f,g**) standing X-rays showing correction of combined imbalance. Postoperative CT showing T11 (*closed arrow*) and T12 (*curved arrow*) lateral breaches and L1 medial (*open arrow*) breach. S1 anterior breach (*circle*) in axial and sagittal views (**h**).

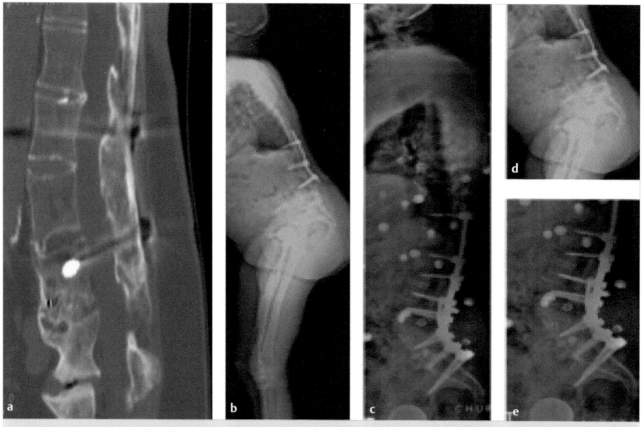

Fig. 13.3 Treatment of flat back syndrome with extension of fusion instrumentation and L4 PSO using navigation. Preoperative CT, sagittal view showing obliteration of normal anatomical landmarks within the posterior elements **(a)**. Preoperative **(b,d)** and postoperative **(c,e)** lateral standing X-rays showing correction of sagittal alignment. (Reproduced with permission from Vital et al.[37])

As in the lumbar spine, conventional strategies for placing pedicle screws have been associated with a breach rate that is not insignificant. Preoperative comorbidities such as rheumatoid arthritis have been found to contribute to higher breach rates[39,40] as well as the spinal level of interest with more cranial levels at risk due to smaller pedicle size.[40,41] Image-guided navigation has therefore been proposed to improve accuracy not only in the setting of first-time surgical correction in the cervical spine but also in cases of revision.[19,41,42,43]

13.5 Conclusion

Revision spinal surgeries can be technically challenging due to loss of anatomical landmarks such as in the presence of a fusion mass. The use of navigation or image-guided assistance is an excellent tool to potentially aid in the placement of instrumentation during revision surgery. The objective for improving accuracy is not only to prevent neurovascular injury but also to decrease the chances of recurrent surgical failure as success rates of revisions significantly decrease with each reoperation. Though the reported data suggests an accuracy advantage with navigation in the arthrodesed spine, clinical results have not shown significant improvement despite this technology. Therefore, more prospective studies with larger sample size, improved control cohorts, standardized breach classification, and longer follow-up are warranted.

References

[1] Adogwa O, Parker SL, Shau DN, et al. Cost per quality-adjusted life year gained of revision neural decompression and instrumented fusion for same-level recurrent lumbar stenosis: defining the value of surgical intervention. J Neurosurg Spine. 2012; 16(2):135–140

[2] Sebaaly A, Lahoud MJ, Rizkallah M, Kreichati G, Kharrat K. Etiology, evaluation, and treatment of failed back surgery syndrome. Asian Spine J. 2018; 12 (3):574–585

[3] Turunen V, Nyyssönen T, Miettinen H, et al. Lumbar instrumented posterolateral fusion in spondylolisthetic and failed back patients: a long-term follow-up study spanning 11–13 years. Eur Spine J. 2012; 21(11):2140–2148

[4] Pateder DB, Park YS, Kebaish KM, et al. Spinal fusion after revision surgery for pseudarthrosis in adult scoliosis. Spine. 2006; 31(11):E314–E319

[5] Arts MP, Kols NI, Onderwater SM, Peul WC. Clinical outcome of instrumented fusion for the treatment of failed back surgery syndrome: a case series of 100 patients. Acta Neurochir (Wien). 2012; 154(7):1213–1217

[6] Adogwa O, Owens R, Karikari I, et al. Revision lumbar surgery in elderly patients with symptomatic pseudarthrosis, adjacent-segment disease, or same-level recurrent stenosis. Part 2. A cost-effectiveness analysis: clinical article. J Neurosurg Spine. 2013; 18(2):147–153

[7] Guyer RD, Patterson M, Ohnmeiss DD. Failed back surgery syndrome: diagnostic evaluation. J Am Acad Orthop Surg. 2006; 14(9):534–543

[8] Luther N, Iorgulescu JB, Geannette C, et al. Comparison of navigated versus non-navigated pedicle screw placement in 260 patients and 1434 screws:

screw accuracy, screw size, and the complexity of surgery. J Spinal Disord Tech. 2015; 28(5):E298–E303

[9] Cho W, Cho SK, Wu C, Fellow C. The biomechanics of pedicle screw-based instrumentation. J Bone Joint Surg Br. 2010; 92(8):1061–1065

[10] Nottmeier EW, Seemer W, Young PM. Placement of thoracolumbar pedicle screws using three-dimensional image guidance: experience in a large patient cohort. J Neurosurg Spine. 2009; 10(1):33–39

[11] Xu R, Ebraheim NA, Ou Y, Yeasting RA. Anatomic considerations of pedicle screw placement in the thoracic spine. Roy-Camille technique versus open-lamina technique. Spine. 1998; 23(9):1065–1068

[12] Yoon JW, Nottmeier EW, Rahmathulla G, Fenton DS, Pirris SM. Redirecting pedicle screws: a revision spinal fusion strategy using three-dimensional image guidance. Int J Med Robot. 2016; 12(4):758–764

[13] Laine T, Lund T, Ylikoski M, Lohikoski J, Schlenzka D. Accuracy of pedicle screw insertion with and without computer assistance: a randomised controlled clinical study in 100 consecutive patients. Eur Spine J. 2000; 9(3):235–240

[14] Mirza SK, Wiggins GC, Kuntz C, IV, et al. Accuracy of thoracic vertebral body screw placement using standard fluoroscopy, fluoroscopic image guidance, and computed tomographic image guidance: a cadaver study. Spine. 2003; 28(4):402–413

[15] Hsieh JC, Drazin D, Firempong AO, Pashman R, Johnson JP, Kim TT. Accuracy of intraoperative computed tomography image-guided surgery in placing pedicle and pelvic screws for primary versus revision spine surgery. Neurosurg Focus. 2014; 36(3):E2

[16] Aoude A, Ghadakzadeh S, Alhamzah H, et al. Assess pedicle screw breach. Asian Spine J. 2018; 12(1)

[17] Ughwanogho E, Flynn JM. Current navigation modalities in spine surgery with a focus on the use of the O-arm in Deformity Surgery Expert commentary. Univ Pa Orthop J. 2010; 20:65–69

[18] Silbermann J, Riese F, Allam Y, Reichert T, Koeppert H, Gutberlet M. Computer tomography assessment of pedicle screw placement in lumbar and sacral spine: comparison between free-hand and O-arm based navigation techniques. Eur Spine J. 2011; 20(6):875–881

[19] Richter M, Cakir B, Schmidt R. Cervical pedicle screws: conventional versus computer-assisted placement of cannulated screws. Spine. 2005; 30(20):2280–2287

[20] Rivkin MA, Yocom SS. Thoracolumbar instrumentation with CT-guided navigation (O-arm) in 270 consecutive patients: accuracy rates and lessons learned. Neurosurg Focus. 2014; 36(3):E7

[21] Theologis AA, Burch S. Safety and efficacy of reconstruction of complex cervical spine pathology using pedicle screws inserted with stealth navigation and 3d image-guided (O-arm) technology. Spine. 2015; 40(18):1397–1406

[22] Holly LT, Foley KT. Intraoperative spinal navigation. Spine. 2003; 28(15) Suppl:S54–S61

[23] Gebhard FT, Kraus MD, Schneider E, Liener UC, Kinzl L, Arand M. Does computer-assisted spine surgery reduce intraoperative radiation doses? Spine. 2006; 31(17):2024–2027, discussion 2028

[24] Kim YW, Lenke LG, Kim YJ, et al. Free-hand pedicle screw placement during revision spinal surgery: analysis of 552 screws. Spine. 2008; 33(10):1141–1148

[25] Kraus MD, Krischak G, Keppler P, Gebhard FT, Schuetz UHW. Can computer-assisted surgery reduce the effective dose for spinal fusion and sacroiliac screw insertion? Clin Orthop Relat Res. 2010; 468(9):2419–2429

[26] Drazin D, Al-Khouja L, Shweikeh F, Pashman R, Johnson JP, Kim T. Economics of image guidance and navigation in spine surgery. Surg Neurol Int. 2015; 25(6):2024–2027

[27] Zausinger S, Scheder B, Uhl E, Heigl T, Morhard D, Tonn JC. Intraoperative computed tomography with integrated navigation system in spinal stabilizations. Spine. 2009; 6(Suppl 10):S323–S326

[28] Hecht AC, Koehler SM, Laudone JC, Jenkins A, Qureshi S. Is intraoperative CT of posterior cervical spine instrumentation cost-effective and does it reduce complications? Clin Orthop Relat Res. 2011; 469(4):1035–1041

[29] Lu Y, Qureshi SA. Cost-effective studies in spine surgeries: a narrative review. Spine J. 2014; 14(11):2748–2762

[30] Amiot LP, Lang K, Putzier M, Zippel H, Labelle H. Comparative results between conventional and computer-assisted pedicle screw installation in the thoracic, lumbar, and sacral spine. Spine. 2000; 25(5):606–614

[31] Ling JM, Dinesh SK, Pang BC, et al. Routine spinal navigation for thoraco-lumbar pedicle screw insertion using the O-arm three-dimensional imaging system improves placement accuracy. J Clin Neurosci. 2014; 21(3):493–498

[32] Yu T, Mi S, He Y, et al. Accuracy of pedicle screw placement in posterior lumbosacral instrumentation by computer tomography evaluation: a multi-centric retrospective clinical study. Int J Surg. 2017; 43:46–51

[33] Austin MS, Vaccaro AR, Brislin B, Nachwalter R, Hilibrand AS, Albert TJ. Image-guided spine surgery: a cadaver study comparing conventional open laminoforaminotomy and two image-guided techniques for pedicle screw placement in posterolateral fusion and nonfusion models. Spine. 2002; 27(22):2503–2508

[34] Lim MR, Girardi FP, Yoon SC, Huang RC, Cammisa FP, Jr. Accuracy of computerized frameless stereotactic image-guided pedicle screw placement into previously fused lumbar spines. Spine. 2005; 30(15):1793–1798

[35] Rampersaud YR, Lee KS. Fluoroscopic computer-assisted pedicle screw placement through a mature fusion mass: an assessment of 24 consecutive cases with independent analysis of computed tomography and clinical data. Spine. 2007; 32(2):217–222

[36] Obeid I, Bourghli A, Boissière L, Vital JM, Barrey C. Complex osteotomies vertebral column resection and decancellation. Eur J Orthop Surg Traumatol. 2014; 24 Suppl 1:S49–S57

[37] Vital JM, Boissière L, Bourghli A, Castelain JE, Challier V, Obeid I. Osteotomies through a fusion mass in the lumbar spine. Eur Spine J. 2014; 24(1). DOI: 10.1007/s00586-014-3657-4

[38] Rienmüller A, Buchmann N, Kirschke JS, et al. Accuracy of CT-navigated pedicle screw positioning in the cervical and upper thoracic region with and without prior anterior surgery and ventral plating. Bone Joint J. 2017; 99-B(10):1373–1380

[39] Ishikawa Y, Kanemura T, Yoshida G, et al. Intraoperative, full-rotation, three-dimensional image (O-arm)-based navigation system for cervical pedicle screw insertion. J Neurosurg Spine. 2011; 15(5):472–478

[40] Hojo Y, Ito M, Suda K, Oda I, Yoshimoto H, Abumi K. A multicenter study on accuracy and complications of freehand placement of cervical pedicle screws under lateral fluoroscopy in different pathological conditions: CT-based evaluation of more than 1,000 screws. Eur Spine J. 2014; 23(10):2166–2174

[41] Abumi K, Shono Y, Ito M, Taneichi H, Kotani Y, Kaneda K. Complications of pedicle screw fixation in reconstructive surgery of the cervical spine. Spine. 2000; 25(8):962–969

[42] Yoshimoto H, Sato S, Hyakumachi T, Yanagibashi Y, Masuda T. Spinal reconstruction using a cervical pedicle screw system. Clin Orthop Relat Res. 2005 (431):111–119

[43] Ludwig SC, Kowalski JM, Edwards CC, II, Heller JG. Cervical pedicle screws: comparative accuracy of two insertion techniques. Spine. 2000; 25(20):2675–2681

14 Navigated Minimally Invasive Transforaminal Lumbar Interbody Fusion

Bradley C. Johnson and Thomas J. Errico

Abstract:

Navigated minimally invasive transforaminal lumbar interbody fusion combines the benefits of minimally invasive surgery, decreased tissue damage, and expedited recovery, with the increased implant accuracy and decreased radiation exposure of navigation. It is a safe and effective surgical option for many degenerative lumbar pathologies.

Keywords: navigation, minimally invasive surgery, transforaminal lumbar interbody fusion, spine, lumbar fusion

14.1 Introduction

Navigated minimally invasive transforaminal lumbar interbody fusion (TLIF) evolved from the posterior interbody technique. By utilizing a more lateral approach, TLIF allows access to the intervertebral disk while minimizing the need for neural retraction, decreasing the frequency of accidental durotomy and postoperative radiculitis.[1] The addition of interbody arthrodesis to posterior fusion increases arthrodesis rates and potentially restores sagittal alignment.[2,3]

Over the last two decades, there has been a trend toward minimally invasive surgery (MIS) when performing TLIF. Studies have consistently demonstrated that relative to open TLIF, MIS TLIF is associated with reduced blood loss, less postoperative pain, shorter hospital stay, less soft-tissue trauma, earlier mobilization, improved cosmesis, and decreased infection rates.[4,5,6] At the same time, MIS surgery has a steep learning curve and significantly higher radiation exposure than open surgery.[7]

Computer-assisted navigation (CAN) was introduced in spine surgery in the 1990s in an effort to improve surgical accuracy and reduce radiation exposure.[8] CAN systems combine intraoperative three-dimensional (3D) fluoroscopy or cone-beam computed tomography (CT) with real-time precision instrument tracking to allow 3D stereotactic guidance. Navigation expands on the promise of MIS by decreasing radiation exposure, improving accuracy, and potentially easing the MIS learning curve.[9]

14.2 Indications

Indications for navigated MIS TLIF are similar to open TLIF,[10] which include spondylolisthesis with associated stenosis or mechanical back pain, recurrent disk herniation, foraminal stenosis or a synovial cyst which cannot be safely addressed without destabilizing the facet joint, pseudarthrosis, and postlaminectomy kyphosis or instability.[6,10,11] Navigation is particularly useful in cases where visualization is compromised, anatomy is distorted, or safe implant corridors are limited. For example, navigation is beneficial in cases of obesity, oncology, revision surgery, complex deformity, pediatric surgery, iliac fixation, and cervical or thoracic pedicle screw placement.[6,12]

14.3 Contraindications

There are few absolute contraindications to TLIF except active local infection. Relative contraindications include systemic infection, aberrant anatomy such as a foraminal conjoined nerve root, severe spondylolisthesis, spinal metastases, acute fracture, extensive scarring, severe osteoporosis, or ankylosis of the affected level.[10,13] Wound healing risk factors such as poor nutritional status or diabetes mellitus should be optimized; however, if surgery is necessary, MIS may provide a more appropriate option due to limited wound size.[13] Metallic implants from previous surgery may distort imaging and make MIS unsafe or navigation inaccurate. Multilevel surgery may be technically more challenging to perform with an MIS technique. Unlike posterior lumbar interbody fusion, TLIF can be performed in the lumbar spine at the level of the conus; however, injury to neural structures in the upper lumbar spine remains a concern. Interbody fusion for diskogenic back pain has not shown significantly better outcomes than nonoperative management[14] and surgery should be carefully considered in this population. Patients with impaired ability to follow postoperative restrictions may not be appropriate for operative intervention.

14.4 Preoperative Planning

A thorough history and examination is mandatory in all patients. Particular attention should be paid to the side of most prominent radicular symptoms, as this will dictate the side of the TLIF approach. Patients without emergent findings should have symptoms refractory to at least 3 months of conservative management prior to surgical consideration.

Anteroposterior and lateral radiographs of the lumbar spine are used to evaluate sagittal and coronal alignment, extent of disk disease, and bone quality. Sagittal flexion and extension radiographs can reveal dynamic instability. Comparing standing plain films to supine imaging such as CT or magnetic resonance imaging (MRI) may also reveal subtle instability. MRI is used to confirm the diagnosis, plan surgery, and assess neural anatomy. CT myelography is ordered if MRI is contraindicated. CT can help distinguish bony neural compression from soft-tissue pathology and help plan implant size, type, and position. The CT scan should be optimized for the planned CAN system if preoperative fine-cut CT scan is required.

A surgical plan should be formulated preoperatively and all members of the surgical team should be briefed. A preemptive multimodal analgesia regimen is administered in the preoperative holding area[15] and antibiotics are administered prior to incision.

14.5 Operating Room Setup and Positioning

Deliberate operating room (OR) preparation is critical for safe and efficient surgery. A large OR is helpful to accommodate the imaging unit, surgical microscope, and navigation system including cameras and monitors (▶ Fig. 14.1). The patient is positioned prone on a radiolucent table such as a Jackson cradle which allows preservation of lumbar lordosis. The abdomen hangs free to prevent venous congestion and pressure points are well padded. The anesthesiologist should be instructed to turn the head frequently to decrease pressure on the face. When working in the lower lumbar spine, a reverse Trendelenburg table position decreases forces on the face and chest while allowing a more vertical trajectory for pedicle screws and disk preparation. The patient is secured to the bed with tape which helps decrease patient movement and increase navigation accuracy. For CT scanning–based CAN, the scanner is typically positioned at the patient's head with leads, cords, and suction tubes extending cephalad through the gantry. Neuromonitoring is initiated prior to transferring the patient prone; changes in somatosensory evoked potentials and motor evoked potentials after flipping may indicate a need to adjust positioning.

14.6 Registration and Localization

Navigation systems require registration of the patient's bony anatomy with the system's 3D anatomic reconstruction. After standard sterile draping, the operation begins by embedding the reference array firmly in the posterior superior iliac crest through a stab incision. The navigation camera is then registered with the reference array and surgical instruments are

calibrated. At this time, most CAN systems utilize an intraoperative scan to register patient position and reconstruct 3D anatomy. In CAN systems which utilized preoperative CT, coregistration is performed with fluoroscopy or bony point matching with a navigable probe.

14.7 Pedicle Preparation and Pedicle Screw Insertion

Posterior pedicle screw instrumentation supports the interbody construct. Incisions should be planned using a navigable probe to mark pedicle trajectories on the skin. By confirming retractor and pedicle screw trajectories, a smaller and more accurate incision may be utilized, resulting in less skin retraction. The incision is located approximately 3 cm lateral to the palpable midline spinous processes at the disk level. Surgery generally follows the transmuscular paraspinal (Wiltse) plane between the multifidus and longissimus portion of the sacrospinalis muscles[16]; however, dilator tubes invariably result in some muscle splitting. After the incision is made, the initial, navigable dilator is advanced to dock on the lateral facet in a trajectory coaxial with the pedicle and a K-wire is advanced into bone.

Pedicle screws may be placed before or after the TLIF. Placing screws prior to interbody work facilitates distraction between the screw heads, increasing visualization and easing insertion of the interbody device. However, pedicle screws may limit the working space during disk preparation and distraction may weaken pedicle screw fixation. If TLIF is to be performed first, wires are retracted out of the field.

When placing pedicle screws, sequential dilators are advanced over the K-wire until the final retractor is positioned and affixed firmly to the operative table. A navigable tap

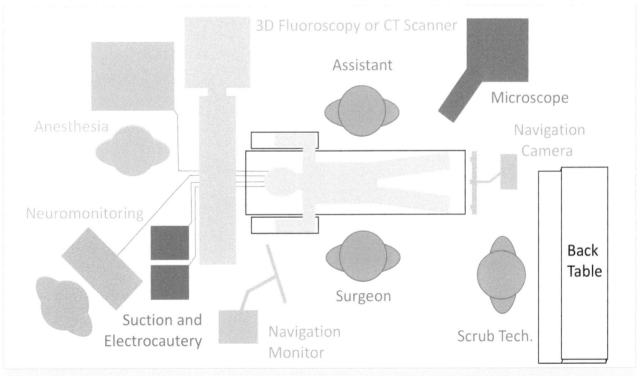

Fig. 14.1 Operating room setup diagram.

undersized 1 mm from the desired screw diameter is then used to cannulate the pedicle and is advanced into the vertebral body under live guidance. If electromyography neuromonitoring is being utilized, this tap may be stimulated to identify wall breaches in the pedicle. An appropriately sized pedicle screw is then placed with guidance.

14.8 Accessing the Facet

The neural foramen can be efficiently located using the cannulated pedicles as guides, aiming slightly caudal to the midpoint between them (▶ Fig. 14.2). Successive dilators are advanced with the final retractor attached to the contralateral bedrail using an articulating arm. Care should be taken to avoid penetration of the interlaminar space when advancing the initial dilators. The final retractor position and trajectory are confirmed using navigation or fluoroscopy. An operative microscope is used to enhance visualization and illuminate the field. Overlying muscle and capsuloligamentous attachments are removed from bone with bayonetted Bovie electrocautery.

14.9 Facetectomy

After soft-tissue removal, the inferior articular process is removed using an osteotome or high-speed burr. First, a longitudinal cut is made just medial to the facet inferiorly and extended cephalad to the superior border of the facet. A second cut is then made in the transverse plane directed laterally through the pars interarticularis. Retaining a portion of the pars protects the exiting nerve root during interbody work (▶ Fig. 14.3). The loose inferior articular process is freed of soft-tissue attachments using a curved curette and removed with a Kerrison rongeur.

The superior articular process (SAP) is removed with a transverse cut just rostral to the pedicle of the inferior vertebra. A Woodson elevator is used to palpate the pedicle and can be left within the foramen to protect deep structures during the cut. Soft tissue is freed with a curved curette and bone is removed with a Kerrison rongeur. If working space is limited, the SAP can be removed in two fragments using two parallel transverse cuts. Bleeding is often encountered during SAP removal, as a

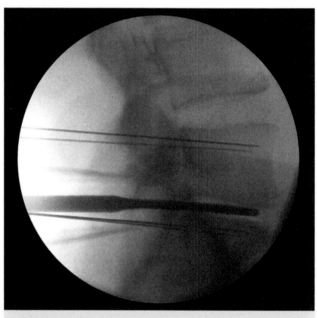

Fig. 14.2 Fluoroscopy image showing transforaminal lumbar interbody fusion (TLIF) retractor trajectory between cannulated pedicles. The instrument is being used to gauge the depth of disk removal.

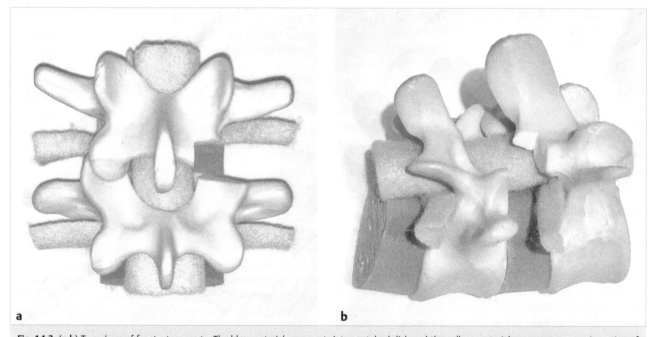

a   b

Fig. 14.3 (a,b) Two views of facetectomy cuts. The blue material represents intervertebral disk and the yellow material represents nerve. A portion of the pars interarticularis is preserved to protect the exiting nerve root.

consistent venous plexus traverses the disk at the level of the foramen. These vessels can be safely ligated with bipolar electrocautery at the rostral border of the inferior pedicle.

During disk preparation, ligamentum flavum is preserved to protect the thecal sac and traversing root, although it can be released from the lamina to allow retraction or resected to increase visualization. The exiting nerve root superiorly and the traversing root medially may be protected with nerve root retractors as needed. After interbody work is complete, the flavum can be resected if stenosis is present. For central stenosis, the retractor is rotated medially toward the junction of the spinous process and lamina. Bony resection is carried to the contralateral side with a burr and the entire flavum is removed.

14.10 Disk Preparation

A 1-cm rectangular annulotomy is made lateral to the posterior longitudinal ligament using a scalpel. The annular window can be enlarged during disk preparation as needed using a Kerrison, being sure to clear overlying tissues to avoid inadvertent durotomy. Resection of the posterior lips of the superior and inferior end plates with an osteotome facilitates access to the disk.

Disk preparation is initiated with a straight cup curette or narrow Cobb elevator working sequentially down each end plate. Care should be taken if sequential paddle reamers are used for initial disk preparation, as high distraction forces may lead to end plate violation. A straight pituitary is used to remove loose disk fragments, taking care not to disrupt the anterior longitudinal ligament. Angled cup curettes are then used to elevate disk across the midline to the contralateral side, working one end plate at a time and clearing disk material with an up-biting pituitary rongeur. Rasps or ring curettes can be used to complete the diskectomy if desired. Disk decompression can be checked by palpating the inside of the prepared interbody space using a navigable probe[17] or by taking a lateral fluoroscopic image with a metal instrument inserted into the disk space (▶ Fig. 14.2).

14.11 Interbody Device and Rod Placement

Sizing the disk space is performed by inserting sequential implant trials until the trial is snug but passes easily into the disk space with a mallet. An undersized trial can lead to instability, nonunion, and loss of lordosis, while an oversized implant can disrupt the end plate or be difficult to insert, increasing the risk of nerve injury. Morselized bone graft is packed anteriorly and medially using a funnel. The interbody device is inserted across the midline and the implant position is checked with orthogonal fluoroscopic images, although the use of a CAN probe to check implant position has been described.[17,18]

Appropriately sized and contoured rods are then placed using the manufacturer's technique. Mild compression across the construct improves lordosis and decreases the likelihood of interbody device back out. Prior to removing navigation trackers, the position of implants is checked with two-dimensional (2D) fluoroscopy or a 3D scan.[10,19]

14.12 Contralateral Facet Preparation

The contralateral facet at the level of fusion is approached through a separate incision. After exposing the joint, articular cartilage is removed with a burr or osteotome. The facet is then packed with morselized bone graft. A posterolateral fusion is not mandatory as interbody fusion provides ample surface area for fusion[6,20]; however, one may be performed if desired. First, the retractor is directed laterally toward the transverse process of the caudal vertebra which is dissected of soft tissue and decorticated using a burr. The tube is then angled superiorly and the preparation is repeated at the superior transverse process. The posterolateral gutter is then grafted.

14.13 Closure

The wound is copiously irrigated with normal saline. Though not typically necessary, the annulotomy opening can be sealed with bone wax[10] or fibrin glue to prevent posterior egress of graft material. This is particularly important if the surgeon has chosen to use BMP-2 which can irritate neural structures. A drain is rarely used. The lumbodorsal fascia is closed with a heavy gauge braided absorbable suture. Soft tissues are infiltrated with 0.25% bupivacaine to augment postoperative pain control.[21] Skin is closed in layers, followed by a sterile, occlusive dressing.

14.14 Postoperative Protocol

A multimodal analgesia protocol is essential to facilitate early mobilization and decrease medication side effects.[22] Mobilization begins on the day of surgery with physical therapy followed by ambulation with nursing assistance. Postoperative restrictions include no bending at the waist while upright, no twisting, and a 5 pound lifting limit. Bracing is not routinely used.[23] Patients are discharged on the first or second postoperative day, although there is increasing evidence supporting same-day discharge.[24] Full activities are resumed at bony fusion, at least 3 months from surgery.

14.15 Technical Pearls

- The patient should be prepared for the possibility of an open surgery. In a prospective multicenter registry of O-Arm navigation, the system failed to work as expected in 5.1% of cases.[25]
- The posterior, central disk is often missed during disk preparation, especially with MIS.
- Be cognizant of where CAN reference arrays are located, as an inadvertent bump will necessitate rescanning the patient, slowing the surgery and increasing the patient's radiation exposure.
- An in-line suction bone trap is useful to collect autograft bone.
- There is a significant learning curve for MIS. Surgeons new to MIS should choose the largest available MIS tube or an expandable retractor.

- Minimize MIS retractor adjustment to help reduce muscle creep into the surgical field.
- When using navigation, it is helpful to confirm accuracy at each step by palpating a landmark such as a transverse process. If the patient's anatomy is incongruous with the 3D reconstruction, registration should be repeated.

14.16 Complications

Potential complications of navigated MIS TLIF include the risks of general anesthesia, hardware malposition, pain, infection, nerve injury, fracture, failure to improve, bleeding, durotomy, and pseudarthrosis.[10,26] Correction of intraoperative complications is more difficult in MIS, as the working corridor is small and visibility is limited. Navigation may decrease the rate of hardware complications.[26] Due to the lack of dead space in MIS, if direct repair of a dural leak is not possible, a collagen sponge and dural sealant followed by meticulous fascial closure is often sufficient to tamponade leaks and allow healing.[10]

14.17 Outcomes

MIS TLIF has comparable fusion rates to open TLIF, generally above 95%.[6,20] In a systematic review and meta-analysis comparing MIS versus open TLIF, MIS was found to have similar operative times with significantly lower intraoperative blood loss and infection rates. Additionally, VAS back pain scores and postoperative ODI scores were significantly lower in the MIS group.[6] A prospective comparison by Peng et al found that early surgical outcomes favored MIS, while outcomes were similar at 2 years postoperatively.[27]

Navigated pedicle screws are safe and highly accurate.[9,12,25,28,29] A meta-analysis of 599 patients undergoing MIS surgery with 3D navigation found a breach rate of 0.33% (2 of 2,132 screws) compared to a breach rate of 13.1% using 2D fluoroscopic guidance.[29] Mason et al reviewed pedicle screw accuracy in 30 studies and found an accuracy of 68.1% with conventional fluoroscopy compared to 95.5% with 3D fluoroscopic navigation.[28] In deformity-free cadavers, however, Tabaraee et al found that pedicle screws placed with navigation had similar accuracy rates to those placed with conventional fluoroscopy.[30] A retrospective multivariate analysis of 15,222 patients undergoing lumbar pedicle screw fixation found that CAN resulted in significantly fewer major and minor adverse events and less blood transfusion with significantly longer operative times.[26]

14.18 Conclusion

Navigated MIS TLIF is a safe and effective surgical option for many degenerative lumbar pathologies. MIS surgery decreases blood loss and tissue damage, expedites recovery, and decreases costs. The addition of navigation increases implant placement accuracy and can decrease radiation exposure.

References

[1] Liu J, Deng H, Long X, Chen X, Xu R, Liu Z. A comparative study of perioperative complications between transforaminal versus posterior lumbar interbody fusion in degenerative lumbar spondylolisthesis. Eur Spine J. 2016; 25(5):1575–1580

[2] Mobbs RJ, Phan K, Malham G, Seex K, Rao PJ. Lumbar interbody fusion: techniques, indications and comparison of interbody fusion options including PLIF, TLIF, MI-TLIF, OLIF/ATP, LLIF and ALIF. J Spine Surg. 2015; 1(1):2–18

[3] Jalalpour K, Neumann P, Johansson C, Hedlund R. a randomized controlled trial comparing transforaminal lumbar interbody fusion and uninstrumented posterolateral fusion in the degenerative lumbar spine. Global Spine J. 2015; 5(4):322–328

[4] Lee KH, Yue WM, Yeo W, Soeharno H, Tan SB. Clinical and radiological outcomes of open versus minimally invasive transforaminal lumbar interbody fusion. Eur Spine J. 2012; 21(11):2265–2270

[5] Parker SL, Adogwa O, Witham TF, Aaronson OS, Cheng J, McGirt MJ. Postoperative infection after minimally invasive versus open transforaminal lumbar interbody fusion (TLIF): literature review and cost analysis. Minim Invasive Neurosurg. 2011; 54(1):33–37

[6] Phan K, Rao PJ, Kam AC, Mobbs RJ. Minimally invasive versus open transforaminal lumbar interbody fusion for treatment of degenerative lumbar disease: systematic review and meta-analysis. Eur Spine J. 2015; 24(5):1017–1030

[7] Yu E, Khan SN. Does less invasive spine surgery result in increased radiation exposure? A systematic review. Clin Orthop Relat Res. 2014; 472(6):1738–1748

[8] Schlenzka D, Laine T, Lund T. Computer-assisted spine surgery. Eur Spine J. 2000; 9 Suppl 1:S57–S64

[9] Kim TT, Drazin D, Shweikeh F, Pashman R, Johnson JP. Clinical and radiographic outcomes of minimally invasive percutaneous pedicle screw placement with intraoperative CT (O-arm) image guidance navigation. Neurosurg Focus. 2014; 36(3):E1–A27

[10] Pelton MA, Nandyala SV, Marquez-Lara A, Singh K. Minimally invasive transforaminal lumbar interbody fusion. In: Minimally Invasive Spine Surgery. New York, NY: Springer New York; 2014:151–158

[11] Kim JY, Park JY, Kim KH, et al. Minimally invasive transforaminal lumbar interbody fusion for spondylolisthesis: comparison between isthmic and degenerative spondylolisthesis. World Neurosurg. 2015; 84(5):1284–1293

[12] Gelalis ID, Paschos NK, Pakos EE, et al. Accuracy of pedicle screw placement: a systematic review of prospective in vivo studies comparing free hand, fluoroscopy guidance and navigation techniques. Eur Spine J. 2012; 21(2):247–255

[13] Louie PK, Massel DH, Mayo BC, et al. TLIF/PLIF MIS option. In: Minimally Invasive Spine Surgery. New York, NY: Springer; 2017:416

[14] Bydon M, De la Garza-Ramos R, Macki M, Baker A, Gokaslan AK, Bydon A. Lumbar fusion versus nonoperative management for treatment of discogenic low back pain: a systematic review and meta-analysis of randomized controlled trials. J Spinal Disord Tech. 2014; 27(5):297–304

[15] Kim S-I, Ha K-Y, Oh I-S. Preemptive multimodal analgesia for postoperative pain management after lumbar fusion surgery: a randomized controlled trial. Eur Spine J. 2016; 25(5):1614–1619

[16] Lehman RA, Jr, Vaccaro AR, Bertagnoli R, Kuklo TR. Standard and minimally invasive approaches to the spine. Orthop Clin North Am. 2005; 36(3):281–292

[17] Lian X, Navarro-Ramirez R, Berlin C, et al. Total 3D Airo® Navigation for Minimally Invasive Transforaminal Lumbar Interbody Fusion. BioMed Res Int. 2016; 2016(6):5027340

[18] Drazin D, Liu JC, Acosta FL, Jr. CT navigated lateral interbody fusion. J Clin Neurosci. 2013; 20(10):1438–1441

[19] Wang Y, Hu Y, Liu H, Li C, Li H, Yi X. Navigation makes transforaminal lumbar interbody fusion less invasive. Orthopedics. 2016; 39(5):e857–e862

[20] Karikari IO, Isaacs RE. Minimally invasive transforaminal lumbar interbody fusion: a review of techniques and outcomes. Spine. 2010; 35(26) Suppl: S294–S301

[21] Perera AP, Chari A, Kostusiak M, Khan AA, Luoma AM, Casey ATH. Intramuscular local anesthetic infiltration at closure for postoperative analgesia in lumbar spine surgery: a systematic review and meta-analysis. Spine. 2017; 42(14):1088–1095

[22] Kurd MF, Kreitz T, Schroeder G, Vaccaro AR. The role of multimodal analgesia in spine surgery. J Am Acad Orthop Surg. 2017; 25(4):260–268

[23] Yee AJ, Yoo JU, Marsolais EB, et al. Use of a postoperative lumbar corset after lumbar spinal arthrodesis for degenerative conditions of the spine. A prospective randomized trial. J Bone Joint Surg Am. 2008; 90(10):2062–2068

[24] Eckman WW, Hester L, McMillen M. Same-day discharge after minimally invasive transforaminal lumbar interbody fusion: a series of 808 cases. Clin Orthop Relat Res. 2014; 472(6):1806–1812

[25] Van de Kelft E, Costa F, Van der Planken D, Schils F. A prospective multicenter registry on the accuracy of pedicle screw placement in the thoracic, lumbar, and sacral levels with the use of the O-arm imaging system and StealthStation Navigation. Spine. 2012; 37(25):E1580–E1587

[26] Nooh A, Aoude A, Fortin M, et al. Use of computer assistance in lumbar fusion surgery: analysis of 15 222 patients in the ACS-NSQIP database. Global Spine J. 2017; 7(7):617–623

[27] Peng CWB, Yue WM, Poh SY, Yeo W, Tan SB. Clinical and radiological outcomes of minimally invasive versus open transforaminal lumbar interbody fusion. Spine. 2009; 34(13):1385–1389

[28] Mason A, Paulsen R, Babuska JM, et al. The accuracy of pedicle screw placement using intraoperative image guidance systems. J Neurosurg Spine. 2014; 20(2):196–203

[29] Bourgeois AC, Faulkner AR, Bradley YC, et al. improved accuracy of minimally invasive transpedicular screw placement in the lumbar spine with 3-dimensional stereotactic image guidance: a comparative meta-analysis. J Spinal Disord Tech. 2015; 28(9):324–329

[30] Tabaraee E, Gibson AG, Karahalios DG, Potts EA, Mobasser J-P, Burch S. Intraoperative cone beam-computed tomography with navigation (O-ARM) versus conventional fluoroscopy (C-ARM): a cadaveric study comparing accuracy, efficiency, and safety for spinal instrumentation. Spine. 2013; 38(22):1953–1958

15 Robotic Instrumentation for Lumbosacral Spondylolisthesis

Michael R. Conti Mica, Michael P. Silverstein, R. Alden Milam IV, and Eric B. Laxer

Abstract:

Instrumentation for the surgical treatment of lumbosacral spondylolisthesis can be performed with the use of a surgical robotic guidance system. This chapter discusses the use of the Mazor Renaissance Guidance System for posterior instrumentation of isthmic and degenerative spondylolisthesis. We describe an approach to preoperative planning, building the appropriate frame construct, registration, and the execution of percutaneous conventional pedicle screws or open cortical pedicle screws in combination with either an anterior lumbar interbody fusion or transforaminal lumbar interbody fusion. Pearls to avoid common complications and pitfalls are presented.

Keywords: robotics, spondylolisthesis, Mazor Renaissance, cortical screws, percutaneous pedicle screws

15.1 Introduction

The most common type of spondylolisthesis that occurs at L5–S1 is isthmic.[1] While the vast majority of patients are asymptomatic, symptomatic patients tend to present with mechanical back, buttock, and referred posterior thigh pain due to segmental instability. Patients may also present with L5 radicular symptoms due to foraminal stenosis caused by fibrous tissue emanating from the pars defect and spondylosis of the disk. Less frequently, degenerative spondylolisthesis may occur, with a similar presentation of back and leg pain in the L5 or S1 distributions.

This chapter describes the techniques for robotic-assisted instrumentation for the treatment of lumbosacral spondylolisthesis using the Mazor Renaissance Guidance System (MRGS; MAZOR Robotics, Inc., Orlando, FL).

15.2 Surgical Indications, Contraindications, and Options

The primary surgical indications for lumbosacral spondylolisthesis are persistent symptoms refractory to nonsurgical care, neurological deficit, and slip progression. Contraindications include, but are not limited to, active infection and uncontrolled medical comorbidities. Patients with such conditions should be medically optimized prior to surgery.[2]

Surgical options include the following:
1. Anterior lumbar interbody fusion (ALIF) combined with posterior percutaneous pedicle screws.
2. Transforaminal lumbar interbody fusion (TLIF) combined with cortical screws or conventional pedicle screws.

3. Pars repair with direct screw insertion and bone grafting. While robotic guidance can be used for this technique in the setting of spondylolysis, this technique is not discussed in this chapter.

Options 1 and 2 provide for stabilization of the segmental instability and indirect foraminal decompression. Foraminotomy can be added if direct decompression is preferred by the surgeon; however, this is typically not the approach of the authors. The role of the robot during these cases is to assist the surgeon with safe and accurate screw placement.

This chapter will focus on the general steps common to all procedures using the Mazor Renaissance Guidance System, followed by additional details on the first two surgical options listed earlier based on the techniques we use.

15.3 Steps for Use of the Mazor Renaissance Guidance System

There are four steps that are common to all cases when using the MRGS:
1. *Preoperative planning.* A preoperative thin section CT scan from the lower thoracic spine to the sacrum is performed following the manufacturer's protocol. This is typically obtained prior to the day of surgery, but may be done on the day of surgery with an intraoperative CT scanner. The images are then loaded into a computer with Mazor's proprietary planning software. Planning is based on full details of vertebral, spinal canal, and foraminal anatomy. The software allows for the assessment and selection of optimal screw position and trajectory. Additionally, planning is useful for screw head alignment to facilitate the seating of the rods. The plan is then transferred to Mazor's intraoperative computer workstation.
2. *Frame construct.* Once the patient is placed under anesthesia, positioned, prepped, and draped for surgery, a frame is constructed using several different options based on the surgical plan. The frame requires a cephalad spinous process pin, and either a set of caudad pelvic pins or table-mounted posts called "Condors." The frame is completed by attaching a bridge to these cephalad and caudad anchoring points to which the robotic device will be attached.
3. *Registration.* Intraoperative fluoroscopy is used to register the patient's spine anatomy with the preoperative CT scan. This allows the planning software to recognize the patient's spine and execute the operative plan.
4. *Screw preparation and insertion.* The surgical team works with the manufacturer's intraoperative staff and uses the robotic guidance system to sequentially drill a pathway, insert guidewires, and place screws.

15.4 Details of the ALIF and TLIF Techniques

15.4.1 Anterior Lumbar Interbody Fusion Combined with Posterior Percutaneous Conventional Pedicle Screws Using the Mazor Bed Mount Assembly

Following completion of a standard ALIF, the patient is subsequently positioned prone on a Jackson table.

The following steps are then performed:

1. The cephalad anchoring point is attached. A spinous process pin is drilled into the L1 or L2 spinous process. Fixation of this pin must be secure. Fluoroscopy is used to confirm the correct level, pin depth, and orientation. The entrance point usually corresponds to the level of the disk space just caudad to the spinous process. For example, the L1 spinous process pin will usually be in line with the L1–L2 disk space.

2. The caudad anchoring point is attached. A single Condor is connected to the table using a table clamp. Fixation of the clamp to the Jackson table and fixation of the Condor to the clamp must be secure. Any toggle of the Condor could result in inaccurate screw insertion.

3. The bed mounted platform and bridge are connected to the spinous process pin cephalad, and the Condor caudad (▶ Fig. 15.1, ▶ Fig. 15.2).

4. Registration is performed by securing the yellow three-dimensional (3D) marker on the bridge at the level of surgery and taking 60- and 90-degree fluoroscopic images, which are then sent to the workstation and used to match the operative plan to the patient's intraoperative position.

5. A pedicle is selected for screw insertion. The robotic device is secured to the bridge (▶ Fig. 15.3); the workstation sends the screw trajectory coordinates to the robotic device which then positions itself to the desired starting point and trajectory. There are several attachment options to the robotic device and the surgeon assembles those designated by the workstation onto the robot. There is a short arm that extends from these attachments that represents the planned trajectory.

6. The surgeon passes a scalpel through the arm and makes a small skin incision at the point of entry based on the screw trajectory. This is extended slightly and deepened past the lumbodorsal fascia. A trocar and cannula are passed through the arm, tissues, and docked onto bone. Tactile awareness is important to audit for any potential skive. If that is a concern, the surgeon may remove the trocar and use the Peteron device through the sleeve to flatten the point of bone contact and minimize the skive risk. The drill guide is then inserted and a lateral fluoroscopic image is obtained to verify that the trajectory is consistent with what was planned. The screw pathway is then drilled. A reduction tube and safety guidewire are then passed together through the drill guide and seated into bone, passing through the pedicle and into the back of the vertebral body. The surgeon can feel the crepitus of the cancellous bone, as this occurs until a firm endpoint is reached. The reduction tube is then removed, and care must be taken to protect the guidewire. This is repeated for the three other screws.

7. Anteroposterior (AP) and lateral fluoroscopic images are obtained to confirm all four guidewires are well placed.

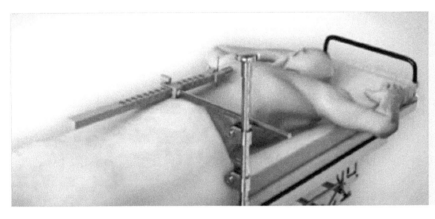

Fig. 15.1 Illustration of the bed mount frame, platform, and bridge. Note the spinous process pin cephalad and the bed mount Condor caudad with the large tightening knob on top. (From the Mazor Renaissance Surgical Technique guide for Hover-T, Bed Mount, and Multidirectional Bridge. Image provided by Medtronic.)

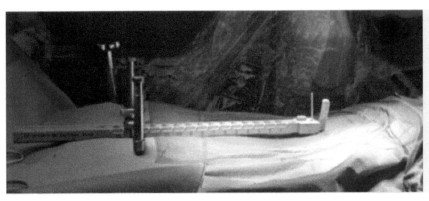

Fig. 15.2 Assembled bed mount frame, platform, and bridge. Cephalad is to the right. Note the spinous process pin cephalad and the bed mount Condor caudad on the far side of the table, with the large tightening knob at the top.

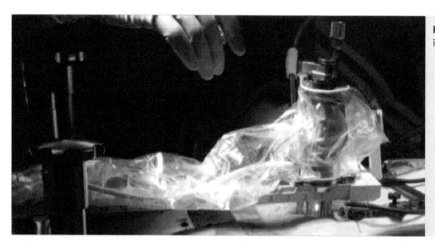

Fig. 15.3 Robotic device (blue, right side of image) attached to frame and ready for use.

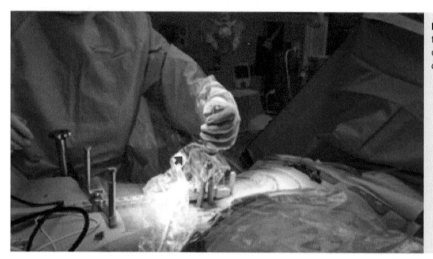

Fig. 15.4 Screw preparation and insertion. Note the blue Mazor robotic device is on the other side of the screwdriver (just to the right of the *blue arrow*).

8. The screws are then inserted and the wires removed (▶ Fig. 15.4).

9. Incisions are extended as needed and the construct is completed by inserting rods and caps.

10. The incisions are irrigated and hemostasis is obtained. The fascia is closed with 0 Vicryl suture as needed; the subcutaneous tissues approximated with 2–0 Vicryl suture; and the skin is closed with a buried, running 3–0 Monocryl subcuticular suture. Sterile dressings are placed.

15.4.2 Transforaminal Lumbar Interbody Fusion Combined with Cortical Bone Screws Using the Mazor Multidirectional Bridge

The technique described later in this section uses cortical-based trajectory screws. This is our preference for these cases, as it can be done through a smaller incision with less soft-tissue dissection. Although a finite element analysis study has suggested that cortical screws demonstrate inferior fixation strength compared to conventional pedicle screws when done through the pars defect, this has not been identified as a clinical concern.[3]

Traditional open techniques for cortical screw insertion follow the guidelines described by Santoni et al, with a starting point roughly at the midpoint of the pars interarticularis and with a trajectory about 10 degrees cephalad and 25 degrees lateral.[4] The goal of this trajectory is to maximize the four-point contact described by Matsukawa et al, which is composed of the laminar portion of the pars, the medial wall of the dorsal portion of the pedicle, the lateral wall of the ventral portion of the pedicle, and the lateral aspect of the vertebral body.[5] While the location and anatomic guidelines are similar using the Mazor system, the advantage of the robotic technique is that it allows for the most optimal placement of screws to reduce neurologic injury and maximize mechanical purchase while accommodating the nuances of the patient's particular anatomy. For example, the surgeon can plan screw placement such that the L5 screw heads avoid the L4–L5 facet joint, and planning can help the surgeon decide if a slightly longer screw at L5 is needed to facilitate seating of the rods.

The patient is positioned prone on a Jackson table with a padded leg board to maximize lordosis and indirectly reduce the slip. The spine is exposed through a midline approach and bilateral dissection is carried out to the pars and facet joints, which are denuded of their soft tissue. At this point, it is important to make sure the pars surface will not promote skiving of the drill. If this is the case, the starting point on the pars may be burred to create a more secure docking point for the drill. Also, any bone around the facet joints that could cause a deviation of the trocar, cannula, or drill sleeve must be trimmed with a burr or osteotome. We are careful not to remove more bone than is necessary until the screw pathways have been drilled because doing so may interfere with the registration process preventing use of the robot or resulting in screw malposition.

Once the exposure is completed, all metallic retractors from the surgical field are removed as their presence may interfere with the registration process.

The following steps are then performed:

1. The cephalad anchoring point is attached. A spinous process pin is drilled into the L1 or L2 spinous process. See step 1 in section "Anterior Lumbar Interbody Fusion Combined with Posterior Percutaneous Conventional Pedicle Screws Using the Mazor Bed Mount Assembly."

2. The caudad anchoring point is attached. A Condor is attached to each side of the table using a table clamp. The same clamps as described earlier are used. Fixation of the clamps to the Jackson table and fixation of the Condors to the clamps must be secure. The Condors are further fixed by adding a patient stabilizer which is a round flat attachment that pushes against the bilateral greater trochanters and further limits patient movement. This is needed because cortical screws require use of the multidirectional bridge which has several station options that may require manual adjustments between screws. The multidirectional bridge is connected to the spinous process pin cephalad and the Condors caudad. An alternative option is to use the Hover-T platform where the caudad anchoring points are via pins drilled into the patient's posterior-superior iliac spine. We like to leave 2 to 3 cm of space between the bridge and skin incision to allow for use of handheld retractors if needed (see step 5 below).

3. Registration is done by securing the yellow 3D marker on the bridge at the level of surgery, and taking 60- and 90-degree fluoroscopic images, which are then sent to the Mazor workstation and used to match the preoperative plan to the patient's intraoperative position.

4. A pedicle is selected for screw insertion. There are several station options on the bridge, and the surgeon positions the bridge to the correct station based on instructions from the workstation. The robotic device is secured to the bridge; the workstation sends the screw trajectory coordinates to the robotic device which then orients itself to the desired trajectory. There are several attachment options to the robotic device and the surgeon assembles those selected by the workstation onto the robot. There is a short arm that extends from these attachments that represents the planned trajectory.

5. Handheld retractors may be gently used for visualization and to avoid soft-tissue deflection of the trocar, cannula, or drill sleeve if needed. Care must be taken to not forcefully retract in one direction and displace the patient as this can result in screw malposition. A trocar and sleeve are passed through the arm and docked onto the bone. Tactile feel and direct visualization are critical to audit for potential skive or deviation. If that is a concern, the surgeon can remove the trocar, and repeat the earlier steps of burring the pars or facet. If the deflection is from soft tissue, simple counterforce applied to the trocar, cannula, or drill sleeve with a finger or cobb may suffice. The drill guide is then inserted, and a lateral fluoroscopic image is obtained to verify that the trajectory is consistent with what was planned. The screw pathway is then drilled. A reduction tube and safety guidewire are then passed together through the drill guide and seated into bone, passing through the pedicle and into the back of the vertebral body. The surgeon can feel the crepitus of the cancellous bone as this occurs until a firm endpoint is reached. The reduction tube is then removed, and care must be taken to protect the guidewire. For L5, the screw holes are tapped, and the screw inserted. For S1, we prefer to drill, tap, remove the guidewires, and place bone wax on the holes. This allows for easier decompression and TLIF insertion, as the S1 screws can get in the way of the TLIF instruments. An alternative is to use modular screws with isolated insertion of the shank, then adding the polyaxial heads after the TLIF is complete.

6. The frame is disassembled, retractors can now be reinserted, and the TLIF is performed using the surgeon's preferred technique.

7. The S1 screws are inserted. AP and lateral images are taken to confirm screw position if needed.

8. The construct is completed by inserting rods and caps.

9. The incision is irrigated, and hemostasis is obtained; a drain is inserted if needed and vancomycin powder is placed within the wound. The fascia is closed with 0 Vicryl suture; the subcutaneous tissues approximated with 2–0 Vicryl suture; and the skin is closed with a running, subcuticular 3–0 Monocryl suture. A sterile dressing is placed.

If the surgeon prefers instrumentation with conventional pedicle screws, this can be done as well. The technique we use with pedicle screws is similar to pedicle screw insertion described in section "Details of the ALIF and TLIF Techniques," except that after the screws have been inserted we use a pedicle-based retractor system to perform a minimally invasive TLIF.

15.5 Case Examples

See ▸ Fig. 15.5, ▸ Fig. 15.6, and ▸ Fig. 15.7 for specific case examples.

15.6 Postoperative Care

We do not use a brace. Intravenous and oral pain medication are provided as needed. Patients are mobilized with physical therapy on postoperative day 0 and are usually discharged home the day after surgery.

15.7 Avoiding Pitfalls and Complications

There are potential challenges with the use of the robot. Skiving at the starting point can be identified by feel and watching for any displacement of the drill guide. Contouring or removing bone at or near the drill site and holding the guide to counter this displacement can help maintain the correct starting point. It is important to have good fluoroscopic images, as this can

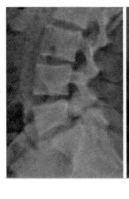
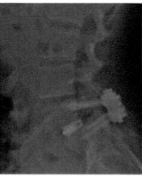
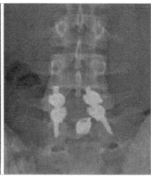

Fig. 15.5 Case illustration. Pre-op and post-op images of patient with grade I spondylolisthesis at L5–S1. Transforaminal lumbar interbody fusion with cortical screws inserted with robotic assistance.

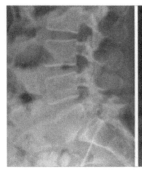
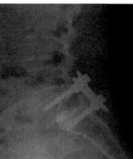
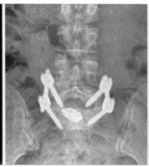

Fig. 15.6 Case illustration. Pre-op and post-op images of patient with grade II spondylolisthesis at L5–S1. Transforaminal lumbar interbody fusion with conventional pedicle screws inserted with robotic assistance.

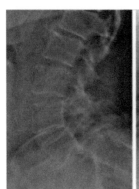
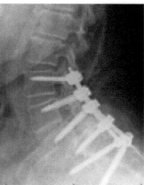
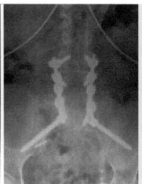

Fig. 15.7 Case illustration. Pre-op and post-op images of patient with grade IV spondylolisthesis at L5–S1. The patient was treated with a partial reduction and fusion with L3–S1 pedicle and S2–A1 screws inserted with robotic assistance. Interbody placement was aborted.

limit the ability to perform registration. The position of the patient should not change following registration, as this will completely change the orientation of the anatomy relative to the bridge. On occasion, there is failure to register, and traditional insertion techniques, such as screw insertion with bony landmarks or fluoroscopy, must ensue. The surgeon must be prepared for this.

All staff involved with the case such as the surgeon, scrub techs, circulators, Mazor team, implant reps must have ongoing excellent communication and be fully engaged. We have a strict policy for utilizing repeat back dialogue for all individual steps throughout the procedure. Any deficiency of the aforementioned may lead to improper instrumentation.

References

[1] Wiltse LL, Newman PH, Macnab I. Classification of spondylolysis and spondylolisthesis. Clin Orthop Relat Res. 1976(117):23–29
[2] Hikata T, Iwanami A, Hosogane N, et al. High preoperative hemoglobin A1c is a risk factor for surgical site infection after posterior thoracic and lumbar spinal instrumentation surgery. J Orthop Sci. 2014; 19(2):223–228
[3] Matsukawa K, Yato Y, Imabayashi H, Hosogane N, Asazuma T, Chiba K. Biomechanical evaluation of lumbar pedicle screws in spondylolytic vertebrae: comparison of fixation strength between the traditional trajectory and a cortical bone trajectory. J Neurosurg Spine. 2016; 24(6):910–915
[4] Santoni BG, Hynes RA, McGilvray KC, et al. Cortical bone trajectory for lumbar pedicle screws. Spine J. 2009; 9(5):366–373
[5] Matsukawa K, Yato Y, Nemoto O, Imabayashi H, Asazuma T, Nemoto K. Morphometric measurement of cortical bone trajectory for lumbar pedicle screw insertion using computed tomography. J Spinal Disord Tech. 2013; 26(6): E248–E253

16 The Role of Navigation in the Resection of Primary Spinal Tumor

Taolin Fang, Jian Dong, and Stefano Boriani

Abstract

The primary spinal tumor can be effectively treated with total *en bloc* spondylectomy (TES) to achieve margin-free resection of the tumor. However, *en bloc* resection of spine tumors is a technically demanding surgery. Although more and more surgeons have started to perform *en bloc* resections in the recent two decades, the complication rate is reportedly as high as 35%. These complications include but are not limited to the injury of the vena cava, late aortic dissections, intraoperative hemorrhage, and other less severe complications. The emerging navigation and robotic assistance focus on the precision of the spine surgery, decreasing of the surgical errors, and improving the patient outcomes. With showing a difficult surgical case of an advanced-staged spinal tumor, step by step, from preoperative and intraoperative surgical planning to accurate osteotomy and reconstruction, this chapter illustrates how spine navigation technology provides a high level of accurate visualization to facilitate the *en bloc* resection of the primary spinal tumor with a full circumferential tumor-free margin. Although *en bloc* resection still carries a high complication profile, the application of navigation and robotics has made it safer and more efficient.

Keywords: primary spinal tumor, desmoplastic fibroma of bone, 3D-printing, 3D CT-based navigation, total en bloc spondylectomy, intraoperative cone-beam CT

16.1 Introduction

The treatment of primary spinal tumors has evolved over the past four decades. The development of an oncological staging system for spinal tumors[1,2] has afforded a better understanding of the biological behavior of single histotypes and, in turn, more advanced surgical planning.

Stener[3] was the first to coin and develop the concept of *en bloc* tumor resection in the spine and Roy-Camille et al[4] and Tomita et al[5] then systemized the procedure by single posterior approach. But these techniques, known as TES (total en bloc spondylectomy) can achieve an appropriate margin-free tumor resection only if the tumor is located inside the vertebral body. If the tumor grows extracompartmentally, a combination of approaches is generally required for a full margin control. Subsequent modifications of the technique for the treatment of vertebral neoplasm according to the tumor extension has provided a chance for oncological appropriate resection margins, thereby improving tumor control and overall survival.[4,5] In a series reported by Boriani et al, 70.4% of the patients were free from recurrence at mid/long term after en bloc resections.[6] Up to 83.4% of patients were in remission when treated for de novo disease.

Today, en bloc resections are more commonly performed and a large series of studies have been published in the spine literature. However, there is still a high complication rate associated with the procedure, with reported rates of approximately 35%, including intraoperative death due to injury of the vena cava, late aortic dissections, massive intraoperative hemorrhage, and other less severe complications. The complication rate has been reported at 10.6% for the single posterior approach and much higher for a double-approach resection.[6]

Surgical decision-making in cases of primary spinal tumors can be complicated and nuanced. The extent of tumor resection needs to be tailored based on a shared decision-making model between patient and physician. Sometimes, for a true wide margin en bloc tumor resection, vital structures including nerve roots, dura, or vascular structures must be sacrificed. Other times, oncological principles of wide dissection may be violated, the so-called intentional transgression,[7] potentially placing the patient at higher risk for recurrence, but likely sparing some other dysfunction (e.g., neurologic). In this setting, a multidisciplinary approach (medical and radiation oncology) for adjuvant therapy can sometimes compensate for margin violation according to the specific tumor histotypes. Sometimes, tumor extension can exceed the anatomical criteria to perform a tumor-free margin en bloc resection.[8] This so-called incidental transgression[7] requires adjuvant therapy as well.

This is the case reported here: the extension of the tumor (desmoplastic fibroma of bone, ICD-O code 8823/0: a low-grade locally aggressive tumor) was so huge that it was considered impossible to perform an en bloc resection with a full circumferential tumor-free margin. The major constraint was considered the intrathoracic extension under the scapula. Therefore, an intentional transgression to separate the huge tumor in two major pieces was planned as the best possible oncologically appropriate surgery. On the operative field, however, the spine navigation technology allowed such a high level of accurate visualization to make possible the en bloc resection with a full circumferential tumor-free margin.

The image-based technology creates a virtual, three-dimensional (3D) model of the patient's spine, essentially a digital roadmap or blueprint to help guide the surgeon. It is especially useful to the complex spine surgery like en bloc resection of spine tumors. Over the past decade, 3D navigation system is reported to have assisted surgeons to perform complex spine surgeries in a much safer manner.[9] Computed tomography (CT)-based image-guidance technology represents one of the most recent advancements in 3D navigation in spine surgery. Intraoperative cone-beam CT (O-arm, Medtronic, Minneapolis, MN), frequently coupled with stereotactic navigation (StealthStation, Medtronic), is increasingly used in the surgical management of spine surgery. It is gaining popularity due to the ability to provide automated registration with an intraoperative, post-positioning CT scan with the theoretical benefit of enhanced safety and accuracy.[10,11] It is one of the options advocated to limit instrumentation misplacement. The use of 3D CT-based navigation in TES treating primary neoplasm, however, has not been well studied or reported.[12] In this chapter, we will introduce our experience based on the

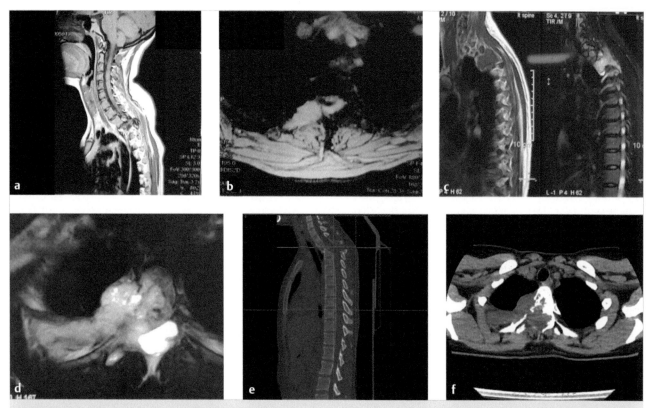

Fig. 16.1 **(a)** The MRI image 10 years ago showed destruction of the third vertebral body, Th2 spondylolisthesis. **(b)** Transaxial MRI scan showed compression on the spinal cord. **(c,d)** Current MRI showed the whole vertebral body of T3 was destructed. Both intrathecal and intrathoracic tumor grew significantly. The progressive compression of the spinal cord was observed. The posterior element was affected. **(e,f)** 3D CT showed severe osteolytic lesion of the spine.

previously introduced tumor resection, performed under O-arm navigation.

16.2 Relative Indication and Contraindication

Tomita classified spinal tumors into seven types according to the extent of tumor invasion.[5,13,14] TES was mainly indicated in Tomita lesion types 2 to 5, and lesion types 1 and 6 were only relatively indicated. With the improvement of the surgical techniques, more and more Tomita type 1 and 6 lesions have been reported to be successfully resected en bloc. Multisegmental resection of more than three levels in a single procedure has been reported in recent years, and although reportedly successful, increasing numbers of resected segments has been shown to be an independent predictor of major complications,[6] with 100% complications in four-level resection compared with 50% in three-level resection, 45.5% in two-level resection, and 34.9% in single-level resection.[15]

16.3 Case Example

A 46-year-old female presented with a history of back pain and numbness on lower part of the torso for 9 years and was admitted after progressive girdle band sensation around the waist for 1 month. She started to have back pain and mild numbness around the waist and bilateral leg pain, numbness, and tingling. MRI revealed multiple osteolytic lesions from the second and the third thoracic vertebrae expanding through the transverse processes to the ribs on the right side, with the spinal canal involvement and spinal cord compression. Physical examination demonstrated back pain in the area of the second and third thoracic vertebrae and decreased mobility of the thoracic spine with moderate-to-severe neurological deficit, including perineal hypoesthesia, bilateral hyperreflexia, bilateral patellar and ankle clonus, and reduced sensorium. Computed tomography showed a tumor at the described thoracic level Th2–Th3, involving the third rib on the right side, with the second and the third thoracic spondylolisthesis (▶ Fig. 16.1).

16.3.1 Navigation Techniques

Preparation before the Surgery

Surgical preparation for navigation started several days prior to the surgery. Cytology from a preoperative CT-guided needle aspiration of the paraspinal mass showed a myofibroblast type tumor. No evidence of distant metastasis was found on PET-CT and bone scintigraphy. Using patient's MRI and CT scans and the help of the 3D printing technology, a 3D model of the tumor and its surrounding area was created. This model allowed better understanding of the exact positioning of the tumor and

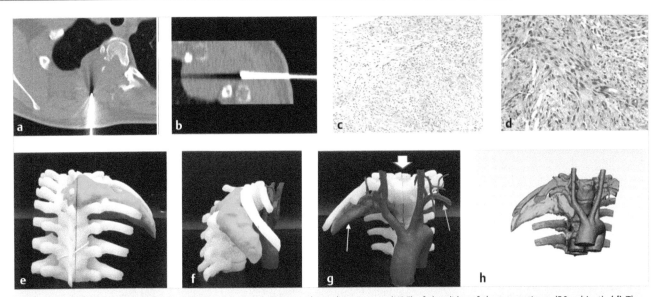

Fig. 16.2 (a,b) CT-guided aspiration of the tumor. **(c)** The hematoxylin and eosin stain (H&E) of the slides of the tumor tissue (20x object). **(d)** The hematoxylin and eosin stain (H&E) of the slides of the tumor tissue (40x object). The pathology report showed that the diagnosis was desmoplastic fibroma of bone. **(e,f)** Preoperative 3D printing of the tumor, according which the surgical plan was made. **(g)** The green mass in the 3D model indicated by the thin white arrow is the tumor. The thick white arrow indicates the spinal cord. The yellow arrow indicates the large vessels around the tumor.

how it interfered with the blood vessels and nerves. An en bloc resection of the second to fourth thoracic vertebral level followed by a second-stage intrathoracic tumor resection through thoracotomy was planned (▶ Fig. 16.2).

Preparation in the Operating Room

The patient was positioned prone on a Jackson table. The design of the O-arm allows it to work ideally with the Jackson table, which does not have a base obstructing movement along the long axis of the patient and table. The Jackson table enables the O-arm to be positioned along any level of the spinal axis.[16] The table is well designed for imaging purposes, with its core structure containing minimal radio-dense metal, resulting in minimal radiographic artifact.

A three-pronged Mayfield head clamp was used to position the head in the usual fashion at the accepted anatomic landmarks and all pressure points were well padded. The O-arm is then used to take fluoroscopy image in anteroposterior and lateral views to assure that the Th2, Th3 vertebrae are in the center of the O-arm gantry. The reference frame is attached. A "spin" is acquired and the 3D reconstructed images are obtained and transmitted to the StealthStation. The O-arm is then removed and the surgical site is prepped and draped in the usual fashion, avoiding any disturbance to the sterile reference pin.

O-arm Techniques

During the surgery, the sterile draped O-arm is also used to take a 3D CT with medium dose of radiation. The sterile cover for O-arm can be cumbersome, at times getting caught between the shields.[16] An alternate draping of the patient in a 360-degree circumferential manner is more efficient and avoids problems,

while the O-arm opens and closes around the patient and operating table.[16]

The O-arm images are then coupled to the navigation system and the registration process is automated with rare issues. The coupling of intraoperative imaging to navigation systems saves a large amount of time and improves accuracy of navigation. The images acquired are rapidly transferred to the navigation workstation, where multiplanar reconstructions of the anatomy are generated. At this stage the navigation is ready and the surgery can continue. From the start of image acquisition through image registration generally takes less than 2 minutes. Given the potential for motion or other sources of error, sometimes frequent validation and accuracy assessment on a continuous basis are necessary. In our example, a conventional open midline incision was made and image acquisition and registration were performed after completing the approach to eliminate motion-related inaccuracy.

Placement of the Reference Arc

Preoperative planning with proper placement of the reference arc is crucial. The reference arc must be placed in a position that can be seen by the camera, close enough to the operative field to maintain accuracy, but out of the line of sight to the operative tools. Maintaining navigation accuracy following cone-beam CT registration must be constantly monitored throughout the surgery.[10] We believe the most stable reference fixation in the thoracolumbar spine is found on the spinous process. The spikes on the clamp of the reference arc should penetrate the cortical bone of the spinous process to prevent the spikes from sliding on the bone. Interspinous placement of the reference arc should be avoided. Before registration, the reference arc may gently be tugged to confirm secure fixation. Extra care should

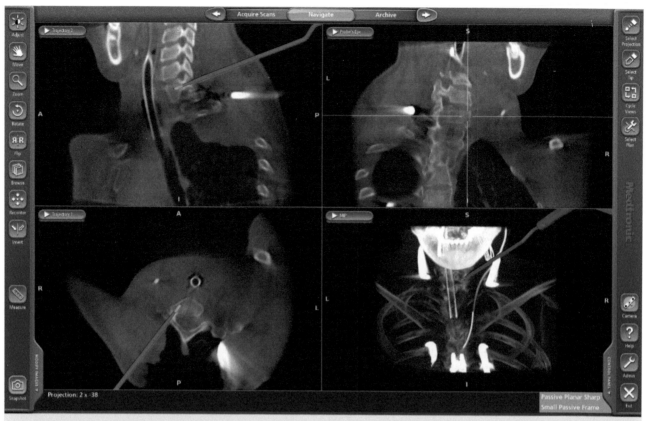

Fig. 16.3 Pedicle screw placement under navigation.

be taken to prevent fracture of the spinous process when screwing the clamp onto the spinous process.

In our case, the reference arc was placed on the spinous process of the eighth thoracic vertebra. Ideally, radiolucent retractors should be used to avoid imaging artifacts, but if no such instruments are available, standard retractors will need to be removed to obtain clear images without distortion.

Placement of the Pedicle Screws

In long-level structural fixation like this case, we prefer reference arc placement on the most inferiorly exposed spinous process, although some groups prefer the most superior one. In this case we placed instrumentation beginning distal to the arc (C6–Th1) and moving proximal (Th5–Th7), as instrumentation placement inevitably results in some movement of the spine and the image-guided system is less accommodating in maintaining navigation accuracy at the levels most distal to the reference arc (▶ Fig. 16.3). It is critical to confirm navigation accuracy prior to placement of each screw, which can be easily and quickly accomplished by touching the spine anatomy and confirming accuracy on the image-guided system. Avoiding Trendelenburg and rotational changes in bed position after cone-beam CT registration helps limit movement of the spine relative to the reference arc and also helps maintain navigation accuracy in long-level reconstruction procedures after resections of bone tumors of the spine.

After placement of all pedicle screws, a 3D scan (O-arm) was performed to confirm the position of all the screws. In this present case, using ball-tipped navigation probe to evaluate the size and the location of the intrathoracic lesion, we found that the intrathoracic part of the tumor could be fully exposed with the protraction of the right scapula. Therefore, after discussion with the family, a one-staged intrathoracic tumor resection was performed (▶ Fig. 16.4).

En Bloc Spondylectomy

Surgical field for the en bloc surgery must be wide enough to allow adequate dissection. After confirmation of placement of all the screws, navigation is particularly helpful in identifying the correct start point and orientation for planned osteotomies, in this case, of the Th2, Th3, and Th4 vertebral bodies. After registration of the ultrasonic osteotome (▶ Fig. 16.5), the device is used to perform the osteotomy beginning with an initial cut of the ribs at the affected Th2–Th4 levels, transecting them 3 to 4 cm lateral to the costotransverse joint. In this case, the thecal sac was then gently retracted to the right until the medial edge of the tumor within the vertebral bodies was identified. The osteotomies were initiated to the right of this location. The supraspinous ligaments of Th1–Th2 and Th4–Th5 were then resected and laminectomies were performed with the ultrasonic osteotome. The tumor was thereby exposed and destruction of bilateral pedicles was observed. Trajectory views were then utilized to determine the appropriate angle of the osteotome cuts. Once the osteotomies were in progress, the navigation probe was placed within the cut created by the osteotome to confirm that the resection was accurately proceeding beyond

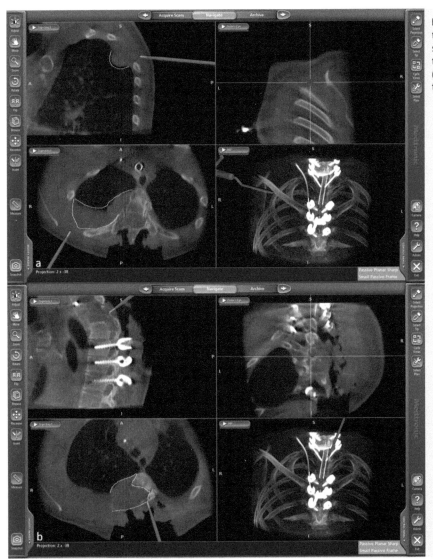

Fig. 16.4 Using ball-tipped probe to investigate the adjacent relationship between the tumor and scapula. **(a)** Confirmation of the margin of the tumor and involvement of the posterior element. **(b)** The yellow line shows the margin of the tumor.

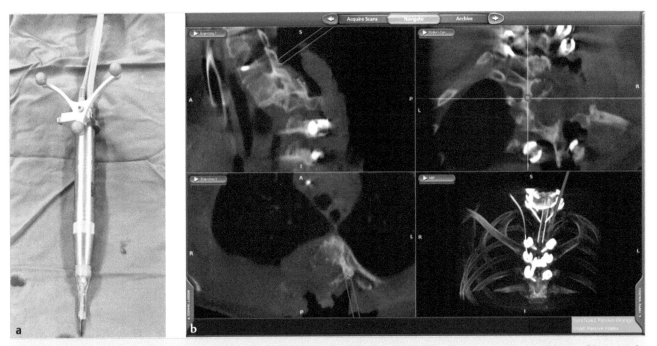

Fig. 16.5 **(a)** Customer registration of the ultrasonic osteotome intraoperatively. **(b)** With the aid of the navigation, accurate osteotomy of lamina and pedicle is performed to protect the neural and vascular structure as well as the tumor tissue.

the edge of the tumor. CT windows were utilized for this portion of the procedure, to visualize the neoplastic involvement of the bone. The restoration of the pulsatile movement of the spinal cord should be assessed after decompression is completed.

In our experience, at the lower thoracic spine, only one rib on each side needs to be cut; at the upper thoracic spine, two ribs on each side need to be cut. The pleura is carefully separated from the vertebra. The superior articular process of the uppermost vertebra is exposed.[13] The spinous and inferior articular processes of the neighboring vertebra are osteotomized and removed with dissection of the attached soft tissues, including the ligamentum flavum allowing the entire posterior element of the spine to be removed in one piece. The segmental vessels are then identified and ligated bilaterally with bipolar electrocautery. The residual stump of the ligated intercostal vessels can be used as a marker to trace to the aorta, which is then separated from the vertebrae.

The intercostal nerve roots are transected on both sides at 0.5 cm distal to the branching from the spinal cord at Th2–Th3 level. Blunt dissection through the plane between the pleura and the vertebral bodies is performed on both the sides. The important structures like aorta and esophagus are carefully separated posteriorly from the anterior aspect of the spinal column until fingertips meet each other directly at the anterior aspect of the affected vertebral bodies without any soft tissue intervening. Afterward, the ultrasonic osteotome and scalpel are used to remove both intervertebral disks in above (Th1/2) and below (Th4/5) levels. A pair of long curved protective retractors is inserted with their anterior tips overlapping at the anterior aspect of the affected body. The total en bloc resection of the vertebral tumor is achieved by pushing the Th2–Th4 vertebra to the anterior and rotate the whole bloc out from the left side, and a cage and two rods are used for the final reconstruction (► Fig. 16.6). The patient started to walk under the protection of cervicothoracic orthosis (CTO) brace on postoperative day 5, with low extremity muscle strength totally recovered to 5 and a VAS of 3 (► Fig. 16.7).

Final pathology for the immunohistochemical diagnosis in this case was desmoplastic fibroma of bone, ICD-O code 8823/0: a low-grade locally aggressive tumor. The margins

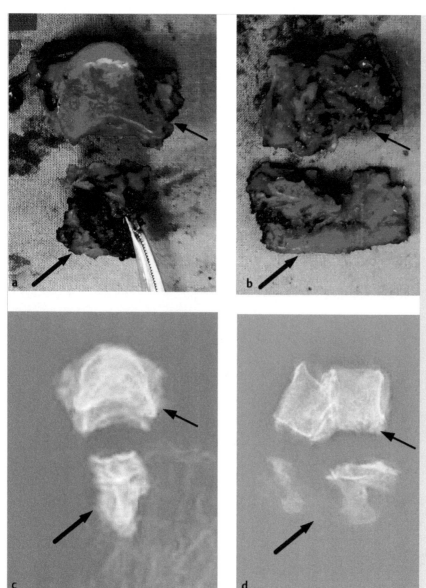

Fig. 16.6 (a,b) Specimen of Th2–Th4-vertebral desmoplastic fibroma of bone after total en bloc excision. **(c,d)** Fluoroscopy of the specimen. The thin black arrow indicates the anterior vertebral body, thick black arrow posterior element.

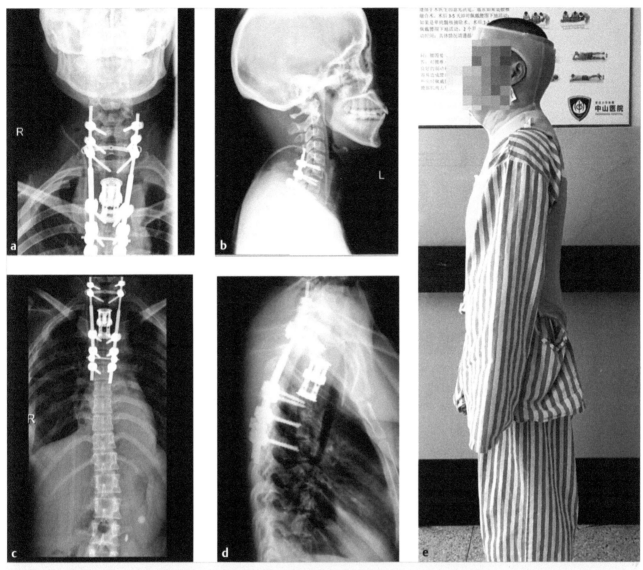

Fig. 16.7 (a–d) Postoperative biplanar radiographs spinal instrumentation. **(e)** The patient started to walk under the protection of cervicothoracic orthosis (CTO) brace on postoperative day 5, with low extremity muscle strength totally recovered and a VAS of 3.

were reported tumor-free (wide/marginal) at both specimens.

16.4 Advantages of Navigation in TES Surgery

16.4.1 Validation of Planned Resection or Resection Margin

Assessment of the resection margin for oncological surgery is critical and is traditionally confirmed with the use of frozen sections. A positive result may be used to guide further resection, whereas a negative result does not necessarily add additional information about the distance from the tumor's edge. By positioning the ball tip of the navigation probe at the achieved bone resection, surgeons can measure the distance between the virtual tip of the navigation probe and the planned resection on

the preoperative virtual images and the actual resection achieved intraoperatively.[17]

16.4.2 Superior Accuracy Rates for the Pedicle Screw

Pedicle screw placement with the use of navigation (e.g., O-arm/Stealth system) has been associated with low rates of malposition.[18] The time for screw placement has been improved and is likely less than previously reported with CT navigation, but longer than conventional techniques. It is important to be aware of the potential discrepancy between snapshot navigation images and actual screw placement on final O-arm images. Rivkin[19] reported 5.3% breach rate for the pedicle screws in patients who underwent thoracolumbar pedicle screw fixation utilizing the O-arm imaging system in conjunction with StealthStation navigation. Cervical pedicle screw placement is even more challenging as even minor screw malposition can therefore result in severe neurovascular injury. Moreover, sub-axial cervical pedicles are typically narrow in width and height, making placement even more difficult. The use of O-arm and navigation can potentially make screw placement safer, allowing measurement of several parameters including pedicle screw entry point, direction, angle, length, and diameter.

16.4.3 To Enhance the Accuracy of the Osteotomy

During the TES surgery, in order to fully expose the superior vertebral articular processes, the inferior articular processes and the lamina of the level above must be resected. However, the extent of osteotomy is somewhat variable. Too large an osteotomy may affect the stability of the superior vertebral body after spinal reconstruction, thus influencing the patient's recovery; while insufficient osteotomy may require multiple other smaller osteotomies, which will significantly extend the operation time. With aid of the navigation and the ultrasonic osteotome, the osteotomy of the superior vertebral lamina and the inferior articular processes become more accurate, and the operation time is shortened. Furthermore, the navigation helped surgeons easily find the target intervertebral space, avoiding accidentally cutting into the vertebral body.

16.4.4 Intraoperative Surgical Planning

Real-time intraoperative navigation in TES surgery helps the surgeon study the anatomy of the tumor during the surgery and makes it possible to tailor the surgical strategy intraoperatively more precisely for the specified patient. O-arm assisted navigation can overcome anatomical challenges and broaden the available stabilization options in the management of spine reconstruction.

Other advantages include protecting the surgical team from cumulative fluoroscopic radiation exposure and patients from repeat surgery due to implant malposition. There is now extensive evidence confirming decreased radiation exposure using 3D CT-based spinal navigation compared with fluoroscopy.[11]

16.5 Limitations

The potential for increased radiation exposure to the patient is a limitation of spinal navigation with intraoperative 3D image acquisition. The radiation dose generated by the O-arm for 3D image acquisition was approximately one-half of that produced by a 64-slice CT scanner imaging the same area.[20] In another study evaluating the effective radiation dose of the O-arm in thoracolumbar spinal surgery, it was found that dose was dependent on patient size.[21] A single scan was defined as image acquisition up to four spinal levels. It was noted that six scans on small patients would approximate a single abdominal CT scan dose, whereas three scans in larger patients could potentially exceed the dose from a single abdominal CT scan. The decision to use the O-arm for increased accuracy and decreased surgeon and staff radiation exposure should be weighed against the potential for increased patient radiation exposure.

16.6 Future Development of the Navigation in En Bloc Resections for Bone Tumors of the Spine

Navigation has advanced rapidly in the field of orthopedic oncology, and its workflow is maturing. In the near future, the technology will allow more accurate performance of complex resections and reconstructions. With real-time instant visual feedback, intraoperative navigation enables surgeons to locate anatomic and pathologic structures precisely, but there are still barriers to overcome; the technology involves cumbersome navigation facilities, long setup time, and lacks reliable navigational cutting tools. More studies are needed to better define its feasibility and clinical results in orthopedic oncology before the field sees more widespread adoption.

On the horizon, integration of augmented reality (AR) technology may provide valuable assistance to the performance of computer-aided navigated surgery.[22] Some examples of AR-based surgical applications have been presented in the literature, for example, a hybrid tracking method for spine surgery augmented reality,[23] an integral videography system,[24] and an alternative biopsy guidance. A thorough description of AR technologies is beyond the scope of this chapter and is detailed elsewhere in this text. A method for calibrating an optical see-through head mounted display (HMD) has been introduced and validated on an optical see-through system, and a surgical navigation system based on this AR has been developed.[25] Unlike virtual reality (VR), AR captures real world images with two miniature video cameras mounted on the head gear. The real world can be seen through semitransparent mirrors placed in front of the user's eyes with the optical see-through HMD superimposed on advanced imaging pictures so that one can simultaneously see the real and virtual worlds with only slight distortion of the field of view.

AR can allow simultaneous visualization of potential preoperative plans and critical 3D anatomical structures with the optical see-through HMD, along with whatever the surgeon is currently viewing in the real world before him. Techniques for registering patient position and synthesizing the data for the HMD through a series of spatial transformations can ensure that the position and orientation of the virtual model will match the real anatomical structures throughout the intraoperative navigation procedure. The hope for AR technology is to improve the safety, accuracy, and reliability of surgery. Unfortunately, no advantages have so far been realized. Recently, a comparison of the accuracy of a navigation system using either a head-mounted display or a monitor as a device for visualization demonstrated no benefits to the use of a HMD over traditional display mounts.[26]

16.7 Conclusion

En bloc resection of spine tumors is technically demanding and requires a high level of ability and knowledge of spinal anatomy and physiology. Although the operation carries a high complication profile, recurrence rates in expert hands can be quite low. With the advent of navigation and robotics, TES has been made safer and more efficient. Newer technologies such as AR have been recently introduced but, as of yet, have not demonstrated improved outcomes.

References

[1] Enneking WF, Spanier SS, Goodman MA. A system for the surgical staging of musculoskeletal sarcoma. Clin Orthop Relat Res. 1980(153):106–120

[2] Boriani S, Weinstein JN, Biagini R. Primary bone tumors of the spine: terminology and surgical staging. Spine. 1997; 22(9):1036–1044

[3] Stener B. Total spondylectomy in chondrosarcoma arising from the seventh thoracic vertebra. J Bone Joint Surg Br. 1971; 53(2):288–295

[4] Roy-Camille R, Mazel CH, Saillant G, Lapresle PH. Treatment of malignant tumors of the spine with posterior instrumentation. Tumors Spine Diagnosis Clin Manag 1990:473–487

[5] Tomita K, Kawahara N, Baba H, Tsuchiya H, Nagata S, Toribatake Y. Total en bloc spondylectomy for solitary spinal metastases. Int Orthop. 1994; 18(5): 291–298

[6] Boriani S, Bandiera S, Colangeli S, Ghermandi R, Gasbarrini A. En bloc resection of primary tumors of the thoracic spine: indications, planning, morbidity. Neurol Res. 2014; 36(6):566–576

[7] Fisher CG, Saravanja DD, Dvorak MF, et al. Surgical management of primary bone tumors of the spine: validation of an approach to enhance cure and reduce local recurrence. Spine. 2011; 36(10):830–836

[8] Demura S, Kawahara N, Murakami H, et al. Giant cell tumor expanded into the thoracic cavity with spinal involvement. Orthopedics. 2012; 35(3):e453–e456

[9] Bolger C, Wigfield C. Image-guided surgery: applications to the cervical and thoracic spine and a review of the first 120 procedures. J Neurosurg. 2000; 92 (2) Suppl:175–180

[10] Attia W, Orief T, Almusrea K, Alfawareh M, Soualmi L, Orz Y. Role of the O-arm and computer-assisted navigation of safe screw fixation in children with traumatic rotatory atlantoaxial subluxation. Asian Spine J. 2012; 6(4):266–273

[11] Gelalis ID, Paschos NK, Pakos EE, et al. Accuracy of pedicle screw placement: a systematic review of prospective in vivo studies comparing free hand, fluoroscopy guidance and navigation techniques. Eur Spine J. 2012; 21(2):247–255

[12] Ammirati M, Salma A. Placement of thoracolumbar pedicle screws using O-arm-based navigation: technical note on controlling the operational accuracy of the navigation system. Neurosurg Rev. 2013; 36(1):157–162, discussion 162

[13] Guo C, Yan Z, Zhang J, et al. Modified total en bloc spondylectomy in thoracic vertebra tumour. Eur Spine J. 2011; 20(4):655–660

[14] Kawahara N, Tomita K, Murakami H, Demura S. Total en bloc spondylectomy for spinal tumors: surgical techniques and related basic background. Orthop Clin North Am. 2009; 40(1):47–63, vi

[15] Amendola L, Cappuccio M, De Iure F, Bandiera S, Gasbarrini A, Boriani S. En bloc resections for primary spinal tumors in 20 years of experience: effectiveness and safety. Spine J. 2014; 14(11):2608–2617

[16] Rahmathulla G, Nottmeier EW, Pirris SM, Deen HG, Pichelmann MA. Intraoperative image-guided spinal navigation: technical pitfalls and their avoidance. Neurosurg Focus. 2014; 36(3):E3

[17] Wong K-C, Kumta S-M. Use of computer navigation in orthopedic oncology. Curr Surg Rep. 2014; 2(4):47

[18] Patil S, Lindley EM, Burger EL, Yoshihara H, Patel VV. Pedicle screw placement with O-arm and stealth navigation. Orthopedics. 2012; 35(1):e61–e65

[19] Rivkin MA, Yocom SS. Thoracolumbar instrumentation with CT-guided navigation (O-arm) in 270 consecutive patients: accuracy rates and lessons learned. Neurosurg Focus. 2014; 36(3):E7

[20] Zhang J, Weir V, Fajardo L, Lin J, Hsiung H, Ritenour ER. Dosimetric characterization of a cone-beam O-arm imaging system. J XRay Sci Technol. 2009; 17 (4):305–317

[21] Lange J, Karellas A, Street J, et al. Estimating the effective radiation dose imparted to patients by intraoperative cone-beam computed tomography in thoracolumbar spinal surgery. Spine. 2013; 38(5):E306–E312

[22] Chen X, Xu L, Wang Y, et al. Development of a surgical navigation system based on augmented reality using an optical see-through head-mounted display. J Biomed Inform. 2015; 55 Suppl C:124–131

[23] Elmi-Terander A, Nachabe R, Skulason H, et al. Feasibility and accuracy of thoracolumbar minimally invasive pedicle screw placement with augmented reality navigation technology. Spine (Phila Pa 1976). 2018; 43(14):1018–1023

[24] Suenaga H, Hoang Tran H, Liao H, et al. Real-time in situ three-dimensional integral videography and surgical navigation using augmented reality: a pilot study. Int J Oral Sci. 2013; 5(2):98–102

[25] Suzuki N, Hattori A, Iimura J, et al. Development of AR surgical navigation systems for multiple surgical regions. Stud Health Technol Inform. 2014; 196: 404–408

[26] Vigh B, Müller S, Ristow O, et al. The use of a head-mounted display in oral implantology: a feasibility study. Int J CARS. 2014; 9(1):71–78

17 Surgical Management of Thoracolumbar Spinal Metastases Using Navigation

Zach Pennington, A. Karim Ahmed, Camilo A. Molina, and Daniel M. Sciubba

Abstract

Given the significant frailty observed in many patients with spinal metastases, there has been increased emphasis on reducing surgical morbidity. One potential means of achieving this goal is by using minimally invasive surgery (MIS) techniques, such as mini-open approaches with percutaneous instrumentation, as they promise lower intraoperative blood loss and faster postoperative recovery. With advancements in intraoperative navigation, e.g., CT-guided navigation, more and more surgeons are able to add these techniques to their operative armamentarium. Here we describe the use of intraoperative navigation for the surgical treatment of spinal metastases and provide a comparison of open and MIS techniques for the treatment of this clinical pathology.

Keywords: spinal metastases, minimally invasive surgery, intraoperative navigation, CT-guided navigation, percutaneous instrumentation, SINS score, operative morbidity

17.1 Introduction

Each year some 1.7 million Americans will be diagnosed with cancer[1] and 40 to 70% of these patients[2,3,4,5,6,7] will experience one or more spinal metastases. The majority of these lesions remain clinically silent; however, a small minority of patients—18,000 to 25,000 per year[8,9,10,11,12,13,14]—will present with some indication for surgery, whether it be neurological dysfunction[5,15,16,17,18,19,20,21,22,23,24,25,26] or gross spinal instability.[8,15,27] For these patients, surgical management has been demonstrated to provide superior treatment outcomes as compared to radiation or chemotherapy alone.[8] However, many patients within this population are particularly frail, and may not have the physical reserve to stand up to conventional surgery. As a result, there has been greater emphasis on applying minimally invasive techniques to this patient population. However, minimally invasive techniques are technically very difficult and have the disadvantage of poor/suboptimal visualization. To compensate for this limited visualization, there has been increased use of fluoroscopy and CT-guided navigation technologies. The latter allow correlation of patient intraoperative anatomy with preoperative anatomy in three dimensions, which may be especially beneficial in patients with metastatic disease, where tumor proliferation leads to disruption of normal anatomic landmarks. The objectives of this chapter are to provide an overview of the management of metastatic spine disease, to describe current intraoperative navigation techniques with a focus on intraoperative CT-guided navigation, and to describe how these navigation techniques can be applied to surgery for spinal metastases.

17.2 Overview of Management of Metastatic Spine Disease

Unlike primary spinal neoplasms, which are commonly characterized by local disease only, all spinal metastases are stage IV systemic disease, by definition. As a result, the goal of surgery in patients with metastatic spine disease is very different than that in patients with primary neoplasms: mainly, symptom palliation and improvement in patient quality of life, rather than oncologic cure. In some rare cases, where the patient is confirmed to have disease isolated to the spinal metastasis, it may be acceptable to perform en bloc tumor resection, as some literature has suggested that it provides clinically significant survival benefit for these patients.[16,28] Such patients represent the vast minority of patients though—2 to 3% per some estimates—and as such will not be considered here.[29]

For the majority of patients with metastatic spine disease—those in whom disease is systemic and surgery is palliative—there are four considerations that need to be made in surgical planning, emphasized in the neurologic-oncologic-mechanical-systemic (NOMS) assessment paradigm.[30] The first of these components is expected patient survival (systemic assessment). As surgery in this patient population is designed to improve patient quality of life, surgery is restricted to only those patients who are expected to survive long enough to rehabilitate from surgery and therefore realize the functional and symptomatic benefits conferred by surgery. Current consensus is that in order for a patient to be considered surgical, they must have a residual life expectancy of at least 3 months, though more conservative groups recommend that life expectancy exceed 6 months.[8,17,19,21,22,31,32,33,34,35,36,37] As can be seen, the consideration of a patient for surgery is then highly dependent upon the ability of the surgeon and rest of the oncologic care team to accurately predict patient survival. Previous literature has indicated that patient prognosis is negatively associated with male sex,[34,38,39,40] increasing age,[5,10,22,34] lung[5,34,41,42] or GI primary pathology,[40] polyvertebral disease,[5,18,41,42,43,44] visceral metastases,[5,22,38,41,42,45,46] decreasing time between diagnosis of primary and metastasis,[47,48] and preoperative neurological deficit[8,34,35,38,44,47] or nonambulatory status.[18,43,44,48,49] In accordance with these, several predictive scales have been generated to aid in patient selection, the most popular of which are the Tomita[16] and revised Tokuhashi scales.[50] However, none of these scales has been demonstrated to predict patient survival across primary pathologies with great accuracy,[19,31,46,50,51,52] and so they are recommended as decision aids, as opposed to definitive treatment guides.[15,21,37,53,54,55,56,57] Additionally, some evidence also suggests that preoperative cachexia, assessed by body morphometry and fat distribution, may negatively predict postoperative survival (authors' unpublished results).

The decision to operate on a patient with metastatic spine disease requires thoughtful consideration of the indications for surgery, potential benefits/risks of surgery, prognosis and likelihood of appreciable benefit from surgery, and patient expectations.[19,20,21] Surgical indications may include the treatment of pain, spinal instability, and neurologic dysfunction.[30] Metastatic epidural spinal cord compression with neurologic deficit, estimated to occur in 2.5 to 14% of patients with spinal metastases,[5,6,8,18,19,20,32,44,58,59,60,61,62,63] is perhaps the strongest indication for surgical decompression. These patients present with any of a variety of neurological symptoms, of which the most common are isolated or radicular pain (83–95%),[18,27,32,60,63,64,65] sensory disturbances (50–70%),[18,48,66,67] and weakness (35–75%),[9,18,27,31,32,48] though patients may also present with an inability to walk (11–68%),[8,18,20,43,44,60,68,69] autonomic dysfunction, and/or incontinence (50–60%).[18]

From the late 1970s to early 2000s, the standard of care for these patients was radiotherapy, as class III evidence up to that point had identified it as being clinically equivalent to surgical decompression, but with lower associated morbidity.[8,18,32,70,71,72] However, in 2005, Patchell and colleagues[8] presented level I evidence demonstrating superior neurological outcomes and superior survival in patients treated with surgical decompression and adjuvant radiotherapy compared to radiotherapy alone. As such, standard of care for patients with metastatic spine disease is now surgical decompression with stabilization where necessary, and adjuvant radiotherapy to address the tumor margins in radiosensitive pathologies. The extent of the margin that is left depends highly upon the radiosensitivity of the tumor (oncologic assessment).[30] Radiosensitive tumors with high-grade epidural spinal cord compression, such as lymphoma, seminoma, and myeloma, can be treated with minimal decompression followed by stereotactic radiation (SRT) to the site of compression. The initial decompression prevents progression of neurological deficits and the radiation leads to rapid regression of the tumor. This more limited resection is known as separation surgery and is popular among frailer patients and those with relatively limited survival, as it has a lower associated morbidity.[73,74,75,76,77] In contrast with the aforementioned pathologies, thyroid, colorectal, renal, NSCLC, sarcoma, hepatocellular, and melanoma metastases are considered radioresistant and require more extensive surgical decompression, as they are unlikely to regress significantly with SRT.[30]

Like neural element compression, mechanical instability in patients with metastatic spine disease can be treated with one of two interventions: surgical stabilization or vertebroplasty.[78] Vertebroplasty may be advantageous for patients with borderline instability, limited life expectancy, or multiostotic disease not amenable to surgical intervention. However, in patients with gross instability who are considered healthy enough for surgery, surgical stabilization is the treatment of choice. Additionally, surgery is the only option for patients with involved levels lacking intact posterior cortices, as the intact cortical bone is necessary to prevent extravasation of the cement into the vertebral column. To help aid with this decision process, the Spinal Oncology Study Group developed the Spinal Instability Neoplastic Score (SINS), which categorizes the stability of the pathologic vertebra based upon spinal level (junctional, semirigid, rigid, or mobile spine level), pain (mechanical, nonmechanical, or no pain), lytic/blastic tumor quality, extent of

vertebral body collapse, and extent of posterior element involvement.[79,80] Stabilization is recommended in lesions presenting with significant vertebral body collapse, mechanical pain, and tricolumnar involvement, whereas medical management with possible vertebroplasty is recommended for patients with more limited or asymptomatic disease.

17.2.1 Minimally Invasive Surgery for Spinal Metastases

As stated, two of the most important considerations for surgical intervention in patients with metastatic spine disease are the expectations that the patient (1) will survival long enough to appreciate symptomatic relief afforded by surgery, and (2) the patient is medically healthy enough to undergo surgery. Patients with systemic disease are a complex population with increased risk for postoperative complications (i.e., pulmonary and liver dysfunction).[81,82] Two widely accepted means for risk stratifying this population include the Charlson Comorbidity Index (CCI)[83,84] and Anesthesiologist Society of America Score,[85,86] both of which assign a cumulative comorbidity to patients based upon their preexisting medical conditions. Higher scores on both of these indices have been previously associated with postoperative complications in patients with spinal metastases.[83,84,85,86] However, not all inputs utilized in scoring for these systems have been demonstrated to impact postoperative outcome, and neither system is designed specifically for patients with metastatic spine disease or spinal oncology patients, in general. A score specifically designed for this population was recently published by de la Garza-Ramos and colleagues,[87,88] who developed a frailty score specifically designed to address surgical risk among patients operated for spinal metastases. They found that patients with greater degrees of frailty had higher complication rate and a 30-day mortality of 25%. This significant risk profile may tilt the risk-benefit profile of surgical intervention in such a manner as to preclude frailer patients from being offered surgical intervention. However, many of these patients would undoubtedly derive clinical benefit from surgical management. For these patients, the best surgical option may be use of minimally invasive techniques.

There are two widely accepted techniques for minimally invasive spine surgery (MISS) in the treatment of spinal metastases: video-assisted thoracic surgery (VATS); and mini-open/minimal access posterior decompression. The latter[89] makes use of a familiar, posterior midline approach utilizing a 2-cm incision as opposed to a more conventional 5-cm incision. VATS is similarly related to a familiar approach—thoracotomy—albeit differing by the use of indirect versus direct visualization. As these techniques are still relatively new, the majority of reports have been published within the past decade. Evidence comparing minimally invasive and open approaches is expectedly limited, with only a handful of reports directly comparing open and MISS procedures.[20,90,91,92,93,94,95,96,97] However, a recent review of this evidence by our group[98] found the minimally invasive techniques to offer similar outcomes in terms of neurological recovery and pain improvement, while having shorter operative times, lower complication rates, shorter operating times, and shorter lengths of stay (▶ Table 17.1, ▶ Table 17.2). Despite this

Table 17.1 Summary of studies directly comparing minimally invasive and open approaches for operative management of metastatic spine disease

Study	Technique	n	Operative			Clinical		
			BL	OT	LOS	NI	PR	CR
Chou and Lu (2011)[90]	Open	5	3,120	408	–	100%	–	20%
	MIS	5	1,320	468	–	100%	–	20%
Fang et al (2012)[91]	Open	17	1,721	403	–	76.5%	7.2	11.8%
	MIS	24	1,058	175	–	91.7%	6.6	29.2%
Hansen-Algenstaedt et al (2017)[92]	Open	30	2,062	220	21.1	33.3%	5.6	40.0%
	MIS	30	1,156	191	11.0	20%	5.2	23.3%
Hikata et al (2017)[93]	Open	25	714	189	–	56%	4.6	44%
	MIS	25	340	205	–	56%	4.3	12%
Huang et al (2006)[94]	Open	17	1,162	180	–	70.8%	–	23.5%
	MIS	29	1,100	179	–	69.2%	–	20.7%
Kumar et al (2017)[95]	Open	18	961	269	13	50.0%	3.5	16%
	MIS	27	184	253	9	56%	5.2	3%
Lau and Chou (2015)[96]	Open	28	1,697	414	11.4	42.9%	–	21.4%
	MIS	21	917	452	7.4	42.9%	–	9.5%
Miscusi et al (2015)[20]	Open	19	900	192	9.3	63%	–	0%
	MIS	23	240	132	7.2	65%	–	4.3%
Stoker et al (2013)[97]	Open	4	1,250	518	24	–	–	100%
	MIS	4	813	367	5.8	–	–	100%

Abbreviations: BL, mean blood loss in mL; CR, complication rate; LOS, mean hospital length of stay in days; MIS, minimally invasive approach; NI, percentage of patients improving by 1 or more ASIA/Frankel grades following surgical intervention; OT, mean operative time in minutes; PR, mean pain relief in points on numeric pain rating scale.
Source: **Pennington** et al (2018).[98]

Table 17.2 Meta-analysis of studies directly comparing MIS and open approaches to management of metastatic spine disease

Endpoint	MIS		Open		Result	p
	n	N	n	N	$\delta\bar{x}$	
BL (mL)	115	6	100	6	−608.3	<0.00001
OT (min)	115	6	100	6	−69.6	<0.00001
LOS (d)	61	3	52	3	−0.55	<0.0001
PR (NRS pt)	106	4	90	4	0.12	0.66
Endpoint	*n*	*N*	*n*	*N*	OR	*p*
NI	130	9	122	9	0.98	0.94
CR	188	9	164	9	0.58	0.05

Abbreviations: BL, mean blood loss in mL; CR, complication rate; $\delta\bar{x}$, difference in means between open and MIS groups ($\delta\bar{x}$ = MIS − open); LOS, mean hospital length of stay in days; MIS, minimally invasive approach; n, number of patients in group; N, number of studies in group; NI, percentage of patients improving by 1 or more ASIA/Frankel grades following surgical intervention; OR, odds ratio (>1 = more common in MIS group); OT, mean operative time in minutes; PR, mean pain relief in points on numeric pain rating scale.

apparently favorable complication profile, minimally invasive techniques are not without their drawbacks. First, minimally invasive techniques, especially VATS have steep learning curves, and second, the smaller incision and operating corridor employed by these techniques reduces visualization of the spine pathology. Intraoperative fluoroscopy can aid in indirect visualization by assisting with assessment of intraoperative instrument location. Moreover, it can be used to assist in vertebral instrumentation. But, given that many of the patients operated for spinal metastases have epidural cord compression as their primary indication, the key endpoint to surgery is adequate decompression of the neural elements. Such decompression generally requires expansive visualization, which can be challenging with minimally invasive approaches. Additionally, the soft tissue mass compressing the neural elements is not visible using standard fluoroscopy and so determination of adequate decompression in non-navigated MIS procedures is based upon surgeon experience. To overcome this issue and allow for superior outcomes, CT-guided navigation can be employed, effectively expanding the visible window in MIS procedures. CT-guided navigation may also aid in the surgical treatment of complex spinal pathologies, or in patients with anomalous anatomic structures.

17.3 Navigation Modalities and Spine Surgery

Intraoperative navigation includes all techniques that allow for correlation of instrument position with patient anatomy. The most familiar of these technologies is two-dimensional fluoroscopy, which makes use of low-dose serial radiographs to allow for instantaneous analysis of the spatial relationship between the physician's instrument and the patient's bony anatomy. It has been successfully used for more than five decades, with its first application to the spine having been described by Rabinov and colleagues, who used fluoroscopy to guide biopsy of vertebral body lesions.[99] Since then, fluoroscopy has become increasingly popular, with numerous groups describing its use in percutaneous pedicle screw placement,[100,101] vertebroplasty,[102, 103,104,105] and lumbar interbody fusion.[106] Several studies have also been performed, comparing the accuracy of screw placement with freehand and fluoroscopy-guided techniques. Though some report superior accuracy within the fluoroscopy-assisted group,[107,108] others report no clinically significant difference in the accuracy of screws placed freehand and those placed under fluoroscopy, at least among patients with uncomplicated anatomy.[109,110] There is the potential for fluoroscopy to improve accuracy in patients with abnormal anatomy, such as those with metastatic spine disease, and it has also been a standard part of percutaneous pedicle screw instrumentation, as the superficial soft tissues hide landmarks necessary for proper pedicle cannulation and instrumentation.

One of the greatest disadvantages associated with fluoroscopy is the increased radiation exposure to the patient and operating room personnel.[111,112] Although there are no longitudinal studies documenting the relative risk for various oncologic malignancies, among spinal surgeons who employ fluoroscopy, a previous report by Perisinakis and colleagues estimated that the risks of fatal cancer and genetic defects were 115 and 4 per million, respectively, among patients undergoing two-level lumbar fusions.[113] Additionally, extensive literature exists documenting radiation as a risk factor for a multitude of malignancies, suggesting that surgeons who utilize fluoroscopy also have an increased risk of cancer. These risks can be minimized through the use of personal protective equipment, such as lead-lined vests and thyroid shields,[114,115] and the use of intermittent versus continuous fluoroscopy, which reduces overall doses, as well as doses to radiation sensitive areas, notably the gonads, eye, and hand. Additionally, at least one study[116] suggests that the use of biplanar fluoroscopy may reduce radiation exposure to the operating staff. This alternative 3D fluoroscopy technique has also been reported to improve pedicle screw placement accuracy relative to conventional 2D fluoroscopy,[100] suggesting that it may be a superior option for intraoperative navigation.

17.3.1 CT Image-Guided Intraoperative Navigation

Perhaps the most promising intraoperative technology, and the one that will serve as the focus of the rest of this section, is CT image-guided intraoperative navigation, which is supported by systems from a number of manufacturers, including Medtronic

(SteathStation), Brainlab (VectorVision), Ziehm (Vision FD Vario 3D), and Stryker (SpineMap 3D). These systems are particularly exciting because they allow for real-time intraoperative navigation that utilizes preoperative CT imaging, thereby eliminating the need for fluoroscopy and its excess radiation. Additionally, as CT-based imaging with the capability for MR expansion, they allow for visualization of hard and soft tissues, the latter of which are most commonly the cause of metastatic epidural spinal cord compression (MESCC).

All intraoperative CT image-guided platforms work in the same fashion. Preoperatively the patient is imaged using high-resolution computer tomography to generate a 3D image volume to which the patient's anatomy can be registered. Some systems now allow for the use of MR as the pre-procedural imaging modality, which may offer superior results in patients requiring visualization of soft tissues (e.g., those undergoing intradural neoplasm resection, diskectomy, or tumor debulking). But CT remains the gold standard for fusion operations due to its superior visualization of bone. After acquiring the image volume, the patient is brought to operating room, where anesthesia is induced and the patient is transferred to the table, positioned, and draped in sterile fashion. At this point, a reference frame is affixed to the patient, which allows the navigation system to correlate patient anatomy with specific location in the image volume. Registration of the system is then performed, whereby three or more defined points on the patient as well as the markers on the reference frame are tapped with the system wand to correlate the patient's position with the imaging.[117] Either surface or paired-point registration techniques can be used, though no significant difference in accuracy of alignment has been noted. Paired-point registration technique is far quicker.[118] In this system, any anatomic positions can be theoretically used for this process, but the spinous processes of the levels to be instrumented are the most common choice. The reference frame, wand, and all other tools are also registered at this time. Many systems have tools that are automatically detectable by the system, as they are of known size, and are decorated by three or four reflective markers or light-emitting diodes that constitute a single plane. These same markers enable the mapping software to determine the relative orientations of the reference frame and tool to one another and to the patient[119] (▶ Fig. 17.1).

Detection of the markers decorating the detectable tools and reference frame is performed by a stereotactic infrared camera. In the case of the reflective markers, infrared light is emitted from the navigation sensor, which reflects off the markers and is detected by the navigation sensor, whereas LED-based systems use detection of light emitted directly by the markers. After registering the system, the orientation and length of the registered tool should be available on the monitor as a line superimposed on the preoperative imaging volume. At this point, it is recommended that the surgeon perform verification by tapping anatomic landmarks of interest with the tool to confirm that the image–patient alignment is accurate.[117]

In both systems, it is imperative that the reflectors be positioned so that they are in direct line-of-sight of the detector. Disruption of line-of-sight disturbs the correlation of tool and reference frame position with the preoperative scan, though this can be quickly reversed by restoring the line-of-sight. Also, essential to the operation of the system is the avoidance of any contact with the reference device, as this will change the

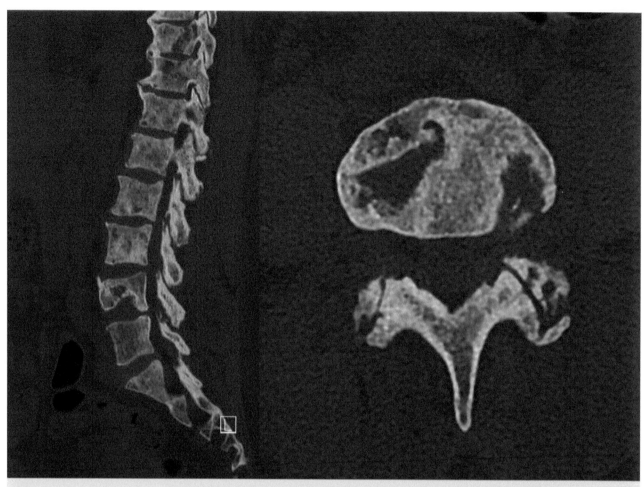

Fig. 17.1 Preoperative imaging of a patient with metastatic spine disease, resulting in a compression fracture of the L4 vertebral body.

relative positioning of patient anatomy and reference frame, resulting in loss of alignment between the image and the patient's anatomy. Again, if recognized, this issue can be resolved by re-registering the reference frame and instrument, but such a solution requires that the operating staff document the disturbance of the reference frame. The SpineMask tracker available from Stryker attempts to bypass this issue by making use of a series of 31 LEDs that are directly affixed to the patient's skin, which allows the reference frame to move with the patient. However, this system is limited by the size of incision that can be made, as the incision must be circumscribed by the reference frame. Additionally, significant skin tension or wide separation of the wound, as occurs with retraction during larger vertical incisions, can distort the relationships between the skin-based reference frame and deeper anatomical structures. This limits the accuracy of the navigation and relegates this technology to minimally invasive and small open approaches.

Despite these hardware differences between systems, there appears to be little to no difference between them regarding operative results. A recent systematic review by Nooh et al[120] compared the accuracy of pedicle screw placement using the Medtronic StealthStation system and Brainlab VectorVision system across 26 included studies reporting the placement of 9,289 total screws in 1,641 patients. The authors found that both systems were highly accurate in terms of screw placement, consistent with previous literature,[108,121,122,123,124] but did not find a clinically meaningful difference between the systems, though the StealthStation placement accuracy was roughly 1% higher. The reason for this similarity likely relates to the fact that all commercially available systems use fundamentally the same technology, and the majority also come equipped with surgical planning software, allowing relative homogeneity in physician experience across devices.

In addition to having similar functionality, most systems have the capacity to include a multitude of different instruments, including various probes, awls, taps, and screwdrivers. Some systems even incorporate adaptors that can be used to align instruments not equipped with their own navigation markers, such as a reciprocating bone scalpel. In the context of spinal metastases, this enables navigation-assisted spinal cord decompression with a wide array of devices. Additionally, the baseline navigation abilities may facilitate separation surgery by helping to define the region of critical compression intraoperatively. Related to this, though, is the concern that CT-guided navigation systems do not incorporate changes in the patient's anatomy that occur throughout the course of an operation, whether because of surgical changes, surgical team contact with the table, patient respiration, or any other cause of a change in patient position relative to the reference frame. As stated, this pitfall is most significant for patients undergoing deformity operation and tumor resection, in whom the goal of surgery constitutes an anatomic change. Systems are currently available, though, that overcome this deficit, such as the O-Arm device, which allow for acquisition of imaging for intraoperative realignment and reevaluation. Use of such intraoperative imaging may prolong the case but allows for a high level of navigation system accuracy to be maintained throughout the procedure.

Advantages and Disadvantages of CT-Guided Navigation Systems

Several benefits have been associated with the use of CT-guided navigation, including higher instrumentation accuracy, reduced blood loss, and reduced patient radiation exposure. Perhaps the best documented of these is the improvement in pedicle screw accuracy.[125,126,127,128,129,130] Over the course of the past decade, five large systematic reviews have been published comparing the accuracy of navigation-assisted pedicle screw placement with freehand instrumentation (▶ Table 17.3).[108,121,122,124,131]

The first of these published studies was reported by Kosmopoulos and colleagues,[108] who reported the results of 53 studies comparing freehand technique (12,299 total screws) to all navigation-assisted techniques (3,059 total screws). The study

found that in patients undergoing instrumentation of thoracic or lumbar levels, navigation conferred a significant improvement in screw accuracy (91.4 vs. 79.2%), with the accuracy improvement being most pronounced for patients undergoing instrumentation of thoracic vertebrae (85.1 vs. 63.1%).

Similar results were reported in 2010 by Verma et al,[124] who performed a meta-analysis of 23 studies describing the accuracy of 5,992 screws placed in 1,288 total patients. Unlike Kosmopoulos, Verma and colleagues directly compared instrumentation with CT-guided navigation systems to freehand techniques. But like the earlier study, navigation-assisted instrumentation was significantly more accurate (93.3 vs. 84.7%; $p < 0.00001$). Additionally, it was associated with a similar neurological complication rate, suggesting that navigation-assisted systems provide an improvement in biomechanical outcomes without increasing risk of adverse events.

Gelalis[121] and Shin[131] both reported systematic reviews of the literature in 2012. That reported by Gelalis was largely descriptive in nature and summarized the findings of 26 studies comparing freehand, fluoroscopy-assisted, and CT-navigation-assisted pedicle screw techniques. Consistent with the earlier reviews, they found that CT-guided navigation provided superior accuracy relative to freehand techniques. Unlike the prior studies though, they also compared the accuracy of instrumentation with CT-guided navigation to that of fluoroscopy and found that the former provided superior accuracy relative to fluoroscopy. They also observed that misplaced screws in

Table 17.3 Systematic reviews and meta-analyses comparing pedicle screw placement accuracy using freehand and navigated techniques

Study	Design	Findings
Gelalis et al (2012)[121]	• Systematic review of 26 studies (1,105 total patients; 6,617 total screws) comparing accuracy freehand (2,412 screws; 362 patients), fluoroscopy-guided (1,902 screws; 323 patients), and CT-navigation-guided (668 screws; 313 patients) pedicle screw instrumentation using Gertzbein–Robbins system	• CT-guided navigation increases instrumentation accuracy relative to freehand technique and fluoroscopy • CT-guided screws err laterally, whereas freehand screws err medially when pedicle wall is breached
Kosmopoulos and Schizas (2007)[108]	• Systematic review of 32 in vivo patient studies evaluating pedicle screw accuracy in freehand instrumentation (12,299 screws) and 21 in vivo studies examining navigation-assisted pedicle screw placement (3,059 screws)	• In thoracolumbar groups only, navigation had higher geometric mean accuracy than freehand instrumentation (91.4% vs. 79.2%) • Navigation produced large improvement in accuracy of thoracic pedicle screw placement (85.1% vs. 63.1%)
Shin et al (2012)[131]	• Meta-analysis of 20 studies (8,539 total screws) comparing accuracy of navigation-assisted and freehand pedicle screw instrumentation • Accuracy compared at all three spinal levels: cervical, thoracic, and lumbar	• Overall risk of pedicle violation lower in navigated patients (OR = 0.39; $p < 0.001$). Difference largest in thoracic spine (OR = 0.32; $p < 0.0001$) and smallest in cervical spine (OR = 0.38; $p < 0.0001$) • One pedicle perforation can be spared for every 11.1 screws placed with navigation assistance vs. freehand • No significant difference between groups in terms of neurological complication, operative time, or blood loss
Tang et al (2014)[122]	• Meta-analysis of 12 articles (732 total patients; 4,953 total screws) comparing accuracy of pedicle screw placement via navigation-assisted and freehand techniques	• Navigated technique reported to have a higher rate of perfect screw placement (OR = 3.36; $p < 0.00001$) and clinically acceptable placement (OR = 4.72; $p < 0.0001$) • Navigated technique had significantly lower risk of potentially hazardous screw placement (OR = 0.27; $p = 0.01$), absolutely hazardous placement (OR= 0.09; $p < 0.00001$), and screw-related complication (OR = 0.25; $p = 0.008$)
Verma et al (2010)[124]	• Meta-analysis of 23 papers (1,288 total patients; 5,992 total screws) evaluating accuracy of navigation-assisted pedicle screw placement • 14 studies compared navigated and freehand screw accuracies	• Overall screw accuracy is superior in navigation group (93.3% vs. 84.7%; $p < 0.00001$) • Neurological complication rate overall not significantly different between groups

CT-guided procedures were more likely to err laterally compared to freehand techniques. Though they did not evaluate the risk of neurological injury among groups, the previous association of medially placed screws with neurological complications[132] suggests that CT-navigation may reduce the risk of neurological complication.

In addition to performing a systematic review, Shin and colleagues also performed a meta-analysis of 20 articles directly comparing CT-navigated and freehand techniques for pedicle screw placement. They found CT-navigation was associated with a 60% decrease in the risk of pedicle violation, with the largest reduction in risk being observed in the thoracic spine, where it approached a 70% reduction in risk. This has since been echoed by a large retrospective series by Waschke and colleagues.[130] Like Verma, Shin et al also failed to detect a difference between groups in terms of neurological complication, operative time, or blood loss.

Lastly, Tang[122] and colleagues reported a meta-analysis of 12 articles comparing the accuracy of pedicle screw placement in freehand and CT-navigated techniques. They reported that not only was CT-navigation associated with a higher rate of perfect screw placement (OR = 3.35; $p < 0.0001$), but also with a higher rate of clinically acceptable placement (OR = 4.72; $p < 0.0001$), lower rate of hazardous placement (OR = 0.09; $p < 0.00001$), and lower rate of screw-related complication (OR = 0.25; $p = 0.008$).

Another significant benefit to the use of CT-navigation-based systems is that they reduce the radiation exposure to both patient and care team compared to traditionally fluoroscopy-based intraoperative navigation. Several studies in the past decade have been presented to this point, including those by Gebhard,[133] Kim,[134] and Smith.[135] Gebhard et al performed a prospective nonrandomized study examining patient radiation dose with CT-guided navigation, C-arm fluoroscopy, and traditional fluoroscopy. They found a roughly 60% reduction in radiation exposure with CT-guided navigation relative to conventional fluoroscopy and a 35% reduction relative to C-arm-based fluoroscopy. Kim and Smith both used cadaveric models to measure surgeon radiation doses during lumbar fusion operations. Both groups found significant reductions in overall radiation dosage and total fluoroscopy time with the use of CT-guided navigation. Kim et al reported nearly undetectable radiation doses in the navigation group and a 61% reduction in total fluoroscopy time, while Smith and colleagues reported a 92% reduction in total radiation exposure. Additionally, Kim et al found no significant difference in total operating time between the navigation and fluoroscopy groups, which has reportedly been a barrier to adoption of this technology.[131]

Despite these advantages, intraoperative navigation is not without its drawbacks. Like any new technology, intraoperative navigation has a learning curve to it, as surgeons must gain experience with the system to establish a new workflow that incorporates periodic use of the navigation. However, the most commonly cited drawbacks to this technology are the potential to prolong operating times, the high direct costs of the system, and the potential to increase overall procedural expenses, which represent a significant financial risk in the setting of the increasingly common value-based care models. The first concern, namely the increase in case duration, is one that has not been borne out by the literature, either in retrospective cohorts[136,137,138,139] or in meta-analyses, such as that published by Shin and colleagues.[131] Fewer studies have examined the impact of CT-navigation technologies on operative cost. Undoubtedly, these technologies are associated with an increase in direct costs, as they require purchase of the hardware and software, as well as training of the operating room personnel. However, the data regarding incremental cost differential for each operation is less clear. Two studies that have examined this are those by Costa[136] and Dea.[140] The former reported the results of retrospective cohort of 499 patients treated for degenerative lumbar spondylolisthesis. They found that use of intraoperative CT-guided navigation was associated with a 3.80% reduction in cost per procedure. Additionally, they found that use of the accompanying intraoperative O-arm technology resulted in a significant decrease in the number of CT examinations ordered outside the operating room, thereby reducing total costs of radiologic examinations for their institution. Dea et al reported similar findings in their cohort of 502 patients. Unlike Costa though, they included the cost savings associated with the reduction in reoperation rate conferred by superior pedicle screw placement in navigated procedures. Including this factor, they found that use of navigation was associated with increased overall costs in the context of low utilization, but for centers that routinely perform more than 254 fusions per year, this technology becomes cost saving.

17.4 Spinal Navigation and Minimally Invasive Surgery for Spinal Metastases

Perhaps the biggest potential application of CT-guided navigation in the context of spinal metastases is the field of minimally invasive surgery. These techniques are by their very nature plagued by poor or restricted visualization of the pathological level, which can result in suboptimal spinal cord decompression and a poorer neurological recovery. Though this has not been borne out by the literature to date, at present, a bulk of published studies are level III evidence and the utilization of navigation in these procedures has not been discussed, meaning that navigation may be behind the apparent clinical equipoise of these procedures.

In addition to improving neural element decompression,[141] navigation can also play a key role in pedicle screw instrumentation. As discussed in the preceding section, percutaneous screw placement has classically relied upon fluoroscopy, which provides only a two-dimensional view of the spine and so requires the surgeon to use dead reckoning for the third dimension, leading to potential malalignment of the instrumentation. CT-guided navigation helps to overcome this weakness by providing the surgeon with a complete three-dimensional view of the surgical levels. Additionally, the use of CT-guided navigation helps to reduce the total radiation dose given to patients, which may lead to superior wound-healing in the postoperative period.[142] Furthermore, CT-navigation is unaffected intraoperatively by patients with significant body mass, unlike fluoroscopy, which often renders poorer results in obese individuals due to significant signal attenuation by subcutaneous adipose tissue.[117]

The last big advantage of navigation in the context of spinal metastases is intraoperative evaluation of the tumor in the context of destruction of normal anatomic landmarks. Through the course of the procedure, the navigation wand can serve a role similar to that of a pedicle probe, allowing pedicle screw trajectory to be planned and then verified following cannulation. In a similar vein, it can be used to identify vital structures involved by the neoplastic mass, such as the inferior cava or aorta in instances where the tumor possesses a significant prevertebral mass.[117] This facilitates the ability of the surgeon to preserve these structures throughout decompression and so decreases potential procedural morbidity. Finally, the wand can be used to evaluate the progress of decompression by correlating debulked areas with regions of compression on the preoperative imaging. This improves the odds of circumferential decompression and so improves the odds of achieving an optimal outcome.

17.5 Current Literature

Despite the potential advantages conferred by CT-guided navigation to operative management of spinal metastases, relatively few studies have been published describing the use of CT-guided navigation in the context of this pathology since Kalfas first proposed this application in 2001.[117]

The first published case series describing the use of this technology in metastatic spine disease was published in 2002 by Arand et al, who reported the results of eight patients with metastases of the thoracic spine.[141] They found that spinal navigation enabled them to achieve perfect pedicle screw placement in 86.4% of these thoracic screws, which is comparable or superior to previous reports of fluoroscopy-assisted pedicle screw placement.[143] Additionally, CT demonstrated adequate decompression in all of these patients, suggesting that navigation may be useful in the treatment of tumors in this patient population. A follow-up study published the next year by this group examined an additional four patients treated with navigation-assisted surgical decompression, which again demonstrated sufficient decompression in all patients.[144] They did note that screws had to be placed manually in six pedicles, as the navigation system failed to register to the vertebral body. The authors did not report the reason for registration failure, but it is possible that such a failure occurred secondary to disruption of the native anatomy by the lesion. Although this visualization issue is less likely in navigated cases, due to the ability to distinguish soft tissues and bone on the preoperative CT, it does occur in such cases and therefore must be considered when selecting these patients for surgical intervention.

Another small series examining the use of navigation in spinal column tumors was presented by Bandiera et al, who reported on a heterogeneous group of seven patients, three of who had solid tumor metastases, and one of whom had a primary plasmacytoma.[145] None of the patients experienced an intraoperative complication and the group was able to achieve perfect screw placement for 70% of screws and clinically acceptable placement in 95% of cases. Again, this suggests that navigated surgery can provide safe and successful outcomes in patients with spinal metastases.

The largest and most recent study to examine the use of navigation solely in patients with metastatic spine disease was reported by Nasser et al, who reported the results of navigation-assisted minimally invasive separation surgery in a combined cadaveric and in vivo cohort.[75] After establishing the utility of navigation in the cadaver cohort, the authors applied the technique to seventeen patients presenting with metastatic epidural spinal cord compression, three of whom had complete destruction of normal anatomic landmarks at the surgical level. CT-navigation was used throughout the case to navigate in areas of normal landmark destruction, as well as to gauge the degree of decompression that had been achieved. Additionally, the navigation system was used to aid in percutaneous screw placement. Despite the loss of normal anatomic landmarks, adequate circumferential decompression was achieved in all patients. The authors did not report the overall accuracy of pedicle screw placement but did note that their successful decompression led to neurological stability or improvement in all patients, as well as pain relief in all patients. Nasser and colleagues updated their results in 2016 with a multicenter cohort review of patients with spinal tumors treated with navigation-assisted surgical decompression, of which 25 were being treated for spinal metastases.[146] Again, they reported overall good results, though they did not elaborate on recovery of neurological function or accuracy of instrumentation placement.

The available literature describing the use of intraoperative neuronavigation for spinal tumors, including its utilization in clinical series of primary tumors and various case reports of metastatic spine disease, suggest its evolving and invaluable role in the surgical treatment of metastatic spine disease.[146,147,148,149,150] This is especially true in cases of anomalous anatomic landmarks, minimally invasive surgical resection/instrumentation, and more complex resections. Higher quality evidence is still required to provide a strong recommendation for its use but given the wider availability of these technologies and greater emphasis on minimally invasive treatments, it seems likely that such evidence will become available. Yet even with greater evidence, we must caution that like all new surgical technologies, intraoperative CT-guided navigation has its own learning curve and will require practice to realize the superior outcomes. In ▶ Table 17.4 we provide pearls and pitfalls for the use of CT-guided navigation during the operative management of spinal metastases based upon our own experience.

17.6 Case Illustration

This is a 47-year-old female with a history of left-sided invasive ductal carcinoma of the breast, who presented with intractable mechanical back pain, restricting her function and activities of daily living. Imaging and biopsy was performed, confirming metastatic spine disease resulting in L4 pathologic compression fracture. She was known to have numerous symptomatic visceral, diffuse axial, and multiple brain metastases that, per progressing, failed chemotherapy and radiation. Given the poor prognosis accounting for systemic burden, cognitive/visual changes from intracranial metastasis, and previous failed therapy, minimally invasive stabilization from L3–L5 was determined to be the most appropriate treatment to maximize the patient's remaining quality of life (▶ Fig. 17.1).

She was placed prone on a Jackson table and a skin incision was placed over the right posterior superior iliac spine for the placement of a reference frame. Intraoperative CT was acquired

Table 17.4 Tips and tricks for using intraoperative CT-guided navigation

Period	Consideration	Consequence
Preoperative		
	Obese patient	• Inadequate tissue penetration on preoperative CT leads to failure of intraoperative alignment
	History with machine	• Surgeons less familiar with machine will have poorer results • Moderate learning curve for the machine which is more gradual for those with significant video game experience
	Surgical table	• Table must be narrow enough to accommodate intraoperative CT imaging if real-time imaging is desired; Jackson table is ideal • Table must be radiolucent for acquisition of intraoperative imaging
	Registration	• Patient anatomy shifts during the course of surgical approach, so if open approach is being used, the intra-op CT should be performed post-approach, followed by registration of the system • Body warmer should be rolled back during image acquisition to reduce image artifact • Use of paired-point vs. surface matching technique for registration does not affect navigation accuracy and decreased operative time • Cervical cases: hold patient ventilation during image acquisition
Intraoperative		
	Table position	• Surgeon should avoid changing table position as this can lead to system malalignment • Surgical staff should avoid contact with table to prevent loss of table–image alignment
	Reference frame placement	• Cervical cases: attach reference frame to Mayfield clamp • Thoracic cases: attach to iliac crest; alternatively use fluoroscopy • Lumbar cases: attach to posterior iliac crest (esp. for LLIF/XLIF) • In open cases, place reference frame on most superiorly exposed vertebrae and place camera at head of bed • Surgeon must remain aware of reference frame position to avoid collision during case • Cord/wires/tubes of cautery, suction should not contact reference frame to avoid loss of alignment intraoperatively
	Operating room setup	• Setup must allow surgeon to have continuous line of site with detector • Reference frame must be positioned to avoid overexposure by room lights, which prevents alignment • Register all image-guided instruments to be used prior to case start
	Intraoperative image acquisition	• Imaged volume should always contain reference frame • If intraoperative CT imaging is to be required (e.g., O-arm), then patient should have wound filled with antibiotic irrigation solution and should then be wrapped with disposable drape to avoid contact with O-arm; O-arm cover is difficult to use
	Instrumentation	• Should be done immediately after intraoperative image acquisition as this is when navigation accuracy is highest • For long constructs, begin with segments most distal from reference frame as these are most adversely affected by changes in navigation accuracy
	Surgical changes	• Vertebrectomy and deformity correction can significantly impact accuracy of reference frame and should be avoided until all pedicle screw instrumentation has been placed

Sources: Holly et al. J Neurosurg Spine 2006;4(4): 323–328; Rahmathulla et al. Neurosurg Focus 2014;36(3):E3.

via the O-arm (Medtronic, Minneapolis, MN) for calibration with the StealthStation Surgical Navigation System (Medtronic, Minneapolis, MN) (▶ Fig. 17.2, ▶ Fig. 17.3). Transpedicular screws were percutaneously placed, via stab incisions, under navigated guidance at L3 and L5, bilaterally. Screws' stimulation demonstrated no abnormalities, and neuromonitoring was stable throughout the case. A rod was locked into place and repeat intraoperative CT confirmed accurate hardware placement (▶ Fig. 17.4).

The patient had substantial relief in her back pain, before succumbing to disease 10 months postoperatively.

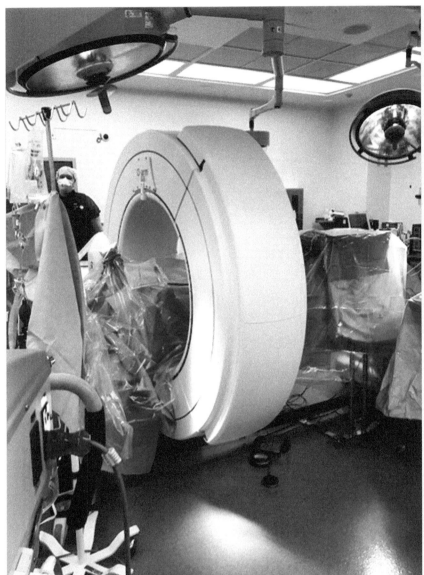

Fig. 17.2 Intraoperative CT scan (O-arm, Medtronic, Minneapolis, MN).

17.7 Conclusion

Though the evidence supporting the use of spinal navigation in metastatic spine disease is sparse, several case series have been published over the past 15 years, describing the ways in which this technology can be applied. Combined, the evidence suggests that the highest impact for this technology will be in patients undergoing minimally invasive techniques. These approaches are associated with poorer visualization relative to open approaches, which when combined with tumor-mediated destruction of normal anatomic landmarks may render circumferential decompression infeasible in the absence of navigation assistance. Given the greater emphasis on minimally invasive procedures, such as minimally invasive separation surgery, it seems that neuronavigation may play a larger role in the treatment of patients with metastatic spine disease.

17.8 Key Points

- CT-guided navigation improves instrumentation accuracy and decreases radiation exposure without increasing operative time.
- CT-guided navigation is optimally suited to metastatic spine cases as it helps to overcome oncologic destruction of normal anatomic landmarks.
- Use of CT-navigation allows surgeon to verify circumferential decompression and an attendant optimal neurological outcome.
- Minimally invasive surgery has biggest possible benefit from intraoperative navigation due to the restricted visualization offered by these techniques.

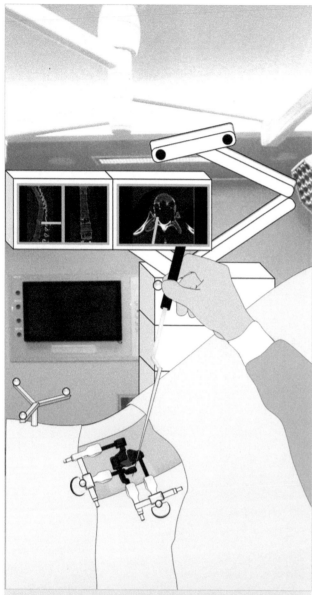

Fig. 17.3 Navigation of transpedicular screws, using the StealthStation Surgical Navigation System (Medtronic, Minneapolis, MN).

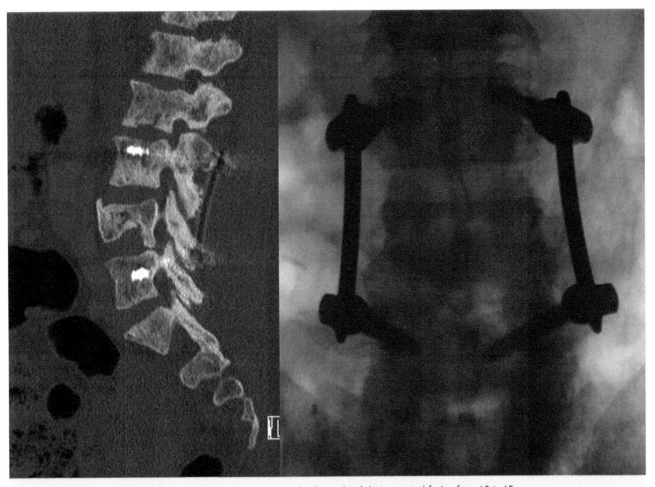

Fig. 17.4 Postoperative imaging demonstrating percutaneous, navigation-assisted, instrumented fusion from L3 to L5.

References

[1] American Cancer Society. Cancer facts & figures 2017. 2017

[2] Arguello F, Baggs RB, Duerst RE, Johnstone L, McQueen K, Frantz CN. Pathogenesis of vertebral metastasis and epidural spinal cord compression. Cancer. 1990; 65(1):98–106

[3] Fornasier VL, Horne JG. Metastases to the vertebral column. Cancer. 1975; 36 (2):590–594

[4] Gezercan Y, Çavuş G, Ökten AI, et al. Single-stage posterolateral transpedicular approach with 360-degree stabilization and vertebrectomy in primary and metastatic tumors of the spine. World Neurosurg. 2016; 95:214–221

[5] Klimo P, Jr, Thompson CJ, Kestle JRW, Schmidt MH. A meta-analysis of surgery versus conventional radiotherapy for the treatment of metastatic spinal epidural disease. Neuro-oncology. 2005; 7(1):64–76

[6] Molina CA, Gokaslan ZL, Sciubba DM. A systematic review of the current role of minimally invasive spine surgery in the management of metastatic spine disease. Int J Surg Oncol. 2011; 2011:598148

[7] Wiggins GC, Mirza S, Bellabarba C, West GA, Chapman JR, Shaffrey CI. Perioperative complications with costotransversectomy and anterior approaches to thoracic and thoracolumbar tumors. Neurosurg Focus. 2001; 11(6):e4

[8] Patchell RA, Tibbs PA, Regine WF, et al. Direct decompressive surgical resection in the treatment of spinal cord compression caused by metastatic cancer: a randomised trial. Lancet. 2005; 366(9486):643–648

[9] Chi JH, Bydon A, Hsieh P, Witham T, Wolinsky JP, Gokaslan ZL. Epidemiology and demographics for primary vertebral tumors. Neurosurg Clin N Am. 2008; 19(1):1–4

[10] Goodwin CR, Khattab MH, Sankey EW, et al. Factors associated with life expectancy in patients with metastatic spine disease from adenocarcinoma of the lung. Global Spine J. 2015; 5(5):417–424

[11] Kan P, Schmidt MH. Minimally invasive thoracoscopic approach for anterior decompression and stabilization of metastatic spine disease. Neurosurg Focus. 2008; 25(2):E8

[12] Patil CG, Lad SP, Santarelli J, Boakye M. National inpatient complications and outcomes after surgery for spinal metastasis from 1993–2002. Cancer. 2007; 110(3):625–630

[13] Ravindra VM, Brock A, Awad AW, Kalra R, Schmidt MH. The role of the mini-open thoracoscopic-assisted approach in the management of metastatic spine disease at the thoracolumbar junction. Neurosurg Focus. 2016; 41(2): E16

[14] Ryken TC, Eichholz KM, Gerszten PC, Welch WC, Gokaslan ZL, Resnick DK. Evidence-based review of the surgical management of vertebral column metastatic disease. Neurosurg Focus. 2003; 15(5):E11

[15] Pointillart V, Vital JM, Salmi R, Diallo A, Quan GMY. Survival prognostic factors and clinical outcomes in patients with spinal metastases. J Cancer Res Clin Oncol. 2011; 137(5):849–856

[16] Tomita K, Kawahara N, Kobayashi T, Yoshida A, Murakami H, Akamaru T. Surgical strategy for spinal metastases. Spine. 2001; 26(3):298–306

[17] Yang SB, Cho W, Chang UK. Analysis of prognostic factors relating to postoperative survival in spinal metastases. J Korean Neurosurg Soc. 2012; 51 (3):127–134

[18] Cole JS, Patchell RA. Metastatic epidural spinal cord compression. Lancet Neurol. 2008; 7(5):459–466

[19] Kaloostian PE, Yurter A, Zadnik PL, Sciubba DM, Gokaslan ZL. Current paradigms for metastatic spinal disease: an evidence-based review. Ann Surg Oncol. 2014; 21(1):248–262

[20] Miscusi M, Polli FM, Forcato S, et al. Comparison of minimally invasive surgery with standard open surgery for vertebral thoracic metastases causing acute myelopathy in patients with short- or mid-term life expectancy: surgical technique and early clinical results. J Neurosurg Spine. 2015; 22(5):518–525

[21] Sciubba DM, Gokaslan ZL, Suk I, et al. Positive and negative prognostic variables for patients undergoing spine surgery for metastatic breast disease. Eur Spine J. 2007; 16(10):1659–1667

[22] Sciubba DM, Goodwin CR, Yurter A, et al. A systematic review of clinical outcomes and prognostic factors for patients undergoing surgery for spinal metastases secondary to breast cancer. Global Spine J. 2016; 6(5):482–496

[23] Eleraky M, Papanastassiou I, Vrionis FD. Management of metastatic spine disease. Curr Opin Support Palliat Care. 2010; 4(3):182–188

[24] Ju DG, Zadnik PL, Groves ML, et al. Factors associated with improved outcomes following decompressive surgery for prostate cancer metastatic to the spine. Neurosurgery. 2013; 73(4):657–666, discussion 666

[25] Katagiri H, Okada R, Takagi T, et al. New prognostic factors and scoring system for patients with skeletal metastasis. Cancer Med. 2014; 3(5):1359–1367

[26] Quraishi NA, Rajagopal TS, Manoharan SR, Elsayed S, Edwards KL, Boszczyk BM. Effect of timing of surgery on neurological outcome and survival in metastatic spinal cord compression. Eur Spine J. 2013; 22(6):1383–1388

[27] North RB, LaRocca VR, Schwartz J, et al. Surgical management of spinal metastases: analysis of prognostic factors during a 10-year experience. J Neurosurg Spine. 2005; 2(5):564–573

[28] Yao KC, Boriani S, Gokaslan ZL, Sundaresan N. En bloc spondylectomy for spinal metastases: a review of techniques. Neurosurg Focus. 2003; 15(5):E6

[29] Rubin P, Brasacchio R, Katz A. Solitary metastases: illusion versus reality. Semin Radiat Oncol. 2006; 16(2):120–130

[30] Laufer I, Rubin DG, Lis E, et al. The NOMS framework: approach to the treatment of spinal metastatic tumors. Oncologist. 2013; 18(6):744–751

[31] Tokuhashi Y, Ajiro Y, Umezawa N. Outcome of treatment for spinal metastases using scoring system for preoperative evaluation of prognosis. Spine. 2009; 34(1):69–73

[32] Quraishi NA, Gokaslan ZL, Boriani S. The surgical management of metastatic epidural compression of the spinal cord. J Bone Joint Surg Br. 2010; 92(8):1054–1060

[33] Smith ZA, Yang I, Gorgulho A, Raphael D, De Salles AA, Khoo LT. Emerging techniques in the minimally invasive treatment and management of thoracic spine tumors. J Neurooncol. 2012; 107(3):443–455

[34] Finkelstein JA, Zaveri G, Wai E, Vidmar M, Kreder H, Chow E. A population-based study of surgery for spinal metastases: survival rates and complications. J Bone Joint Surg Br. 2003; 85(7):1045–1050

[35] Hosono N, Ueda T, Tamura D, Aoki Y, Yoshikawa H. Prognostic relevance of clinical symptoms in patients with spinal metastases. Clin Orthop Relat Res. 2005(436):196–201

[36] Laufer I, Sciubba DM, Madera M, et al. Surgical management of metastatic spinal tumors. Cancer Contr. 2012; 19(2):122–128

[37] Zadnik PL, Hwang L, Ju DG, et al. Prolonged survival following aggressive treatment for metastatic breast cancer in the spine. Clin Exp Metastasis. 2014; 31(1):47–55

[38] Batista N, Tee J, Sciubba D, et al. Emerging and established clinical, histopathological and molecular parametric prognostic factors for metastatic spine disease secondary to lung cancer: helping surgeons make decisions. J Clin Neurosci. 2016; 34(12):15–22

[39] Moon KY, Chung CK, Jahng TA, Kim HJ, Kim CH. Postoperative survival and ambulatory outcome in metastatic spinal tumors : prognostic factor analysis. J Korean Neurosurg Soc. 2011; 50(3):216–223

[40] Sohn S, Kim J, Chung CK, et al. A nationwide epidemiological study of newly diagnosed spine metastasis in the adult Korean population. Spine J. 2016; 16(8):937–945

[41] Bauer HCF, Wedin R. Survival after surgery for spinal and extremity metastases: prognostication in 241 patients. Acta Orthop Scand. 1995; 66(2):143–146

[42] Tokuhashi Y, Matsuzaki H, Toriyama S, Kawano H, Ohsaka S. Scoring system for the preoperative evaluation of metastatic spine tumor prognosis. Spine. 1990; 15(11):1110–1113

[43] Jansson KA, Bauer HCF. Survival, complications and outcome in 282 patients operated for neurological deficit due to thoracic or lumbar spinal metastases. Eur Spine J. 2006; 15(2):196–202

[44] Sioutos PJ, Arbit E, Meshulam CF, Galicich JH. Spinal metastases from solid tumors: analysis of factors affecting survival. Cancer. 1995; 76(8):1453–1459

[45] van der Linden YM, Dijkstra SP, Vonk EJ, Marijnen CA, Leer JW, Dutch Bone Metastasis Study Group. Prediction of survival in patients with metastases in the spinal column: results based on a randomized trial of radiotherapy. Cancer. 2005; 103(2):320–328

[46] Wibmer C, Leithner A, Hofmann G, et al. Survival analysis of 254 patients after manifestation of spinal metastases: evaluation of seven preoperative scoring systems. Spine. 2011; 36(23):1977–1986

[47] Goodwin CR, Sankey EW, Liu A, et al. A systematic review of clinical outcomes for patients diagnosed with skin cancer spinal metastases. J Neurosurg Spine. 2016; 24(5):837–849

[48] Helweg-Larsen S, Sørensen PS, Kreiner S. Prognostic factors in metastatic spinal cord compression: a prospective study using multivariate analysis of variables influencing survival and gait function in 153 patients. Int J Radiat Oncol Biol Phys. 2000; 46(5):1163–1169

[49] Vanek P, Bradac O, Trebicky F, Saur K, de Lacy P, Benes V. Influence of the preoperative neurological status on survival after the surgical treatment of symptomatic spinal metastases with spinal cord compression. Spine. 2015; 40(23):1824–1830

[50] Tokuhashi Y, Matsuzaki H, Oda H, Oshima M, Ryu J. A revised scoring system for preoperative evaluation of metastatic spine tumor prognosis. Spine. 2005; 30(19):2186–2191

[51] Chen H, Xiao J, Yang X, Zhang F, Yuan W. Preoperative scoring systems and prognostic factors for patients with spinal metastases from hepatocellular carcinoma. Spine. 2010; 35(23):E1339–E1346

[52] Schoenfeld AJ, Leonard DA, Saadat E, Bono CM, Harris MB, Ferrone ML. Predictors of 30- and 90-day survival following surgical intervention for spinal metastases: a prognostic study conducted at four academic centers. Spine. 2016; 41(8):E503–E509

[53] Leithner A, Radl R, Gruber G, et al. Predictive value of seven preoperative prognostic scoring systems for spinal metastases. Eur Spine J. 2008; 17(11):1488–1495

[54] Liang T, Wan Y, Zou X, Peng X, Liu S. Is surgery for spine metastasis reasonable in patients older than 60 years? Clin Orthop Relat Res. 2013; 471(2):628–639

[55] Majeed H, Kumar S, Bommireddy R, Klezl Z, Calthorpe D. Accuracy of prognostic scores in decision making and predicting outcomes in metastatic spine disease. Ann R Coll Surg Engl. 2012; 94(1):28–33

[56] Meng T, Chen R, Zhong N, et al. Factors associated with improved survival following surgical treatment for metastatic prostate cancer in the spine: retrospective analysis of 29 patients in a single center. World J Surg Oncol. 2016; 14(1):200

[57] Papastefanou S, Alpantaki K, Akra G, Katonis P. Predictive value of Tokuhashi and Tomita scores in patients with metastatic spine disease. Acta Orthop Traumatol Turc. 2012; 46(1):50–56

[58] Fürstenberg CH, Wiedenhöfer B, Gerner HJ, Putz C. The effect of early surgical treatment on recovery in patients with metastatic compression of the spinal cord. J Bone Joint Surg Br. 2009; 91(2):240–244

[59] Loblaw DA, Laperriere NJ, Mackillop WJ. A population-based study of malignant spinal cord compression in Ontario. Clin Oncol (R Coll Radiol). 2003; 15(4):211–217

[60] Loblaw DA, Perry J, Chambers A, Laperriere NJ. Systematic review of the diagnosis and management of malignant extradural spinal cord compression: the Cancer Care Ontario Practice Guidelines Initiative's Neuro-Oncology Disease Site Group. J Clin Oncol. 2005; 23(9):2028–2037

[61] Mak KS, Lee LK, Mak RH, et al. Incidence and treatment patterns in hospitalizations for malignant spinal cord compression in the United States, 1998–2006. Int J Radiat Oncol Biol Phys. 2011; 80(3):824–831

[62] Tomycz ND, Gerszten PC. Minimally invasive treatments for metastatic spine tumors: vertebroplasty, kyphoplasty, and radiosurgery. Neurosurg Q. 2008; 18(2):104–108

[63] Witham TF, Khavkin YA, Gallia GL, Wolinsky JP, Gokaslan ZL. Surgery insight: current management of epidural spinal cord compression from metastatic spine disease. Nat Clin Pract Neurol. 2006; 2(2):87–94, quiz 116

[64] Holman PJ, Suki D, McCutcheon I, Wolinsky JP, Rhines LD, Gokaslan ZL. Surgical management of metastatic disease of the lumbar spine: experience with 139 patients. J Neurosurg Spine. 2005; 2(5):550–563

[65] Levack P, Graham J, Collie D, et al. Scottish Cord Compression Study Group. Don't wait for a sensory level—listen to the symptoms: a prospective audit of the delays in diagnosis of malignant cord compression. Clin Oncol (R Coll Radiol). 2002; 14(6):472–480

[66] Abrahm JL, Banffy MB, Harris MB. Spinal cord compression in patients with advanced metastatic cancer: "all I care about is walking and living my life". JAMA. 2008; 299(8):937–946

[67] Zaikova O, Giercksky KE, Fosså SD, Kvaløy S, Johannesen TB, Skjeldal S. A population-based study of spinal metastatic disease in South-East Norway. Clin Oncol (R Coll Radiol). 2009; 21(10):753–759

[68] Arrigo RT, Kalanithi P, Cheng I, et al. Predictors of survival after surgical treatment of spinal metastasis. Neurosurgery. 2011; 68(3):674–681, discussion 681

[69] White BD, Stirling AJ, Paterson E, Asquith-Coe K, Melder A, Guideline Development Group. Diagnosis and management of patients at risk of or with metastatic spinal cord compression: summary of NICE guidance. BMJ. 2008; 337:a2538

[70] Chi JH, Gokaslan ZL. Vertebroplasty and kyphoplasty for spinal metastases. Curr Opin Support Palliat Care. 2008; 2(1):9–13

[71] Findlay GF. Adverse effects of the management of malignant spinal cord compression. J Neurol Neurosurg Psychiatry. 1984; 47(8):761–768

[72] Niazi TN, Sauri-Barraza J, Schmidt MH. Minimally invasive treatment of spinal tumors. Semin Spine Surg. 2011; 23(1):51–59

[73] Laufer I, Iorgulescu JB, Chapman T, et al. Local disease control for spinal metastases following "separation surgery" and adjuvant hypofractionated or high-dose single-fraction stereotactic radiosurgery: outcome analysis in 186 patients. J Neurosurg Spine. 2013; 18(3):207–214

[74] Turel MK, Kerolus MG, O'Toole JE. Minimally invasive "separation surgery" plus adjuvant stereotactic radiotherapy in the management of spinal epidural metastases. J Craniovertebr Junction Spine. 2017; 8(2):119–126

[75] Nasser R, Nakhla J, Echt M, et al. Minimally invasive separation surgery with intraoperative stereotactic guidance: a feasibility study. World Neurosurg. 2018; 109:68–76

[76] Moussazadeh N, Laufer I, Yamada Y, Bilsky MH. Separation surgery for spinal metastases: effect of spinal radiosurgery on surgical treatment goals. Cancer Contr. 2014; 21(2):168–174

[77] Zuckerman SL, Laufer I, Sahgal A, et al. When less is more: the indications for MIS techniques and separation surgery in metastatic spine disease. Spine. 2016; 41 Suppl 20:S246–S253

[78] Choi MH, Oh SN, Lee IK, Oh ST, Won DD. Sarcopenia is negatively associated with long-term outcomes in locally advanced rectal cancer. J Cachexia Sarcopenia Muscle. 2018; 9(1):53–59

[79] Fisher CG, DiPaola CP, Ryken TC, et al. A novel classification system for spinal instability in neoplastic disease: an evidence-based approach and expert consensus from the Spine Oncology Study Group. Spine. 2010; 35(22):E1221–E1229

[80] Fourney DR, Frangou EM, Ryken TC, et al. Spinal instability neoplastic score: an analysis of reliability and validity from the spine oncology study group. J Clin Oncol. 2011; 29(22):3072–3077

[81] Ethun CG, Bilen MA, Jani AB, Maithel SK, Ogan K, Master VA. Frailty and cancer: implications for oncology surgery, medical oncology, and radiation oncology. CA Cancer J Clin. 2017; 67(5):362–377

[82] Handforth C, Clegg A, Young C, et al. The prevalence and outcomes of frailty in older cancer patients: a systematic review. Ann Oncol. 2015; 26(6):1091–1101

[83] Luksanapruksa P, Buchowski JM, Zebala LP, Kepler CK, Singhatanadgige W, Bumpass DB. Perioperative complications of spinal metastases surgery. Clin Spine Surg. 2017; 30(1):4–13

[84] Arrigo RT, Kalanithi P, Cheng I, et al. Charlson score is a robust predictor of 30-day complications following spinal metastasis surgery. Spine. 2011; 36(19):E1274–E1280

[85] Sebaaly A, Shedid D, Boubez G, et al. Surgical site infection in spinal metastasis: incidence and risk factors. Spine J. 2018; 18(8):1382–1387

[86] Atkinson RA, Davies B, Jones A, van Popta D, Ousey K, Stephenson J. Survival of patients undergoing surgery for metastatic spinal tumours and the impact of surgical site infection. J Hosp Infect. 2016; 94(1):80–85

[87] De la Garza Ramos R, Goodwin CR, Jain A, et al. Development of a metastatic spinal tumor frailty index (MSTFI) using a nationwide database and its association with inpatient morbidity, mortality, and length of stay after spine surgery. World Neurosurg. 2016; 95::555.e4

[88] Ahmed AK, Goodwin CR, De la Garza-Ramos R, et al. Predicting short-term outcome after surgery for primary spinal tumors based on patient frailty. World Neurosurg. 2017; 108:393–398

[89] Donnelly DJ, Abd-El-Barr MM, Lu Y. Minimally invasive muscle sparing posterior-only approach for lumbar circumferential decompression and stabilization to treat spine metastasis—technical report. World Neurosurg. 2015; 84(5):1484–1490

[90] Chou D, Lu DC. Mini-open transpedicular corpectomies with expandable cage reconstruction: technical note. J Neurosurg Spine. 2011; 14(1):71–77

[91] Fang T, Dong J, Zhou X, McGuire RA, Jr, Li X. Comparison of mini-open anterior corpectomy and posterior total en bloc spondylectomy for solitary metastases of the thoracolumbar spine. J Neurosurg Spine. 2012; 17(4):271–279

[92] Hansen-Algenstaedt N, Kwan MK, Algenstaedt P, et al. Comparison between minimally invasive surgery and conventional open surgery for patients with spinal metastasis: a prospective propensity score-matched study. Spine. 2017; 42(10):789–797

[93] Hikata T, Isogai N, Shiono Y, et al. A retrospective cohort study comparing the safety and efficacy of minimally invasive versus open surgical techniques in the treatment of spinal metastases. Clin Spine Surg. 2017; 30(8):E1082–E1087

[94] Huang TJ, Hsu RW, Li YY, Cheng CC. Minimal access spinal surgery (MASS) in treating thoracic spine metastasis. Spine. 2006; 31(16):1860–1863

[95] Kumar N, Malhotra R, Maharajan K, et al. Metastatic spine tumor surgery: a comparative study of minimally invasive approach using percutaneous pedicle screws fixation versus open approach. Clin Spine Surg. 2017; 30(8):E1015–E1021

[96] Lau D, Chou D. Posterior thoracic corpectomy with cage reconstruction for metastatic spinal tumors: comparing the mini-open approach to the open approach. J Neurosurg Spine. 2015; 23(2):217–227

[97] Stoker GE, Buchowski JM, Kelly MP, Meyers BF, Patterson GA. Video-assisted thoracoscopic surgery with posterior spinal reconstruction for the resection of upper lobe lung tumors involving the spine. Spine J. 2013; 13(1):68–76

[98] Pennington Z, Ahmed AK, Molina CA, Ehresman J, Laufer I, Sciubba DM. Minimally invasive versus conventional spine surgery for vertebral metastases: a systematic review of the evidence. Ann Transl Med. 2018; 6(6):103

[99] Rabinov K, Goldman H, Rosbash H, Simon M. The role of aspiration biopsy of focal lesions in lung and bone by simple needle and fluoroscopy. Am J Roentgenol Radium Ther Nucl Med. 1967; 101(4):932–938

[100] Koktekir E, Ceylan D, Tatarli N, Karabagli H, Recber F, Akdemir G. Accuracy of fluoroscopically-assisted pedicle screw placement: analysis of 1,218 screws in 198 patients. Spine J. 2014; 14(8):1702–1708

[101] Saarenpää I, Laine T, Hirvonen J, et al. Accuracy of 837 pedicle screw positions in degenerative lumbar spine with conventional open surgery evaluated by computed tomography. Acta Neurochir (Wien). 2017; 159(10):2011–2017

[102] Corcos G, Dbjay J, Mastier C, et al. Cement leakage in percutaneous vertebroplasty for spinal metastases: a retrospective evaluation of incidence and risk factors. Spine. 2014; 39(5):E332–E338

[103] Fu TS, Li YD. Fluoroscopy-guided percutaneous vertebroplasty for symptomatic loosened pedicle screw and instrumentation-associated vertebral fracture: an evaluation of initial experiences and technical note. J Neurosurg Spine. 2018; 28(4):364–371

[104] Papp Z, Marosföi M, Szikora I, Banczerowski P. Treatment of C-2 metastatic tumors with intraoperative transoral or transpedicular vertebroplasty and occipitocervical posterior fixation. J Neurosurg Spine. 2014; 21(6):886–891

[105] Yang JS, Chu L, Xiao FT, et al. Anterior retropharyngeal approach to C1 for percutaneous vertebroplasty under C-arm fluoroscopy. Spine J. 2015; 15(3):539–545

[106] Arnold PM, Anderson KK, McGuire RA, Jr. The lateral transpsoas approach to the lumbar and thoracic spine: a review. Surg Neurol Int. 2012; 3 Suppl 3:S198–S215

[107] Agarwal A, Chauhan V, Singh D, Shailendra R, Maheshwari R, Juyal A. A comparative study of pedicle screw fixation in dorsolumbar spine by freehand versus image-assisted technique: a cadaveric study. Indian J Orthop. 2016; 50(3):243–249

[108] Kosmopoulos V, Schizas C. Pedicle screw placement accuracy: a meta-analysis. Spine. 2007; 32(3):E111–E120

[109] Schizas C, Theumann N, Kosmopoulos V. Inserting pedicle screws in the upper thoracic spine without the use of fluoroscopy or image guidance: is it safe? Eur Spine J. 2007; 16(5):625–629

[110] Odgers CJ, IV, Vaccaro AR, Pollack ME, Cotler JM. Accuracy of pedicle screw placement with the assistance of lateral plain radiography. J Spinal Disord. 1996; 9(4):334–338

[111] Mariscalco MW, Yamashita T, Steinmetz MP, Krishnaney AA, Lieberman IH, Mroz TE. Radiation exposure to the surgeon during open lumbar microdiscectomy and minimally invasive microdiscectomy: a prospective, controlled trial. Spine. 2011; 36(3):255–260

[112] Mulconrey DS. Fluoroscopic radiation exposure in spinal surgery: in vivo evaluation for operating room personnel. Clin Spine Surg. 2016; 29(7):E331–E335

[113] Perisinakis K, Theocharopoulos N, Damilakis J, et al. Estimation of patient dose and associated radiogenic risks from fluoroscopically guided pedicle screw insertion. Spine. 2004; 29(14):1555–1560

[114] Bindal RK, Glaze S, Ognoskie M, Tunner V, Malone R, Ghosh S. Surgeon and patient radiation exposure in minimally invasive transforaminal lumbar interbody fusion. J Neurosurg Spine. 2008; 9(6):570–573

[115] Hyun SJ, Kim KJ, Jahng TA, Kim HJ. Efficiency of lead aprons in blocking radiation: how protective are they? Heliyon. 2016; 2(5):e00117

[116] Nascimento A, Carlos Fernando Pereira da Silva H, Helton Luiz Aparecido D, Marina Silva Magalhães V, João de A, Ronaldo Lavôr F. Comparison of exposure to radiation during percutaneous transpedicular procedures, using three fluoroscopic techniques. Coluna/Columna. 2007; 16(2):141–144

[117] Kalfas IH. Image-guided spinal navigation: application to spinal metastases. Neurosurg Focus. 2001; 11(6):e5

[118] Holly LT, Bloch O, Johnson JP. Evaluation of registration techniques for spinal image guidance. J Neurosurg Spine. 2006; 4(4):323–328

[119] Overley SC, Cho SK, Mehta AI, Arnold PM. Navigation and robotics in spinal surgery: where are we now? Neurosurgery. 2017; 80 3S:S86–S99

[120] Nooh A, Lubov J, Aoude A, et al. Differences between manufacturers of computed tomography-based computer-assisted surgery systems do exist: a systematic literature review. Global Spine J. 2017; 7(1):83–94

[121] Gelalis ID, Paschos NK, Pakos EE, et al. Accuracy of pedicle screw placement: a systematic review of prospective in vivo studies comparing free hand, fluoroscopy guidance and navigation techniques. Eur Spine J. 2012; 21(2):247–255

[122] Tang J, Zhu Z, Sui T, Kong D, Cao X. Position and complications of pedicle screw insertion with or without image-navigation techniques in the thoracolumbar spine: a meta-analysis of comparative studies. J Biomed Res. 2014; 28(3):228–239

[123] Shin MH, Ryu KS, Park CK. Accuracy and safety in pedicle screw placement in the thoracic and lumbar spines: comparison study between conventional C-arm fluoroscopy and navigation coupled with O-arm® guided methods. J Korean Neurosurg Soc. 2012; 52(3):204–209

[124] Verma R, Krishan S, Haendlmayer K, Mohsen A. Functional outcome of computer-assisted spinal pedicle screw placement: a systematic review and meta-analysis of 23 studies including 5,992 pedicle screws. Eur Spine J. 2010; 19(3):370–375

[125] Innocenzi G, Bistazzoni S, D'Ercole M, Cardarelli G, Ricciardi F. Does navigation improve pedicle screw placement accuracy? Comparison between navigated and non-navigated percutaneous and open fixations. Acta Neurochir Suppl (Wien). 2017; 124:289–295

[126] Meng XT, Guan XF, Zhang HL, He SS. Computer navigation versus fluoroscopy-guided navigation for thoracic pedicle screw placement: a meta-analysis. Neurosurg Rev. 2016; 39(3):385–391

[127] Shin MH, Hur JW, Ryu KS, Park CK. Prospective comparison study between the fluoroscopy-guided and navigation coupled with O-arm-guided pedicle screw placement in the thoracic and lumbosacral spines. J Spinal Disord Tech. 2015; 28(6):E347–E351

[128] Tian NF, Xu HZ. Image-guided pedicle screw insertion accuracy: a meta-analysis. Int Orthop. 2009; 33(4):895–903

[129] Tian NF, Huang QS, Zhou P, et al. Pedicle screw insertion accuracy with different assisted methods: a systematic review and meta-analysis of comparative studies. Eur Spine J. 2011; 20(6):846–859

[130] Waschke A, Walter J, Duenisch P, Reichart R, Kalff R, Ewald C. CT-navigation versus fluoroscopy-guided placement of pedicle screws at the thoracolumbar spine: single center experience of 4,500 screws. Eur Spine J. 2013; 22(3):654–660

[131] Shin BJ, James AR, Njoku IU, Härtl R. Pedicle screw navigation: a systematic review and meta-analysis of perforation risk for computer-navigated versus freehand insertion. J Neurosurg Spine. 2012; 17(2):113–122

[132] Lonstein JE, Denis F, Perra JH, Pinto MR, Smith MD, Winter RB. Complications associated with pedicle screws. J Bone Joint Surg Am. 1999; 81(11):1519–1528

[133] Gebhard FT, Kraus MD, Schneider E, Liener UC, Kinzl L, Arand M. Does computer-assisted spine surgery reduce intraoperative radiation doses? Spine. 2006; 31(17):2024–2027, discussion 2028

[134] Kim CW, Lee YP, Taylor W, Oygar A, Kim WK. Use of navigation-assisted fluoroscopy to decrease radiation exposure during minimally invasive spine surgery. Spine J. 2008; 8(4):584–590

[135] Smith HE, Welsch MD, Sasso RC, Vaccaro AR. Comparison of radiation exposure in lumbar pedicle screw placement with fluoroscopy vs computer-assisted image guidance with intraoperative three-dimensional imaging. J Spinal Cord Med. 2008; 31(5):532–537

[136] Costa F, Porazzi E, Restelli U, et al. Economic study: a cost-effectiveness analysis of an intraoperative compared with a preoperative image-guided system in lumbar pedicle screw fixation in patients with degenerative spondylolisthesis. Spine J. 2014; 14(8):1790–1796

[137] Khanna AR, Yanamadala V, Coumans JV. Effect of intraoperative navigation on operative time in 1-level lumbar fusion surgery. J Clin Neurosci. 2016; 32:72–76

[138] Wu MH, Dubey NK, Li YY, et al. Comparison of minimally invasive spine surgery using intraoperative computed tomography integrated navigation, fluoroscopy, and conventional open surgery for lumbar spondylolisthesis: a prospective registry-based cohort study. Spine J. 2017; 17(8):1082–1090

[139] Yu X, Xu L, Bi LY. Spinal navigation with intra-operative 3D-imaging modality in lumbar pedicle screw fixation. Zhonghua Yi Xue Za Zhi. 2008; 88(27):1905–1908

[140] Dea N, Fisher CG, Batke J, et al. Economic evaluation comparing intraoperative cone beam CT-based navigation and conventional fluoroscopy for the placement of spinal pedicle screws: a patient-level data cost-effectiveness analysis. Spine J. 2016; 16(1):23–31

[141] Arand M, Hartwig E, Kinzl L, Gebhard F. Spinal navigation in tumor surgery of the thoracic spine: first clinical results. Clin Orthop Relat Res. 2002(399):211–218

[142] Itshayek E, Yamada J, Bilsky M, et al. Timing of surgery and radiotherapy in the management of metastatic spine disease: a systematic review. Int J Oncol. 2010; 36(3):533–544

[143] Nevzati E, Marbacher S, Soleman J, et al. Accuracy of pedicle screw placement in the thoracic and lumbosacral spine using a conventional intraoperative fluoroscopy-guided technique: a national neurosurgical education and training center analysis of 1236 consecutive screws. World Neurosurg. 2014; 82(5):866–871.e1, 2

[144] Gebhard F, Kinzl L, Hartwig E, Arand M. Navigation von tumoren und metastasen im bereich der thorakolumbalen wirbelsäule. Unfallchirurg. 2003; 106(11):949–955

[145] Bandiera S, Ghermandi R, Gasbarrini A, Barbanti Bròdano G, Colangeli S, Boriani S. Navigation-assisted surgery for tumors of the spine. Eur Spine J. 2013; 22 Suppl 6:S919–S924

[146] Nasser R, Drazin D, Nakhla J, et al. Resection of spinal column tumors utilizing image-guided navigation: a multicenter analysis. Neurosurg Focus. 2016; 41(2):E15

[147] Rajasekaran S, Kamath V, Shetty AP. Intraoperative Iso-C three-dimensional navigation in excision of spinal osteoid osteomas. Spine. 2008; 33(1):E25–E29

[148] Van Royen BJ, Baayen JC, Pijpers R, Noske DP, Schakenraad D, Wuisman PI. Osteoid osteoma of the spine: a novel technique using combined computer-assisted and gamma probe-guided high-speed intralesional drill excision. Spine. 2005; 30(3):369–373

[149] Neo M, Asato R, Fujibayashi S, Ito H, Takemoto M, Nakamura T. Navigated anterior approach to the upper cervical spine after occipitocervical fusion. Spine. 2009; 34(22):E800–E805

[150] Jin B, Su YB, Zhao JZ. Three-dimensional fluoroscopy-based navigation for the pedicle screw placement in patients with primary invasive spinal tumors. Chin Med J (Engl). 2016; 129(21):2552–2558

18 Navigated Pelvic Fixation

Haruki Funao, Brian J. Neuman, and Khaled M. Kebaish

Abstract:
Pelvic fixation serves as a rigid distal foundation in various spinal surgeries in the lumbosacral spine, such as spinal deformity, pseudarthrosis, tumor, and infections. In these settings, a secure distal foundation with pelvic instrumentation is critical for maintaining correction and enhancing fusion rates, particularly in spinal deformity requiring long spinal constructs to the sacrum. Iliac screws and S2 alar–iliac screws are the most commonly used with high fusion rates. However, serious complications with pelvic fixation can occur such as neurologic, vascular, or bowel injuries due to the misplacement of pelvic screws. Pelvic screws can be placed with freehand technique or image guidance using either intraoperative fluoroscopy or computed tomography (CT)-based navigation. CT-based navigation can provide three-dimensional (3D) visualization of anatomy not clearly evident through surgical exposure alone. Other advantages include real-time 3D visualization of the screw trajectories and reduction of intraoperative fluoroscopy usage. In the setting of spinal deformity, this may be particularly advantageous, as unusual lumbosacral morphology can make screw insertion challenging. CT navigated pelvic fixation can also make minimally invasive pelvic screw insertion safer and easier without exposing anatomical landmarks. In our review, we describe the navigated pelvic fixation techniques.

Keywords: pelvic fixation, iliac screw, S2 alar–iliac screw, fluoroscopy, navigation

18.1 Introduction

Pelvic fixation can serve as a rigid distal foundation in various spinal surgeries in the lumbosacral spine, such as cases of spinal deformity, pseudarthrosis, tumor, and infections.[1,2,3,4] The sacrum is composed of mostly cancellous bone; thus, S1 screws alone may not achieve adequate fixation, especially in patients with osteoporosis. Secure distal foundation with pelvic instrumentation is critical for maintaining correction and enhancing fusion rates particularly in spinal deformity requiring long spinal constructs to the sacrum with high rates of pseudarthrosis.[5,6] Sacropelvic fixation helps resist the strong flexion moments and cantilever forces present at the lumbosacral junction, preventing fixation failures.

To date, various pelvic fixation techniques have been developed. Allen and Ferguson reported Galveston iliac fixation with advantages of an anchor in the ilium to resist flexion bending moment.[7] Iliac screws and S2 alar–iliac screws are most currently used with high fusion rates.[2,8] McCord et al described the concept of a "lumbosacral pivot point" (▶ Fig. 18.1), a point located at the lumbosacral joint at the intersection of the middle osteoligamentous column and the lumbosacral intervertebral disk, and demonstrated that iliac screws, which cross this point, had a biomechanical advantage at resisting flexion

moments with an improved pullout over the Galveston technique.[9] Accordingly, the pelvic screws should terminate anterior to the pivot point increasing the pullout strength and decreasing the strain on the S1 pedicle screws, reportedly leading to higher fusion rates across the lumbosacral junction. Although iliac screws have secure distal foundation, drawbacks include extensive soft-tissue dissection around the posterior-superior iliac spine and instrumentation prominence. Recently, the S2 alar–iliac technique has been developed for both adults and children requiring pelvic fixation, with the benefits of less soft-tissue disruption, low-profile instrumentation, and in-line rod connection to the proximal constructs[2] (▶ Fig. 18.2). To date, pelvic screws have been placed with freehand technique or image guidance using either intraoperative fluoroscopy or CT-based navigation. The misplacement of pelvic screws can lead to serious complications such as neurologic, vascular, or bowel injuries. Navigated pelvic screw placement can be beneficial when anatomy is not clearly evident.

18.2 Navigated Pelvic Fixation

Inadequate screw length due to a violation of the outer cortex of the ileum or other screw malpositioning, which fails to cross the aforementioned pivot point, can lead to screw failure, as the biomechanical advantages described earlier may not be achieved. Furthermore, serious complications in pelvic screw insertion, such as neurologic, vascular, or bowel injuries, can occur with misplaced pelvic screws that breach the inner or outer cortex of the ileum, acetabulum, or sciatic notch.[10,11,12] Lack of adequate visualization or lack of familiarity with pelvic configuration can be the cause of some of these complications. Several techniques have been reported to reduce the risk of pelvic screw misplacement, including lateral soft-tissue dissection of the ilium to palpate the sciatic notch, using intraoperative fluoroscopy,[13] and CT-based navigation[14,15,16] (▶ Fig. 18.3). Image guidance may provide surgeons more information than surgical exposure alone.

Although pelvic screws can be placed freehand or with image guidance,[14] in cases of complex lumbosacral anatomy, navigated techniques may be particularly useful. Although intraoperative fluoroscopy is useful, radiation exposure has been a source of consternation for many adopters.[17] In addition, fluoroscopy is limited as a two-dimensional representation of a 3D configuration of the pelvis.[18]

Intraoperative CT-based navigation is an innovative technology in spine surgery with the safety and ability to reduce radiation exposure to the surgeon and shorten surgical time with real-time 3D feedback, especially when visibility is suboptimal or anatomic abnormality is present.[19,20,21] Other benefits are the ability for accurate MIS placement and to measure ideal screw length and diameter. A meta-analysis of 3D navigated pedicle screws has demonstrated a screw accuracy rate of 95%.[22]

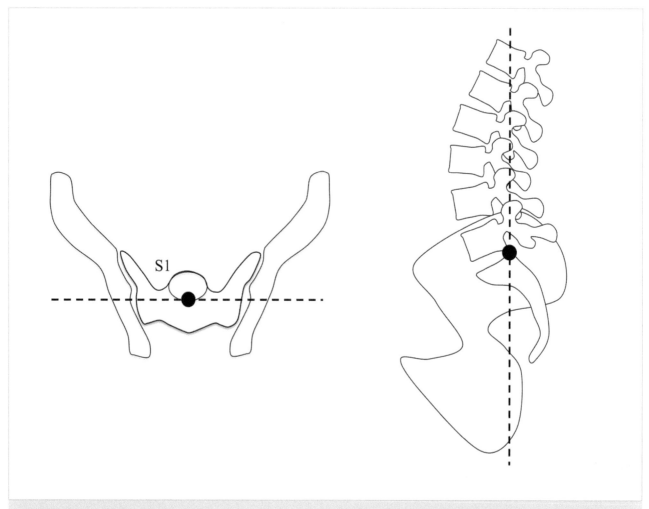

Fig. 18.1 The lumbosacral pivot point (*black dot*) at the lumbosacral joint at the intersection of the middle osteoligamentous column and the lumbosacral intervertebral disk. Pelvic screws should terminate anterior to the pivot point to prevent pullout of S1 pedicle screws with a biomechanical advantage at resisting flexion moments.

18.3 Surgical Technique

The patient is placed in a prone position, and an anatomic registration is performed by an acquired intraoperative CT image. The starting point of the S2 alar–iliac screw is usually located 2 to 4 mm inferior and 2 to 4 mm lateral to the S1 dorsal sacral foramen. The navigated probe was placed at the ideal starting point of S2 alar-iliac screw with the intended trajectory in 3D visualization on the computer screen (▶ Fig. 18.3a), and a burr is used to make a small hole of the starting point. The probe was angled toward the anteroinferior iliac spine; the angle is mostly between 20 and 40 degrees to the caudal and 40 to 50 degrees to the anterior. The trajectory of S2 alar screw was adjusted according to the image reconstructions. "Probe's eye," a view through the screw, enabled us to confirm the position of the navigated probe even in the narrowest part of the pelvis (▶ Fig. 18.3b). The trajectory can be confirmed and adjusted with real time 3D feedback. Then, a hole was tapped until it reached the SI joint, then an S2 alar screw was successfully placed (▶ Fig. 18.3c,d). A previous study recommended using the of S2 alar screw with a diameter of 8 to 10 mm and length

of 80 to 100 mm to avoid screw breakage or failure.[23] The screw on the other side was placed using the same technique. It is advantageous to reduce radiation exposure to surgeons, minimize soft-tissue dissection, and accurate screw placement without cortical breach of the sacrum and ilium.

18.4 Outcomes

Garrido and Wood reported iliac screw placements using intraoperative CT-based navigation.[14] They performed navigated iliac screw placements (range; a width of 7.5–8.5 mm and a length of 85–100 mm) for lumbopelvic fixation in patients with lumbosacral nonunions, a sacral U-type fracture, compromised revision sacral fixation, and as an adjunct to degenerative deformity with multilevel fusion using O-arm system (Medtronic, Inc.). A percutaneous reference frame was placed by minimal soft-tissue exposure without direct notch palpation. Iliac screw placement was within 2 cm of the sciatic notch, and no screw violation was confirmed by intraoperative CT imaging. They concluded that intraoperative CT-based navigation

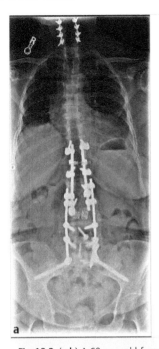
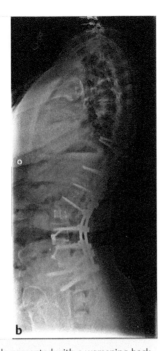

Fig. 18.2 (a,b) A 68-year-old female presented with a worsening back pain with a history of multiple spine surgeries. She underwent a posterior spinal fusion from T10 to the pelvis with bilateral S2 alar–iliac screw fixation. No significant radiographic or clinical signs of distal junctional failure or nonunion were evident on her 1-year postoperative radiographs.

allowed accurate and safe placement of the iliac screws to within 2 cm of the sciatic notch, and radiation exposure could be reduced. In addition, less soft-tissue dissection without direct sciatic notch palpation was required.

Ray et al reported S2 alar–iliac screw placements using intraoperative CT-based navigation.[15] Eighteen patients who underwent posterior spinal fusion from T3–ilium to L4–ilium were included. All patients had computer-assisted stereotactic placement of S2 alar–iliac screws using O-arm system. A second intraoperative CT scan was obtained in all patients to evaluate the S2 alar–iliac screw placement. One patient required repositioning of one of the alar–iliac screws because of an apparent breach in the anterior cortex in the ilium with intraoperative confirmation of correct placement. In their case series, all screws were placed without any vascular or neurological complication. They concluded that S2 alar–iliac fixation was safely performed crossing the sacroiliac joint, choosing trajectory, and ensuring adequate screw length in patients with a variety of pathological conditions by 3D images.

Nottmeier et al also described S2 alar-iliac screw placements using intraoperative CT-based navigation.[16] Twenty patients underwent 32 S2 alar–iliac screw placements with no complications. Five screws penetrated the anterior cortex of the sacrum; however, no clinical consequence was noted. At final follow-up, 15 of 16 patients had achieved a solid fusion at the lumbosacral junction. They concluded that 3D image guidance allows for safe placement of large S2 alar screws that can provide additional biomechanical stability to lumbosacral constructs or

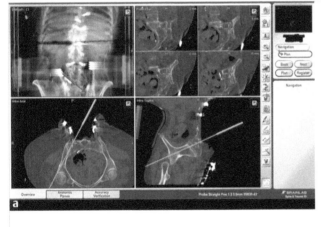
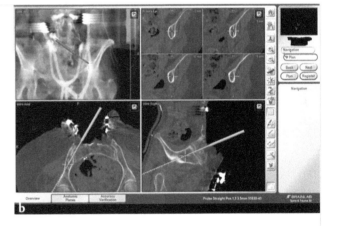
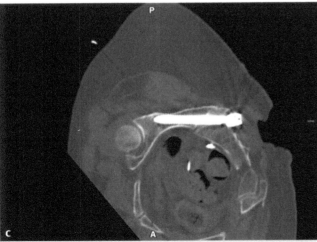
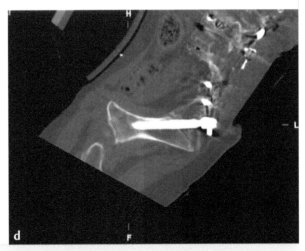

Fig. 18.3 Screen captures from the Brainlab images. The navigated probe is placed at the ideal starting point of S2 alar-iliac screw with the intended trajectory in 3D visualization on the computer screen (a). "Probe's eye," a view through the screw, enables confirmation of the position of the navigated probe even in the narrowest part of the pelvis (b). Screw length can additionally be measured from the three-dimensional images. An S2 alar-iliac screw successfully placed without cortical breach of the sacrum and pelvis (c,d).

serve as an alternate point of sacral fixation when S1 pedicle screws cannot be salvaged or placed.

18.5 Other Technologies

Recently, other technologies have been reported for pelvic screw placements. Jost et al reported inertial measurement units (IMUs) to reproduce the sagittal and axial tilt angles of the S2 alar–iliac screw trajectory.[24] IMUs are electronic systems that power motion-sensitive applications in smartphones or tablet computers. In their study, the IMUs' data output was processed to track the tilt angles of the IMU-mounted pedicle finder and screwdriver in the axial and sagittal planes. They stated that S2 alar–iliac screws can safely and accurately be placed by reproducing preoperatively defined trajectory tilt angles with IMU-equipped surgical tools. The accuracy of the IMU was confirmed to be within 0.5 degree in uniaxial slow motion and within 1 degree in multiaxial slow motion. The IMU-guided navigation is more simple and lightweight compared to 3D navigation. IMUs cost below US $100; thus, IMU guidance may offer an inexpensive and convenient tool for assisting with determining angles for S2 alar–iliac screw placement. IMUs are also clinically used to improve the surgical precision of total knee and hip replacement,[25] and percutaneous placement of lumbosacral pedicle screws.[26] However, the IMU-guided technique in its current version is not applicable to percutaneous screw placement. Potential errors may occur during the surgeon-controlled intraoperative zeroing of the device.

Guarino et al[27] reported utilization of rapid prototyping (RP) models for 13 cases of multiplane spinal or pelvic deformity. RP provides a 3D physical model derived from CT image. They found RP was useful for surgeons in preoperative planning, reference during surgery, communication with patients, and for increasing the safety of the procedure. RP models also led to a reduced surgical time in several surgeries to correct congenital scoliosis and kyphosis. They concluded that RP models could provide significant benefits for complex surgeries of the pediatric spine and pelvis in the areas of preoperative planning, intrasurgical navigation, communication with patients, and a reduced surgical time for congenital scoliosis and kyphosis.

18.6 Limitations of the Navigation System

Intraoperative CT-based navigation has many advantages, but its widespread adoption has been limited by cost and operative suite flow, including adequately trained staff and appropriately equipped and sized operating room suites. Other drawbacks include increased operative time initially during the inevitable learning curve, registration time for patient positioning and operative instruments, and registration inaccuracies if the dynamic reference array is shifted after referencing or is attached too far from the point of interest. Complete reliance on a navigated system is not recommended and a surgeon should always feel comfortable with a freehand technique if needed and have a thorough understanding of surgical anatomy. Lastly, although radiation exposure to the surgical team can be mitigated with navigation, radiation dosage to the patient may

actually be even more than with standard techniques as multiple preoperative and intraoperative CT scans may be used. Ultimately, further high-quality studies are needed before widespread adoption of navigated techniques.

18.7 Conclusion

Iliac screws and S2 alar–iliac screws are the most commonly used for sacropelvic fixation with a high fusion rate; however, serious complications can occur including neurologic, vascular, or bowel injuries due to the misplacement of the screws. These complications may be attributed to the lack of adequate visualization or surgeons' familiarity with pelvic configuration. To date, several techniques of navigated pelvic fixation have been reported. CT-based navigation has several advantages such as 3D visualization of the screw trajectories and reduction of intraoperative radiation exposure. However, there are some limitations in CT-based navigation, and few studies were reported. Further investigation is required, and new technologies for navigation and robotic surgeries will also be demanded in the future.

References

[1] Farcy JP, Rawlins BA, Glassman SD. Technique and results of fixation to the sacrum with iliosacral screws. Spine. 1992; 17(6) Suppl:S190–S195

[2] Chang TL, Sponseller PD, Kebaish KM, Fishman EK. Low profile pelvic fixation: anatomic parameters for sacral alar-iliac fixation versus traditional iliac fixation. Spine. 2009; 34(5):436–440

[3] Martin CT, Witham TF, Kebaish KM. Sacropelvic fixation: two case reports of a new percutaneous technique. Spine. 2011; 36(9):E618–E621

[4] Funao H, Kebaish KM, Isogai N, Koyanagi T, Matsumoto M, Ishii K. Utilization of a technique of percutaneous S2-alar-iliac fixation in immunocompromised patients with spondylodiscitis. World Neurosurg. 2017; 97:757.e11–757.e18

[5] Kostuik JP, Musha Y. Fusion to the sacrum in adult idiopathic scoliosis using C-D instrumentation (1986–1990). Paper presented at the Scoliosis Research Society Annual meeting: Portland, OR, USA; 1994

[6] Boachie-Adjei O, Dendrinos GK, Ogilvie JW, Bradford DS. Management of adult spinal deformity with combined anterior-posterior arthrodesis and Luque-Galveston instrumentation. J Spinal Disord. 1991; 4(2):131–141

[7] Allen BL, Jr, Ferguson RL. The Galveston technique for L rod instrumentation of the scoliotic spine. Spine. 1982; 7(3):276–284

[8] Kuklo TR, Bridwell KH, Lewis SJ, et al. Minimum 2-year analysis of sacropelvic fixation and L5-S1 fusion using S1 and iliac screws. Spine. 2001; 26(18):1976–1983

[9] McCord DH, Cunningham BW, Shono Y, Myers JJ, McAfee PC. Biomechanical analysis of lumbosacral fixation. Spine. 1992; 17(8) Suppl:S235–S243

[10] Kasten MD, Rao LA, Priest B. Long-term results of iliac wing fixation below extensive fusions in ambulatory adult patients with spinal disorders. J Spinal Disord Tech. 2010; 23(7):e37–e42

[11] Miller F, Moseley C, Koreska J. Pelvic anatomy relative to lumbosacral instrumentation. J Spinal Disord. 1990; 3(2):169–173

[12] Altman DT, Jones CB, Routt ML, Jr. Superior gluteal artery injury during iliosacral screw placement. J Orthop Trauma. 1999; 13(3):220–227

[13] Gressot LV, Patel AJ, Hwang SW, Fulkerson DH, Jea A. Iliac screw placement in neuromuscular scoliosis using anatomical landmarks and uniplanar anteroposterior fluoroscopic imaging with postoperative CT confirmation. J Neurosurg Pediatr. 2014; 13(1):54–61

[14] Garrido BJ, Wood KE. Navigated placement of iliac bolts: description of a new technique. Spine J. 2011; 11(4):331–335

[15] Ray WZ, Ravindra VM, Schmidt MH, Dailey AT. Stereotactic navigation with the O-arm for placement of S-2 alar iliac screws in pelvic lumbar fixation. J Neurosurg Spine. 2013; 18(5):490–495

[16] Nottmeier EW, Pirris SM, Balseiro S, Fenton D. Three-dimensional image-guided placement of S2 alar screws to adjunct or salvage lumbosacral fixation. Spine J. 2010; 10(7):595–601

[17] Funao H, Ishii K, Momoshima S, et al. Surgeons' exposure to radiation in single- and multi-level minimally invasive transforaminal lumbar interbody fusion; a prospective study. PLoS One. 2014; 9(4):e95233

[18] Wang MY, Ludwig SC, Anderson DG, Mummaneni PV. Percutaneous iliac screw placement: description of a new minimally invasive technique. Neurosurg Focus. 2008; 25(2):E17

[19] Rajasekaran S, Vidyadhara S, Ramesh P, Shetty AP. Randomized clinical study to compare the accuracy of navigated and non-navigated thoracic pedicle screws in deformity correction surgeries. Spine. 2007; 32(2):E56–E64

[20] Best NM, Sasso RC, Garrido BJ. Computer-assisted spinal navigation using a percutaneous dynamic reference frame for posterior fusions of the lumbar spine. Am J Orthop. 2009; 38(8):387–391

[21] Smith HE, Welsch MD, Sasso RC, Vaccaro AR. Comparison of radiation exposure in lumbar pedicle screw placement with fluoroscopy vs computer-assisted image guidance with intraoperative three-dimensional imaging. J Spinal Cord Med. 2008; 31(5):532–537

[22] Kosmopoulos V, Schizas C. Pedicle screw placement accuracy: a meta-analysis. Spine. 2007; 32(3):E111–E120

[23] Strike S, Hassanzadeh H, Naef F, Sponseller PD, Kebaish KM. Sacro-pelvic fixation using the S2 alar-iliac (S2AI) screws in adult deformity surgery: a prospective study with minimum five-year follow-up. Presented at Scoliosis Research Society 48th Annual Meeting and Course 2013; Lyon, France

[24] Jost GF, Walti J, Mariani L, Cattin P. A novel approach to navigated implantation of S-2 alar iliac screws using inertial measurement units. J Neurosurg Spine. 2016; 24(3):447–453

[25] Nam D, Weeks KD, Reinhardt KR, Nawabi DH, Cross MB, Mayman DJ. Accelerometer-based, portable navigation vs imageless, large-console computer-assisted navigation in total knee arthroplasty: a comparison of radiographic results. J Arthroplasty. 2013; 28(2):255–261

[26] Idler C, Rolfe KW, Gorek JE. Accuracy of percutaneous lumbar pedicle screw placement using the oblique or "owl's-eye" view and novel guidance technology. J Neurosurg Spine. 2010; 13(4):509–515

[27] Guarino J, Tennyson S, McCain G, Bond L, Shea K, King H. Rapid prototyping technology for surgeries of the pediatric spine and pelvis: benefits analysis. J Pediatr Orthop. 2007; 27(8):955–960

19 Navigated Sacroiliac Joint Fusion

Wesley H. Bronson and Joshua E. Heller

Abstract:

Navigated sacroiliac joint (SIJ) fusion has emerged as a novel method of safely and reliably relieving SIJ pain. Recently the SIJ has garnered increased attention as a common source of low back pain. Minimally invasive sacroiliac joint (MIS SIJ) fusion has emerged as an effective and durable procedure, providing lasting relief to patients suffering from sacroiliitis and SIJ dysfunction. While multiple techniques exist, minimally invasive strategies using fluoroscopy to safely place fusion implants and or instrumentation across the SIJ joint is now common practice. The application of 3-D navigation technology to this procedure has enabled surgeons to effectively perform MIS SIJ fusion safely in instances of abnormal (dysmorphic or transitional) SI anatomy as well as decrease occupational exposure to radiation for themselves and OR staff. In this chapter we describe the indications, technique, and preliminary outcomes of navigated SIJ fusion. We also provide case examples to highlight its utility in complicated scenarios.

Keywords: sacroiliac joint, sacroiliitis, sacroiliac joint dysfunction, sacral dysmorphism, minimally invasive surgery, sacroiliac fusion

19.1 Introduction

The sacroiliac joint (SIJ) has recently gained increased attention as a common source of low back pain. In a study of 200 patients presenting to a spine clinic with low back pain, only 65% of patients were found to have pain originating from the spine alone, while 5% had pain coming from the SIJ and 15% had pain from both the SIJ and the spine.[1] Causes of SIJ pain and dysfunction include trauma, osteoarthritis, inflammatory arthritis, infection, and tumors. Degeneration of the SIJ following lumbosacral spinal fusion is also very common.[2] In fact, up to 75% of patients develop SIJ degeneration within 5 years following lumbar fusion.[3]

The burden of SIJ pathology on patients' outcomes is also significant. In a recent analysis, SIJ pain was considered to be as debilitating as other common orthopaedic conditions, including hip and knee osteoarthritis, spinal stenosis, and spondylolisthesis.[4] Additionally, the economic burden of the care for these patients is also significant. Nonoperative management can cost as much as $5,259 per patient per year, with the cost increasing to as much as $30,000 in those with SIJ dysfunction following lumbar spine fusion. The 5-year estimated cost to Medicare beneficiaries is $270 million, with a 3-year cost of $1.6 billion per 100,000 commercial covered lives.[5,6]

Initial treatment for SIJ pathology consists of nonoperative modalities including physical therapy, nonsteroidal anti-inflammatory drugs and pain medications, intra-articular injections, and radiofrequency ablation. Unfortunately, there is little evidence that these nonoperative modalities provide long-lasting relief of SIJ-mediated pain. The only exception to this is radiofrequency ablation of the sacral nerve root lateral branches, which has shown some promise in the short term for providing relief of pain, lasting up to 12 months in some cases.[7,8,9]

While SIJ fusion was initially performed via an open approach, the surgeries were fraught with complications and approach-related morbidity, as well as poor patient-reported outcomes.[10,11,12] Currently, the standard of care for SIJ fusion includes a minimally invasive approach to the SIJ either posteriorly or laterally, with placement of bone or one of several Food and Drug Administration (FDA)-approved porous metal implants to provide stability and bone ingrowth. Our preferred technique is a laterally based approach with placement of three triangular titanium implants. Most surgeons perform the surgery though a minimally invasive approach using fluoroscopic views of the pelvis and sacrum. Now, however, with the use of intraoperative CT scan combined with navigation technology, the same procedure can be performed with increased accuracy in a minimally invasive fashion without the need for intraoperative fluoroscopy.

19.2 Indications

The indications for MIS SIJ fusion include pain attributable to SIJ dysfunction that impacts quality of life and that has failed at least 6 months of nonoperative treatment. The surgeon must perform a thorough history and physical exam to ensure that the pain is not related to another source. SIJ pain should be confirmed with at least three physical examination maneuvers that focus on the SIJ in particular. Pain relief following intra-articular injection is a good prognostic sign that the SIJ is the source of the pain.

While there is no absolute indication for *navigated* SIJ fusion as compared to fluoroscopy-guided techniques, there are several circumstances in which it can be beneficial. The most important of these are in patients with sacral dysmorphism, in whom abnormal sacral morphology may complicate safe implant placement. Radiographically, patients with dysmorphic sacral anatomy can be identified by multiple features, including having the superior aspect of the iliac crests at the level of the L5–S1 disk space, the presence of irregular and large sacral foramen, upper sacral mammillary processes, residual sacral disk spaces, and an acute alar slope that is not collinear with the iliac cortical density on the sacral lateral view. In these patients, the steeper, acute alar slope provides less bone in which to place implants. Additionally, the anterior aspect of the sacrum may also have a deeper groove which contains the L5 nerve root, further restricting the safe osseous pathway across the SIJ into the sacrum. While previously considered to be rare, sacral dysmorphism and upper sacral abnormalities are actually quite common, and some degree of abnormal anatomy is present in about 50% of the population.[13,14] Navigation in these cases permits safe and easy passage of implants in pathways unique to the patient morphology.

Navigated techniques need not be limited to only those patients with abnormal anatomy, for even those with normal anatomy may present challenges in the operating room. The traditional MIS technique relies on radiographic interpretation of the pelvic inlet, pelvic outlet, and sacral lateral views. Doing so requires the surgeon not only to have an understanding of the anatomy and radiographs but also must be able to obtain these views intraoperatively. Studies have shown that while the anatomy is familiar to spine surgeons, it is not always well visualized.[15,16] Large patients or patients with significant amounts of bowel gas may make navigating radiographic trajectories difficult, as it limits the ability to visualize the sacral foramina. Three-dimensional (3D) navigation can circumvent the need to rely on low-quality C-arm images.

Finally, revision cases may be particularly challenging. New implants may need to be placed, and there is limited bone remaining for placement. Navigation in these instances can be helpful to maximize bone purchase in compromised anatomy (see case example 2 later in the chapter).

19.3 Technique

We perform the procedure prone on a Jackson spine table. A wide field is prepped, including as much of the lateral aspect of the hips as possible including the trochanters. First, a small incision is made over the posterior-superior iliac spine (PSIS), usually on the contralateral side, and a pin is placed into the ilium and attached to a reference array. The patient is then draped and a passed into the O-arm intraoperative spin. This generates a 3D CT scan with real-time feedback from the instruments.

A skin incision is marked laterally using a reference probe to determine the appropriate location. The reference probe is then used to determine the ideal trajectory for the first implant into S1. A guidewire is drilled through the ilium, across the SIJ, and into the sacrum with navigation. A soft-tissue dilator followed by tissue protector is placed over the guidewire, and the dilator is then removed. An appropriate-size implant is determined using the navigation to help choose the ideal implant size. The guidewire is overdrilled, the path is broached, and the first implant is placed. A parallel pin guide is used to then place a second guidewire below the first. However, the second guidewire can also be placed freehand using navigation if a better location is determined, especially in cases of abnormal anatomy. The second and third implants are placed using the same technique as the first. To double check that the navigation has resulted in appropriate implant placement, a postimplant intraoperative CT can be obtained. Alternatively, pelvic inlet, outlet, and lateral fluoroscopic views can be obtained to confirm the location of the implants.

The wound is irrigated and hemostasis is achieved if any obvious bleeding is encountered. The layers are closed with Vicryl for the deeper layers and Monocryl for the skin. Patients are given a period of 3 weeks of partial weight bearing and are then progressed to full weight bearing.

19.4 Outcomes

There is a paucity of published literature currently available that specifically analyzes the outcomes of patients following navigated MIS SIJ fusion. Kleck et al performed navigated SIJ fusion with placement of the iFuse implant (SI-Bone, San Jose, CA) using O-arm and StealthStation (Medtronic, Minneapolis, MN) navigation in 47 consecutive patients.[17] Preoperative average Oswestry Disability Index (ODI) was 23.5 compared to 16.2 at 1 year postoperatively. Scores on the Visual Analog Scale (VAS) averaged 6.3 preoperatively compared to 2.8 at 1 year. Two complications occurred due to pin breakage during the procedure, one of which was removed and the other was felt to be contained in bone and was left in place. All patients followed up beyond 1 year were considered to have stable implants and a solid fusion based on radiographic analysis.

Studies of patients following MIS SIJ fusion in general have demonstrated successful outcomes. Polly et al performed a randomized control trial of 148 patients with SIJ dysfunction, separating them into nonoperative or surgical arms with MIS SIJ fusion.[18] At 6 months, patients in the surgical arm exhibited statistically significant higher success rates as well as clinically important improvements in ODI. These improvements were maintained at 12 months, demonstrating the superiority of MIS SIJ fusion over nonoperative treatment. Vanaclocha et al performed a retrospective study of 137 patients who presented with SIJ pain who underwent either conservative management, SIJ denervation, or MIS SIJ fusion.[19] Patients had follow-up between 1 and 6 years. Those who underwent conservative management demonstrated no long-term improvement. However, patients in the SIJ fusion group had improvements in pain, disability, decrease in opioid usage, and good work status.

Several case series have also shown promising results. Duhon et al performed a multicenter prospective trial of 172 patients at 26 sites in the United States undergoing MIS SIJ fusion.[20] At 24 months, opioid usage decreased, and health-related quality-of-life measures improved (SF-36 and EQ-5D). Additionally, CT scans performed at 1 year demonstrated a 97% bone adherence to at least two implants. A study of 144 patients undergoing MIS SIJ fusion followed patients for up to 16 months.[21] They noted a mean operative time of only 73 minutes, minimal blood loss, and hospital length of stay less than 1 day. VAS scores improved by 6 points, clinical benefit was achieved in over 90% of patients, and 96% said they would have the surgery again.

The use of navigation for MIS SI fusion has several advantages demonstrated in the literature. A randomized multicenter study looking at percutaneous sacroiliac screw placement found that 3D CT navigation demonstrates improved accuracy, especially in dysmorphic sacrum. The study analyzed 130 patients who had undergone percutaneous sacroiliac fixation for pelvic trauma. Fifty-eight patients underwent conventional screw placement using fluoroscopy, Eighteen patients underwent two-dimensional (2D) navigation using fluoroscopic images for reference, and 54 patients underwent 3D navigation using CT scan. A total of 109 patients were found to have a normal sacrum and 21 patients had a dysmorphic sacrum. Of the 21 patients, 37 screws were placed. Seven of 22 screws in the conventional group were misplaced, 2/3 screws were misplaced in the 2D navigation group, and 0 screws were misplaced in the 3D navigation group. Including the nondysmorphic sacrums, 3 of 18 patients had misplaced screws in the 2D group and 10 of 58 patients in the fluoroscopic group. No screws were misplaced in the 3D cohort. Thus, the use of 3D navigation appears to provide a safe method of placing iliosacral hardware, especially in dysmorphic anatomy. We believe these results translate to SIJ fusion techniques, as the corridors for hardware placement are nearly identical.

Using navigation during the procedure also has the potential to decrease radiation to the surgeon and operating room team, and potentially even the patient in cases of 2D navigation. The decrease in occupational radiation exposure using computer guidance has been well documented. Multiple studies of lumbar spine procedures have shown that physician doses are high, especially when standing on the ipsilateral side of the C-arm.[22, 23,24] These doses are effectively eliminated by removing the need for intraoperative fluoroscopy. In terms of pelvic surgery, multiple studies of sacroiliac screw placement have shown that 2D navigation use significantly reduces the effective radiation dose to the patient during the procedure, as well as eliminates surgeon radiation.[25,26] Peng et al, however, used intraoperative CT navigation to place sacroiliac screws.[27] They found that the screws were placed with high accuracy using the navigation, and the radiation dose was minimized for the surgeon. For the patient, however, the effective radiation dose was higher than for fluoroscopy-assisted SI screw placement.

19.5 Complications

Complications following MIS SIJ fusion are relatively uncommon. In a systematic review of the literature on SIJ fusion, Zaidi et al analyzed 299 patients who underwent MIS SIJ fusion.[28] The most common complications were new-onset facet joint pain (2.7%), trochanteric bursitis (2.3%), deep wound infection (1.7%), worsening back (1.7%), and knee pain (1.7%). Interestingly, radiculopathy was present in only 1% of patients. In contrast, we have found in our own patients that the most common complications are nerve pain related to implant position, which is now increasingly preventable using navigation. The one study mentioned previously by Kleck et al, which examined a cohort of patients undergoing navigated MIS SIJ fusion, had only two complications related to pin breakage.[17] There were no cases of neurologic injury, and all implants were placed successfully.

19.6 Case Examples

Case 1: This is a 37-year-old female with no past medical history who presented for evaluation of low back pain in the area around her left PSIS. Physical exam was positive for SIJ provocative tests. Injection into her left SIJ provided good, but temporary, relief of her pain. She had exhausted other nonoperative modalities including multiple rounds of physical therapy. She was indicated for a MIS left SIJ fusion (▸ Fig. 19.1). Immediately postoperatively in the PACU, she was endorsing significant new left lower extremity radiculopathy. CT scan demonstrated the proximal most implant was anterior to the ala, and likely contacting the L5 nerve root. Also note the abnormal ala, with likely dysmorphic features, as a standard lateral-medial trajectory cannot be accomplished given her anatomy (▸ Fig. 19.2). The patient was taken back to the operating room, and the proximal implant was removed. Her symptoms improved postoperatively and she did well clinically, with resolution of her left SIJ pain.

The patient presented to the clinic approximately 1.5 years postoperatively with right SIJ mediated pain, and she was indicated for a right SIJ fusion after exhausting nonoperative treatment. Given her abnormal anatomy discovered during the first case, she underwent a CT-navigated SIJ fusion with successful placement of three implants without complication. Note the posterior-anterior direction of the proximal implant to accommodate her anatomy (▸ Fig. 19.3). The use of navigation in this case permitted safe and accurate placement of all 3 implants.

Case 2: This is an 80-year-old female who had undergone a left MIS SIJ fusion at an outside institution several years prior. She initially did well, but had a recurrence of her left SIJ pain. Workup revealed a nonunion of her left SIJ, and CT scan even demonstrated one of her implants did not cross the SIJ (▸ Fig. 19.4). She failed nonoperative treatment and was indicated for a revision left SIJ fusion. Due to the presence of multiple implants, navigation was chosen to help with the limited

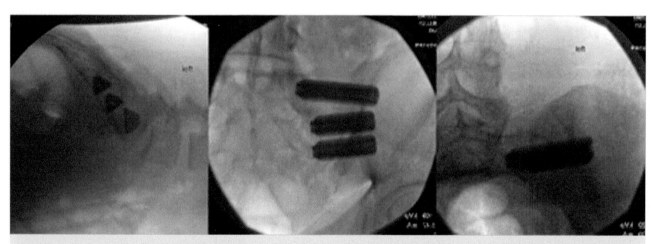

Fig. 19.1 Final intraoperative fluoroscopy lateral, outlet, and inlet views demonstrating placement of three implants across the left sacroiliac joint.

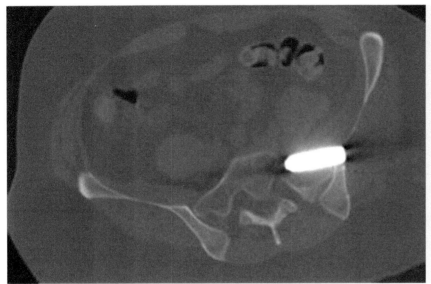

Fig. 19.2 Postoperative CT scan demonstrating anterior placement of the proximal implant with abnormal sacral anatomy.

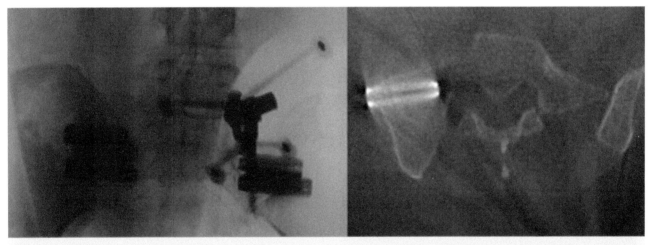

Fig. 19.3 Intraoperative radiograph showing three implants in the right sacroiliac joint and postoperative CT scan showing successful placement of proximal implant.

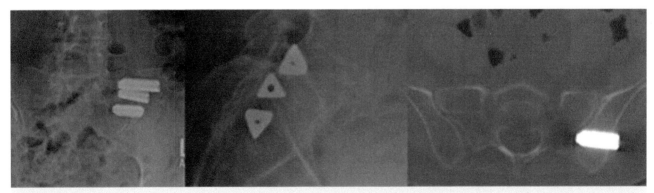

Fig. 19.4 Preoperative radiographs demonstrating dorsal placement of implants. CT scan shows one implant does not even cross the sacroiliac joint.

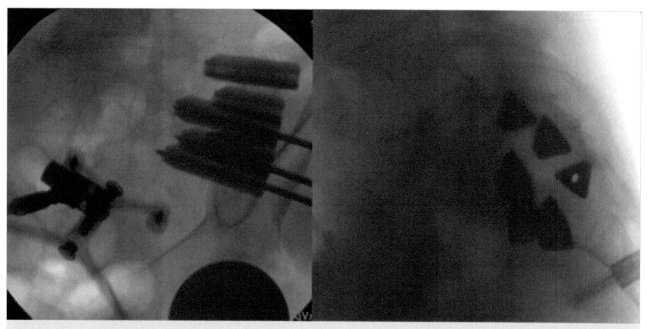

Fig. 19.5 Intraoperative anteroposterior and lateral radiographs demonstrating successful placement of three new additional implants.

available bone stock. Three additional implants were able to be placed ventral to her existing hardware (▶ Fig. 19.5). She did well postoperatively with near-complete elimination of her preoperative pain. This result would likely not have been possible without the use of navigation, as the new implants had little room for error given the presence of old hardware.

19.7 Conclusion

Navigated MIS SIJ fusion is a safe and reliable procedure for patients with SIJ-mediated pain. The current body of literature has demonstrated good long-term outcomes and low complication rates. While the fusion can be performed using intraoperative fluoroscopy, navigation offers several benefits. The surgeon and operating room staff are exposed to less radiation and implants can be optimally placed, especially in cases of abnormal anatomy.

References

[1] Sembrano JN, Polly DW, Jr. How often is low back pain not coming from the back? Spine. 2009; 34(1):E27–E32

[2] Katz V, Schofferman J, Reynolds J. The sacroiliac joint: a potential cause of pain after lumbar fusion to the sacrum. J Spinal Disord Tech. 2003; 16(1):96–99

[3] Ha KY, Lee JS, Kim KW. Degeneration of sacroiliac joint after instrumented lumbar or lumbosacral fusion: a prospective cohort study over five-year follow-up. Spine. 2008; 33(11):1192–1198

[4] Cher D, Polly D, Berven S. Sacroiliac joint pain: burden of disease. Med Devices (Auckl). 2014; 7(12):73–81

[5] Ackerman SJ, Polly DW, Jr, Knight T, Holt T, Cummings J. Management of sacroiliac joint disruption and degenerative sacroiliitis with nonoperative care is medical resource-intensive and costly in a United States commercial payer population. Clinicoecon Outcomes Res. 2014; 6(6):63–74

[6] Ackerman SJ, Polly DW, Jr, Knight T, Holt T, Cummings J, Jr. Nonoperative care to manage sacroiliac joint disruption and degenerative sacroiliitis: high costs

and medical resource utilization in the United States Medicare population. J Neurosurg Spine. 2014; 20(4):354–363

[7] Cohen SP, Hurley RW, Buckenmaier CC, III, Kurihara C, Morlando B, Dragovich A. Randomized placebo-controlled study evaluating lateral branch radiofrequency denervation for sacroiliac joint pain. Anesthesiology. 2008; 109(2):279–288

[8] Patel N, Gross A, Brown L, Gekht G. A randomized, placebo-controlled study to assess the efficacy of lateral branch neurotomy for chronic sacroiliac joint pain. Pain Med. 2012; 13(3):383–398

[9] Patel N. Twelve-month follow-up of a randomized trial assessing cooled radiofrequency denervation as a treatment for sacroiliac region pain. Pain Pract. 2016; 16(2):154–167

[10] Goldstein A, Phillips T, Sclafani SJ, et al. Early open reduction and internal fixation of the disrupted pelvic ring. J Trauma. 1986; 26(4):325–333

[11] Kellam JF, McMurtry RY, Paley D, Tile M. The unstable pelvic fracture. Operative treatment. Orthop Clin North Am. 1987; 18(1):25–41

[12] Painter CF. Excision of the os innominatum. Arthrodesis of the sacroiliac synchondrosis. Boston Med Surg J. 1908; 159(7):205–208

[13] Wu LP, Li YK, Li YM, Zhang YQ, Zhong SZ. Variable morphology of the sacrum in a Chinese population. Clin Anat. 2009; 22(5):619–626

[14] Gardner MJ, Morshed S, Nork SE, Ricci WM, Chip Routt ML, Jr. Quantification of the upper and second sacral segment safe zones in normal and dysmorphic sacra. J Orthop Trauma. 2010; 24(10):622–629

[15] Routt ML, Jr, Simonian PT, Mills WJ. Iliosacral screw fixation: early complications of the percutaneous technique. J Orthop Trauma. 1997; 11(8):584–589

[16] Tonetti J, Carrat L, Lavalleé S, Pittet L, Merloz P, Chirossel JP. Percutaneous iliosacral screw placement using image guided techniques. Clin Orthop Relat Res. 1998(354):103–110

[17] Kleck CJ, Perry JM, Burger EL, Cain CM, Milligan K, Patel VV. Sacroiliac joint treatment personalized to individual patient anatomy using 3-dimensional navigation. Orthopedics. 2016; 39(2):89–94

[18] Polly DW, Cher DJ, Wine KD, et al. INSITE Study Group. Randomized controlled trial of minimally invasive sacroiliac joint fusion using triangular titanium implants vs nonsurgical management for sacroiliac joint dysfunction: 12-month outcomes. Neurosurgery. 2015; 77(5):674–690, discussion 690–691

[19] Vanaclocha V, Herrera JM, Sáiz-Sapena N, Rivera-Paz M, Verdú-López F. Minimally invasive sacroiliac joint fusion, radiofrequency denervation, and conservative management for sacroiliac joint pain: 6-year comparative case series. Neurosurgery. 2018; 82(1):48–55

[20] Duhon BS, Bitan F, Lockstadt H, Kovalsky D, Cher D, Hillen T, SIFI Study Group. Triangular titanium implants for minimally invasive sacroiliac joint fusion: 2-year follow-up from a prospective multicenter trial. Int J Spine Surg. 2016; 10(10):13

[21] Sachs D, Capobianco R, Cher D, et al. One-year outcomes after minimally invasive sacroiliac joint fusion with a series of triangular implants: a multicenter, patient-level analysis. Med Devices (Auckl). 2014; 7(7):299–304

[22] Gebhard FT, Kraus MD, Schneider E, Liener UC, Kinzl L, Arand M. Does computer-assisted spine surgery reduce intraoperative radiation doses? Spine. 2006; 31(17):2024–2027, discussion 2028

[23] Izadpanah K, Konrad G, Südkamp NP, Oberst M. Computer navigation in balloon kyphoplasty reduces the intraoperative radiation exposure. Spine. 2009; 34(12):1325–1329

[24] Kim CW, Lee YP, Taylor W, Oygar A, Kim WK. Use of navigation-assisted fluoroscopy to decrease radiation exposure during minimally invasive spine surgery. Spine J. 2008; 8(4):584–590

[25] Schep NW, Haverlag R, van Vugt AB. Computer-assisted versus conventional surgery for insertion of 96 cannulated iliosacral screws in patients with postpartum pelvic pain. J Trauma. 2004; 57(6):1299–1302

[26] Zwingmann J, Konrad G, Kotter E, Südkamp NP, Oberst M. Computer-navigated iliosacral screw insertion reduces malposition rate and radiation exposure. Clin Orthop Relat Res. 2009; 467(7):1833–1838

[27] Peng KT, Li YY, Hsu WH, et al. Intraoperative computed tomography with integrated navigation in percutaneous iliosacral screwing. Injury. 2013; 44 (2):203–208

[28] Zaidi HA, Montoure AJ, Dickman CA. Surgical and clinical efficacy of sacroiliac joint fusion: a systematic review of the literature. J Neurosurg Spine. 2015; 23(1):59–66

20 Navigation Balloon Kyphoplasty

Richard M. McEntee, Kaitlyn Votta, and I. David Kaye

Abstract:

Kyphoplasty is a commonly performed procedure designed to treat vertebral compression fractures, and seeks to manage pain, decrease spinal deformity, reduce fracture recurrence, and improve quality of life. Kyphoplasty is now being performed utilizing guided navigation systems and has supplanted the traditional fluoroscopic image-guided procedure. Navigated kyphoplasty reduces radiation exposure, and allows surgeons to visualize real-time needle insertion into the pedicle during the procedure, helping to decrease the needle malposition rate. Kyphoplasty utilizing navigation has not been shown to pose any additional risks to the patient compared to traditional kyphoplasty with fluoroscopic guidance.

Keywords: kyphoplasty, navigation, compression fracture, fluoroscopy, vertebral augmentation

20.1 Introduction

Kyphoplasty is a vertebral augmentation procedure designed to treat vertebral compression fractures. The goal of the procedure is to reduce pain, as well as reduce postfracture kyphosis. Kyphoplasty was first performed in 1998 as a minimally invasive procedure to reduce vertebral body fractures.[1] The American Academy of Orthopaedic Surgeons 2010 guidelines indicate that kyphoplasty is currently "an option for patients who present with an osteoporotic spinal compression fracture on imaging with correlating clinical signs and symptoms, and who are neurologically intact."[2]

Vertebral compression fractures commonly result from either trauma (even minor) in the setting of osteoporosis[3,4,5] or pathologic fracture in the setting of malignancy.[3,6,7,8] These types of fractures are associated with spinal deformity, increased pain, compromised pulmonary function, decreased quality of life, and increased mortality.[9,10,11,12] Kyphoplasty can effectively help manage pain in this setting and potentially improve sagittal alignment.[13,14]

Surgical management of compression fractures may involve vertebral augmentation via either vertebroplasty or kyphoplasty. Both surgical procedures have been shown to reduce pain compared to nonsurgical management.[15] While the procedures are similar, kyphoplasty specifically seeks to remediate the resulting kyphosis from vertebral compression.[16] The kyphoplasty procedure involves percutaneous injection of bone cement into a fractured vertebrae under image guidance. Prior to cement injection, inflatable bone tamps are placed into the vertebral body to create a negative pressure cavity which is then filled with cement, reducing the fracture and improving the kyphotic deformity. The procedure can be performed in an outpatient setting that is equipped with proper imagine guidance technology.[17]

20.2 Navigation with Kyphoplasty

Recently, some have supplanted traditional fluoroscopic image-guided kyphoplasty with navigated kyphoplasty. This technique has allowed for more precise needle placement and decreased radiation exposure for both the patient and the surgeon.[1,18,19] Navigation is a relatively new tool that was developed in the hope of creating safer and less-invasive procedures across multiple different fields.[20] Some of the most pertinent applications come in the fields of neurosurgery, otolaryngology, and orthopedics. In these cases, the navigational setup creates a digital rendering of the exact position and orientation of surgical instruments in reference to the patient's anatomy. Some procedures, particularly neurosurgeries, require preoperative MRI scans that are then correlated to intraoperative scans of the patient in his or her current position. Other procedures, mostly orthopedic, do not require special preoperative scans, since the software creates an individualized model of the patient's anatomy based on defined bony landmarks during the intraoperative scans. For both types of surgery, the surgeons receive relevant information throughout the procedure from the navigation system.[20] Use of navigation systems in spine surgery has demonstrated more accurate crew placement, fewer complications, and an overall greater safety profile than traditional fluoroscopic techniques and can lead to increased confidence by the surgeons in their ability to perform the procedures.[20,21,22]

20.3 Technique

To perform a computer-navigated balloon kyphoplasty, the patient is first placed in the prone position on the operating table and the patient is prepped in the usual sterile manner. Surgical instruments may be calibrated during anesthesia and preparation. The vertebral fractures are localized using fluoroscopy in the lateral and anterior–posterior views. An incision is made one vertebral level rostral to the fractured vertebrae, and a reference base is fixed to this spinous process (at the level above the fracture)[1] which allows registration of the advanced 3D image (either CT or fluoroscopically based) (▶ Fig. 20.1). We have used the Siremobil Iso-C3D (Siemens Medical Solutions, Erlangen, Germany), a fluoroscopically based model, to obtain intraoperative multiple axial-plane tomography, which takes an average time of 2 minutes.[1] The images are automatically registered to a navigation platform such as the VectorVisionENT (Brainlab, Munich, Germany) to process the data.[1] This 3D map is then registered to the precalibrated instruments allowing stereotactic guidance of instrumentation (▶ Fig. 20.2). For kyphoplasty, a Jamshidi needle can be calibrated with the system. The needle is then guided into the posterior vertebral column using real-time guidance of the navigation system (▶ Fig. 20.3). By using this method, the need for repetitive

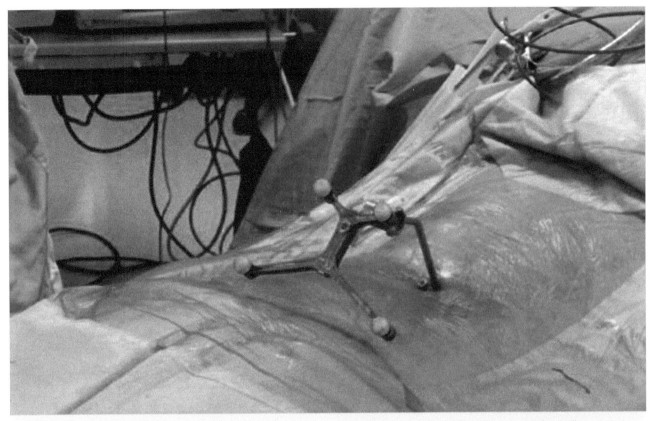

Fig. 20.1 Dissection performed one level cranially, and reference frame is attached to spinous process of vertebrae one level cranially.

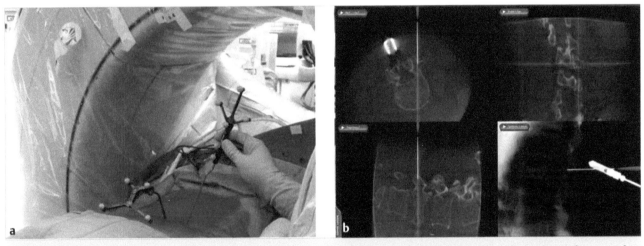

Fig. 20.2 After O-arm spin, localization of appropriate start point is identified with probe and incision then made to allow in line performance of kyphoplasty.

fluoroscopy during this entry step to ensure correct positioning has essentially been eliminated. A guide pin as well as a blunt dissector is then inserted into the posterior third of the fractured vertebral body. A 3-mm working cannula is placed over the blunt dissector into the vertebral body, so that the dissector can be removed and replaced with a 3-mm drill. Drilling into the bone creates a narrow space through which to insert the inflatable bone tamp. An angioplasty injection device equipped

with a pressure monitor is connected to the bone tamp. The drill is removed and the bone tamp inserted into the anterior-most part of the predrilled channel, where it is slowly inflated. Bone cement is then slowly injected into the cavity using a 3-mm filler device, and fluoroscopic visualization or O-arm image acquisition can then be used to ensure adequate filling (▶ Fig. 20.4). After the injection is complete, instruments are removed and the incision closed in a layered fashion.[1,16]

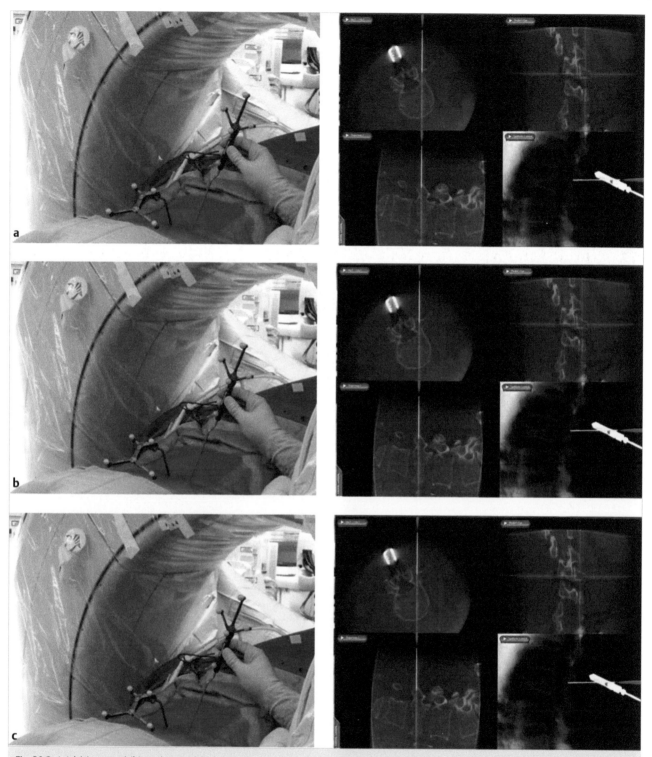

Fig. 20.3 Axial (**a**), sagittal (**b**), and coronal (**c**) localization of trajectory for placement of instruments through pedicle for planned kyphoplasty.

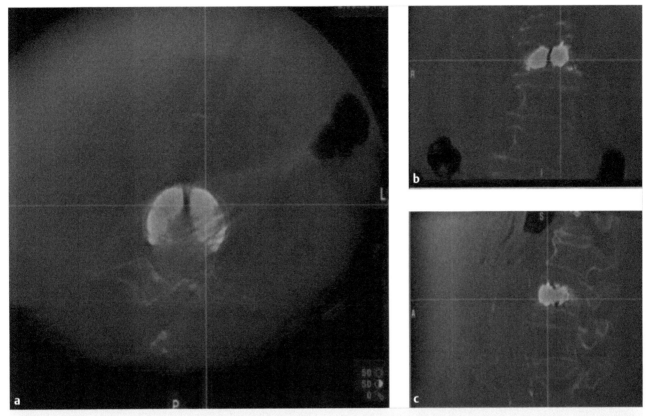

Fig. 20.4 Postprocedure O-arm spin demonstrating axial (**a**), sagittal (**b**), and coronal (**c**) reconstructions with improvement in vertebral body height and alignment and excellent cement fill.

20.4 Outcomes

In many cases, vertebral augmentation procedures are superior to nonsurgical management of vertebral body compression fractures.[15] Balloon kyphoplasty has been shown to provide greater pain relief, greater kyphosis reduction, and fewer fracture recurrences than nonoperative management.[5,15] Kyphoplasty has also been shown to be a safer and more efficacious treatment option than vertebroplasty for osteoporotic vertebral compression fractures.[23] Compared to vertebroplasty, kyphoplasty has been associated with a lower risk of cement extravasation and overall improved quality of life.[15]

Compared to traditional fluoroscopic-based kyphoplasty, navigated kyphoplasty has been shown to have a lower needle malposition rate.[18] A major advantage that navigation conveys to the surgeon is real-time needle insertion into the pedicle during the procedure. In addition to improved accuracy, navigated kyphoplasty has been shown to reduce radiation exposure to both the patient and the surgeon compared to nonnavigated kyphoplasty.[1]

20.5 Complications of Kyphoplasty

Although kyphoplasty is generally considered safe, several potential complications exist. Short-term complications include extravasation of cement from the injection site, which can be insignificant or can lead to devastating sequelae. Cases of pulmonary cement extravasation have led to reported neurologic injuries such as difficulty walking and intractable back pain, as well as cement pulmonary embolisms both symptomatic and asymptomatic.[24,25,26] Use of navigation has not been shown to decrease the historic rates of cement extravasation with traditional fluoroscopic techniques (which only seems to be influenced by factors such as cement viscosity at time of injection, cement volume, and fracture pattern).[18]

Of the two vertebral augmentation procedures, there is a lower rate of cement extravasation in balloon kyphoplasty than with vertebroplasty, with one systematic review by Hulme et al showing rates up to 41% in vertebroplasty, and only 9% in kyphoplasty.[27,28] Cement extravasation can result in patients experiencing pain and damage to spinal cord and nerve roots. Cases of postoperative paraparesis, radiculopathy, and hematoma formation have been described related to cement extravasation.[29,30] Sembrano et al reported a case of nerve root compression during a navigation-guided kyphoplasty procedure, although it is unclear the role navigation played in the development of the complication.[18] Rarely, patients have also experienced life-threatening infectious complications as a result of the surgery.[31] Possible long-term complications include risk for new fracture in adjacent vertebra, and bone resorption acceleration due to a reaction from the cement, although more data is needed to further elucidate these complications.[24] Compared to traditional balloon kyphoplasty with fluoroscopic guidance, it is generally accepted that the use of navigation poses no additional risk.[27,28]

References

[1] Izadpanah K, Konrad G, Südkamp NP, Oberst M. Computer navigation in balloon kyphoplasty reduces the intraoperative radiation exposure. Spine. 2009; 34(12):1325–1329

[2] AAOS Guidelines on the treatment of osteoporotic spinal compression fractures: summary of recommendations. Available at: http://www.aaos.org/research/guidelines/SCFsummary.pdf. Accessed June 27, 2019

[3] Ledlie JT, Renfro MB. Kyphoplasty treatment of vertebral fractures: 2-year outcomes show sustained benefits. Spine. 2006; 31(1):57–64

[4] Schmelzer-Schmied N, Cartens C, Meeder PJ, Dafonseca K. Comparison of kyphoplasty with use of a calcium phosphate cement and non-operative therapy in patients with traumatic non-osteoporotic vertebral fractures. Eur Spine J. 2009; 18(5):624–629

[5] Lieberman IH, Dudeney S, Reinhardt MK, Bell G. Initial outcome and efficacy of "kyphoplasty" in the treatment of painful osteoporotic vertebral compression fractures. Spine. 2001; 26(14):1631–1638

[6] Dudeney S, Lieberman IH, Reinhardt MK, Hussein M. Kyphoplasty in the treatment of osteolytic vertebral compression fractures as a result of multiple myeloma. J Clin Oncol. 2002; 20(9):2382–2387

[7] Fourney DR, Schomer DF, Nader R, et al. Percutaneous vertebroplasty and kyphoplasty for painful vertebral body fractures in cancer patients. J Neurosurg. 2003; 98(1) Suppl:21–30

[8] Lane JM, Hong R, Koob J, et al. Kyphoplasty enhances function and structural alignment in multiple myeloma. Clin Orthop Relat Res. 2004(426):49–53

[9] Lyles KW, Gold DT, Shipp KM, Pieper CF, Martinez S, Mulhausen PL. Association of osteoporotic vertebral compression fractures with impaired functional status. Am J Med. 1993; 94(6):595–601

[10] Kado DM, Duong T, Stone KL, et al. Incident vertebral fractures and mortality in older women: a prospective study. Osteoporos Int. 2003; 14(7):589–594

[11] Silverman SL. The clinical consequences of vertebral compression fracture. Bone. 1992; 13 Suppl 2:S27–S31

[12] Schlaich C, Minne HW, Bruckner T, et al. Reduced pulmonary function in patients with spinal osteoporotic fractures. Osteoporos Int. 1998; 8(3):261–267

[13] Yu CW, Hsieh MK, Chen LH, et al. Percutaneous balloon kyphoplasty for the treatment of vertebral compression fractures. BMC Surg. 2014; 14:3

[14] de Falco R, Bocchetti A. Balloon kyphoplasty for pure traumatic thoracolumbar fractures: retrospective analysis of 61 cases focusing on restoration of vertebral height. Eur Spine J. 2014; 23 Suppl 6:664–670

[15] Papanastassiou ID, Phillips FM, Van Meirhaeghe J, et al. Comparing effects of kyphoplasty, vertebroplasty, and non-surgical management in a systematic review of randomized and non-randomized controlled studies. Eur Spine J. 2012; 21(9):1826–1843

[16] Theodorou DJ, Theodorou SJ, Duncan TD, Garfin SR, Wong WH. Percutaneous balloon kyphoplasty for the correction of spinal deformity in painful vertebral body compression fractures. Clin Imaging. 2002; 26(1):1–5

[17] Wang H, Zhang Z, Liu Y, Jiang W. Percutaneous kyphoplasty for the treatment of very severe osteoporotic vertebral compression fractures with spinal canal compromise. J Orthop Surg Res. 2018; 13(1):13

[18] Sembrano JN, Yson SC, Polly DW, Jr, Ledonio CG, Nuckley DJ, Santos ER. Comparison of nonnavigated and 3-dimensional image-based computer navigated balloon kyphoplasty. Orthopedics. 2015; 38(1):17–23

[19] Schils F. O-arm guided balloon kyphoplasty: preliminary experience of 16 consecutive patients. Acta Neurochir Suppl (Wien). 2011; 109:175–178

[20] Mezger U, Jendrewski C, Bartels M. Navigation in surgery. Langenbecks Arch Surg. 2013; 398(4):501–514

[21] Enchev Y. Neuronavigation: geneology, reality, and prospects. Neurosurg Focus. 2009; 27(3):E11

[22] Meng XT, Guan XF, Zhang HL, He SS. Computer navigation versus fluoroscopy-guided navigation for thoracic pedicle screw placement: a meta-analysis. Neurosurg Rev. 2016; 39(3):385–391

[23] Yang H, Liu T, Zhou J, Meng B, Wang G, Zhu X. Kyphoplasty versus vertebroplasty for painful osteoporotic vertebral compression fractures: which one is better? A systematic review and meta-analysis. Int J Spine Surg. 2013; 7:e45–e57

[24] Watts NB, Harris ST, Genant HK. Treatment of painful osteoporotic vertebral fractures with percutaneous vertebroplasty or kyphoplasty. Osteoporos Int. 2001; 12(6):429–437

[25] Choe DH, Marom EM, Ahrar K, Truong MT, Madewell JE. Pulmonary embolism of polymethyl methacrylate during percutaneous vertebroplasty and kyphoplasty. AJR Am J Roentgenol. 2004; 183(4):1097–1102

[26] Park SY, Modi HN, Suh SW, Hong JY, Noh W, Yang JH. Epidural cement leakage through pedicle violation after balloon kyphoplasty causing paraparesis in osteoporotic vertebral compression fractures: a report of two cases. J Orthop Surg Res. 2010; 5:54

[27] Tarukado K, Tono O, Harimaya K, Doi T. Balloon kyphoplasty and vertebroplasty for vertebral compression fractures: a comparative systematic review of efficacy and safety. J Orthop. 2017; 14(4):480–483

[28] Hulme PA, Krebs J, Ferguson SJ, Berlemann U. Vertebroplasty and kyphoplasty: a systematic review of 69 clinical studies. Spine. 2006; 31(17):1983–2001

[29] Röllinghoff M, Siewe J, Zarghooni K, et al. Effectiveness, security and height restoration on fresh compression fractures: a comparative prospective study of vertebroplasty and kyphoplasty. Minim Invasive Neurosurg. 2009; 52(5-6):233–237

[30] Lovi A, Teli M, Ortolina A, Costa F, Fornari M, Brayda-Bruno M. Vertebroplasty and kyphoplasty: complementary techniques for the treatment of painful osteoporotic vertebral compression fractures. A prospective non-randomised study on 154 patients. Eur Spine J. 2009; 18(01) Suppl 1:95–101

[31] Abdelrahman H, Siam AE, Shawky A, Ezzati A, Boehm H. Infection after vertebroplasty or kyphoplasty: a series of nine cases and review of literature. Spine J. 2013; 13(12):1809–1817

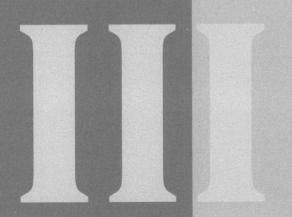

Part III
**Techniques for Robotic-Assisted
Spine Surgery**

21 Outcomes in Robotic Spinal Surgery

Glenn S. Russo, Christopher M. Bono, and James D. Kang

Abstract:

This chapter will review the outcomes of pedicle screw placement in robotic spinal surgery. Several studies have assessed the accuracy of robotically placed pedicle screws and, generally, the literature has supported robotic-assisted pedicle screw placement as a safe and viable technique.

Keywords: robotic spinal surgery, computer-assisted navigation, pedicle screw placement, pedicle screw accuracy

21.1 Introduction

In an effort to improve surgical precision, computer-assisted navigation (CAN) was developed to replace the traditional free-hand technique for pedicle screw placement. While this technology has proved itself to be safe and efficacious, its use still presents several challenges for the operating surgeon. Issues with the obligatory direct line of sight between the tracking system to the instrumentation, maintenance of the relative position of the array to the patient, intraoperative changes in patient position, learning curve, and technical issues have all been identified. The development of robotic-assisted spinal surgery was intended to address some of the shortcomings of CAN. To more readily facilitate their integration, these robotic-assisted technologies were built on the same CAN software platforms.

The two main robotic-assisted surgical devices currently utilized in spinal surgery are the SpineAssist/Renaissance robot (MAZOR Robotics Inc., Orlando, FL) and the ROSA robot (Medtech S.A., Montpellier, France). Integration of the da Vinci Robot (Intuitive Surgical, Sunnyvale, CA) has also been attempted in the field of spinal surgery.

21.2 Mazor Robotics

The Mazor system is the most well studied of the computer-assisted surgical models. Mazor robots function on a predetermined (preoperative or intraoperative) virtual map of the spine that is generated from a computed tomographic (CT) scan. With this map, the surgeon creates an operative template to define the intended position and orientation of each pedicle screw. The robotic software is then able to orient itself to the patient based on intraoperative fluoroscopic images. A robotic arm positions guide tubes in accordance to each pedicle as defined by the operative template. The surgeon is able to cannulate and prepare the pedicle through the guide tubes to place the appropriately planned screw.

21.2.1 Pedicle Screw Accuracy

Early understanding of the accuracy of pedicle screw placement by the Mazor robot was described by Sukovich et al who presented a retrospective review of 98 screws in 14 patients and found that 96% of the screws were within 1 to 2 mm of their planned trajectory. Furthermore, they observed no pedicle breaches from screw malposition.[1]

To more systematically categorize pedicle screw positioning, many of the later studies utilized the CT-based Gertzbein and Robbins classification system (GRS).[2] In this system, the screw's placement is given a grade of A through E. Grade A is no breach; a breach of less than 2 mm is Grade B; a breach of 2 to less than 4 mm is Grade C; a breach of 4 to less than 6 mm is Grade D; a breach of greater than 6 mm is Grade E. To help guide surgeons' decision making, the authors made the determination that Grades A and B were qualified as acceptable placement.

In a retrospective study utilizing the GRS system, Onen et al studied a series of 27 patients in whom 136 robotically assisted screws were placed.[3] They noted 91.2% of screws were deemed Grade A and 7.4% of screws were Grade B. Furthermore, Schatlo et al and van Dijk et al conducted similar retrospective reviews on the placement of 1,265 and 494 robotically assisted screws, respectively. Both studies demonstrated successful placement (GRS Grade A or B) of over 96% of screws.[4,5] The Mazor system was also studied in prospective fashion using the GRS classification for its use in pedicle screw placement in patients undergoing posterior lumbar interbody fusion (PLIF).[6] After a review of 122 screws (31 patients), they determined that over 99% were GRS Grade A or B.

The largest retrospective review to date was performed by Devito et al. They had planned for 3,912 screws to be placed in 682 patients. However, 3,271 screws (83.6%) were placed with full robotic guidance, while the remaining were started with the robot but finished manually.[7] The initial fluoroscopic evaluation determined that 98% of the screws were in an acceptable position. For the 646 screws in patients who had a subsequent CT scan, over 98.3% were designated as either GRS Grade A or B. Of the remaining screws rated Grade C or lower, 1.4% breached between 2 and 4 mm and only 2 screws (0.3%) violated the pedicle wall by more than 4 mm. Neurologic symptoms were found in four patients; however, following revision surgery, no permanent deficits were noted.

In an effort to help optimize usage of the Mazor robot, Kuo et al developed an intraoperative assessment of robotic pedicle screw placement through a secondary registration.[8] The authors used the Mazor robot to place K-wires and their position was subsequently rechecked with biplanar fluoroscopy. This group determined that secondary registration increased the accuracy rate of robotic pedicle screw placement.[8] There were 317 K-wires placed and only 6% (19 wires) were malpositioned by more than 3 mm. Upon repositioning, 15 of 19 were improved. The final four wires required manual placement for an ultimate accuracy rate of 98.7%.

21.2.2 Comparative Studies

In addition to evaluating the accuracy of the Mazor system, several groups have sought to help stratify the utility of robotic guidance by comparing it to a traditional freehand pedicle screw placement and/or CAN.

Perhaps the most well-performed study on the topic was a single-center, prospective, randomized controlled study by Ringel and colleagues. Interestingly, this study produced the only results, to our knowledge, that demonstrate inferiority of pedicle screw placement with the SpineAssist/Mazor robot as compared to the freehand technique.[9] In this study, 60 patients were randomly assigned into a percutaneous robotically assisted instrumentation cohort or an open, freehand technique cohort. The robotically assisted cohort demonstrated acceptably placed screws in 85% of those attempted (146 screws). The freehand cohort showed that 93% of screws were acceptably placed. Furthermore, they noted that the freehand technique showed shorter surgical time (84 vs. 95 minutes). The group also found that when the robotically assisted screws were malpositioned, they tended to be placed laterally. The authors determined that the robotic positioning was vulnerable to lateral deviation due to the fact that there was slippage or skidding of the drill sleeves off the lateral aspect of the facet.

In another randomized controlled trial, Hyun et al randomized 60 patients to receive either robotic or freehand pedicle screws. 100% accuracy was demonstrated in a robotically assisted group as compared to 98.6% in the freehand group.[10] They noted that in the freehand group, there was a violation of one proximal facet, while there were no such instances in the robotic cohort.

A third randomized controlled trial was performed by Kim et al who compared pedicle screw placement using robot and freehand techniques in patients undergoing minimally invasive PLIF.[11] The team demonstrated a 99.4% accuracy rate in both groups; however, they noted proximal joint violations in 15.9% of freehand screws (13 screws) but no joint violations in the robotically placed screws.

Kantelhardt et al demonstrated 94.5% accuracy with the SpineAssist/Mazor model and 91.5% accuracy with a freehand, fluoroscopically assisted technique in a nonrandomized retrospective study.[12] They also noted that those who underwent robotic-assisted surgery required less opioids, had shorter hospitalization, and lower rates of adverse events as compared to conventional screw placement. Furthermore, these benefits were exaggerated in patients who underwent percutaneous robot-assisted procedures.

Schizas and colleagues, in a prospective study, reported 95% accuracy for robot-assisted pedicle screw placement (11 patients, 64 screws) as compared to 92% with fluoroscopically guided insertion (23 patients, 64 screws).[13] Another study, as part of a review on robotic spine surgery, described a preliminary prospectively collected data set that demonstrated a 99% accuracy rate of robotic lumbosacral pedicle screw placement compared to 98% accuracy with a fluoroscopically guided technique and a 92% success rate with CAN.[14]

A retrospective, case-matched study by Schatlo et al found a nonsignificant difference in the proportion of acceptable pedicle screws placed between the Mazor system (91.4%) and conventional freehand technique (87.1%).[15] Notably, in their series, the group had one freehand screw that required a revision procedure due to an iatrogenically induced radiculopathy. Another retrospective cohort study of patients with spondylodiskitis by Keric et al demonstrated superiority in the accuracy of robotically assisted pedicle screw and that they were less likely to require revision for malposition or loosening.[16]

Roser et al performed a randomized controlled trial with three groups: traditional freehand technique, standard neuronavigation, and robotically assisted pedicle screw placement.[14] In this study, an "accurate" screw was defined as GRS Group A, which differed from most of the studies in the literature that denoted both GRS Groups A and B to be considered accurate. The Mazor robot (99% accuracy) was superior to both the freehand technique (97.5% accuracy) and the neuronavigation technique (92% accuracy). When GRS Group B screws were included in what was considered "acceptable," the accuracy rates increased to 99% with the robot, 100% with the freehand technique, and 97.2% with neuronavigation.

21.2.3 Other Uses of Robotic Technology in Spinal Surgery

In the setting of spinal tumor surgery, Hu et al utilized the Mazor system for posterior instrumentation with nine patients without any screw malposition.[17] Furthermore, this series also demonstrated successful use of robotically assisted vertebral augmentation in four patients in the cohort. In a subsequent study, robotic-assisted screw placement was successful in 95 out of 102 patients. In these 95 patients (960 screws), there was accurate implantation of 98.9% of the screws despite significant deformity and revision settings.[18]

Dreval et al studied the Mazor robot in its ability to assist in four different cohort scenarios: transcutaneous transpedicular interdisk fusion using the guided oblique lumbar interbody fusion (GO-LIF) procedure, transpedicular instrumentation in the setting of trauma, vertebroplasty, and biopsy of an unknown lesion.[19] This study included 72 screws (36 patients); one patient required revision due to inadequate screw purchase. In the vertebroplasty group, use of the Mazor robotic system resulted in good results in all 16 patients studied. With regard to the biopsy group, robotic assistance allowed for safe and reliable sampling from all 11 patients.

In the setting of adolescent idiopathic scoliosis, Macke et al studied the utility of the Mazor robot.[20] They determined that of the 662 screws (48 patients) implanted, 92.7% were acceptably placed. Of the 48 misplaced screws, 30 were GRS Grade C, 10 were GRS Grade D, and 8 were GRS Grade E.

Bederman et al investigated the placement of S2-alar-iliac screws in 31 implants (14 patients).[21] With the use of the Mazor robot, they reported 100% accuracy without any breach of the anterior sacrum.

21.3 ROSA

The ROSA robot is similar to the Mazor robotic system. However, it is distinctive in that it is a freestanding device with a rigid arm that moves in concordance with the patient by virtue of real-time camera monitoring. The camera follows the patient by tracking percutaneously placed pins. This technology therefore circumvents the reliance on a secure bone dock for the drill sleeves required in the Mazor system.

Although the literature on the ROSA system is much less robust than that of the Mazor robot, one study regarding the ROSA robot was performed as a prospective case-matched study comparing robotically assisted screw placement to screws placed by an open freehand technique.[22] The 36 screws placed with robotic assistance showed 97.2% accuracy, while the 50 screws placed freehand yielded 92% accuracy. However, it is important to note that four screws intended for robotic placement were unable to be implanted due to technical difficulties with the system.

21.4 da Vinci

The da Vinci robot (Intuitive Surgical) is typically used in the fields of general surgery, obstetrics and gynecology, and urology. However, with regard to spinal surgery, it has been used to perform a laparoscopic anterior lumbar interbody fusion (ALIF). The da Vinci robot functions as an extension of the surgeon whereby the surgeon operates the robot via a remote telesurgical console. However, with regard to length of stay, blood loss, and morbidity, several studies did not demonstrate any advantage to usage of the da Vinci robot as compared to a traditional open procedure.[23,24,25,26] Furthermore, there was a higher incidence of retrograde ejaculation and the need for conversion to an open procedure that was associated with laparoscopic ALIF. Although the technique has largely been abandoned, as robotic surgery has become more sophisticated, there has been a resurgence of the da Vinci use.

21.5 Conclusion

Robotic surgery is a recent addition to the armamentarium of today's spinal surgeon. While much of the early literature is supportive, continued scrutiny will be important to understand when and how it can be cultivated in the best interests of patient safety.

References

[1] Sukovich W, Brink-Danan S, Hardenbrook M. Miniature robotic guidance for pedicle screw placement in posterior spinal fusion: early clinical experience with the SpineAssist. Int J Med Robot. 2006; 2(2):114–122

[2] Gertzbein SD, Robbins SE. Accuracy of pedicular screw placement in vivo. Spine. 1990; 15(1):11–14

[3] Onen MR, Simsek M, Naderi S. Robotic spine surgery: a preliminary report. Turk Neurosurg. 2014; 24(4):512–518

[4] Schatlo B, Martinez R, Alaid A, et al. Unskilled unawareness and the learning curve in robotic spine surgery. Acta Neurochir (Wien). 2015; 157(10):1819–1823, discussion 1823

[5] van Dijk JD, van den Ende RP, Stramigioli S, Köchling M, Höss N. Clinical pedicle screw accuracy and deviation from planning in robot-guided spine surgery: robot-guided pedicle screw accuracy. Spine. 2015; 40(17):E986–E991

[6] Pechlivanis I, Kiriyanthan G, Engelhardt M, et al. Percutaneous placement of pedicle screws in the lumbar spine using a bone mounted miniature robotic system: first experiences and accuracy of screw placement. Spine. 2009; 34 (4):392–398

[7] Devito DP, Kaplan L, Dietl R, et al. Clinical acceptance and accuracy assessment of spinal implants guided with SpineAssist surgical robot: retrospective study. Spine. 2010; 35(24):2109–2115

[8] Kuo KL, Su YF, Wu CH, et al. Assessing the intraoperative accuracy of pedicle screw placement by using a bone-mounted miniature robot system through secondary registration. PLoS One. 2016; 11(4):e0153235

[9] Ringel F, Stüer C, Reinke A, et al. Accuracy of robot-assisted placement of lumbar and sacral pedicle screws: a prospective randomized comparison to conventional freehand screw implantation. Spine. 2012; 37(8):E496–E501

[10] Hyun SJ, Kim KJ, Jahng TA, Kim HJ. Minimally invasive robotic versus open fluoroscopic-guided spinal instrumented fusions: a randomized controlled trial. Spine. 2017; 42(6):353–358

[11] Kim HJ, et al. A prospective, randomized, controlled trial of robot-assisted vs freehand pedicle screw fixation in spine surgery. Int J Med Robot. 2017; 13 (3):Epub September 27, 2016

[12] Kantelhardt SR, Martinez R, Baerwinkel S, Burger R, Giese A, Rohde V. Perioperative course and accuracy of screw positioning in conventional, open robotic-guided and percutaneous robotic-guided, pedicle screw placement. Eur Spine J. 2011; 20(6):860–868

[13] Schizas C, Thein E, Kwiatkowski B, Kulik G. Pedicle screw insertion: robotic assistance versus conventional C-arm fluoroscopy. Acta Orthop Belg. 2012; 78(2):240–245

[14] Roser F, Tatagiba M, Maier G. Spinal robotics: current applications and future perspectives. Neurosurgery. 2013; 72 Suppl 1:12–18

[15] Schatlo B, Molliqaj G, Cuvinciuc V, Kotowski M, Schaller K, Tessitore E. Safety and accuracy of robot-assisted versus fluoroscopy-guided pedicle screw insertion for degenerative diseases of the lumbar spine: a matched cohort comparison. J Neurosurg Spine. 2014; 20(6):636–643

[16] Keric N, Eum DJ, Afghanyar F, et al. Evaluation of surgical strategy of conventional vs. percutaneous robot-assisted spinal trans-pedicular instrumentation in spondylodiscitis. J Robot Surg. 2017; 11(1):17–25

[17] Hu X, Scharschmidt TJ, Ohnmeiss DD, Lieberman IH. Robotic assisted surgeries for the treatment of spine tumors. Int J Spine Surg. 2015; 9:9

[18] Hu X, Ohnmeiss DD, Lieberman IH. Robotic-assisted pedicle screw placement: lessons learned from the first 102 patients. Eur Spine J. 2013; 22(3):661–666

[19] Dreval ON, et al. Results of using Spine Assist Mazor in surgical treatment of spine disorders. Vopr Neirokhir. 2014; 78(3):14–20

[20] Macke JJ, Woo R, Varich L. Accuracy of robot-assisted pedicle screw placement for adolescent idiopathic scoliosis in the pediatric population. J Robot Surg. 2016; 10(2):145–150

[21] Bederman SS, Hahn P, Colin V, Kiester PD, Bhatia NN. Robotic guidance for S2-alar-iliac screws in spinal deformity correction. Clin Spine Surg. 2017; 30(1): E49–E53

[22] Lonjon N, Chan-Seng E, Costalat V, Bonnafoux B, Vassal M, Boetto J. Robot-assisted spine surgery: feasibility study through a prospective case-matched analysis. Eur Spine J. 2016; 25(3):947–955

[23] Inamasu J, Guiot BH. Laparoscopic anterior lumbar interbody fusion: a review of outcome studies. Minim Invasive Neurosurg. 2005; 48(6):340–347

[24] Liu JC, Ondra SL, Angelos P, Ganju A, Landers ML. Is laparoscopic anterior lumbar interbody fusion a useful minimally invasive procedure? Neurosurgery. 2002; 51(5) Suppl:S155–S158

[25] Chung SK, Lee SH, Lim SR, et al. Comparative study of laparoscopic L5-S1 fusion versus open mini-ALIF, with a minimum 2-year follow-up. Eur Spine J. 2003; 12(6):613–617

[26] Kaiser MG, Haid RW, Jr, Subach BR, Miller JS, Smith CD, Rodts GE, Jr. Comparison of the mini-open versus laparoscopic approach for anterior lumbar interbody fusion: a retrospective review. Neurosurgery. 2002; 51(1):97–103, discussion 103–105

22 Robotic Subaxial Cervical Spine Pedicle Screw Instrumentation

Wei Tian, Mingxing Fan, Jingwei Zhao, and Yajun Liu

Abstract:
Robotic subaxial cervical spine pedicle screw instrumentation will talk about the challenges, the indications, the techniques, and cases for robot-assisted subaxial cervical surgery. Subaxial cervical spine pedicle screw instrumentation is difficult due to the complicated anatomy in cervical spine. The navigation may not be satisfied in solving all the questions in subaxial cervical spine surgery. As the robot techniques are becoming more and more popular for orthopaedic surgeries, one way to overcome the drawbacks and face the challenge of the cervical surgeries is to use navigation combined robots, which will make the complicated procedures feasible, safe, and accurate.

Keywords: cervical spine, pedicle screw, robot, real-time navigation, learning curve

22.1 Introduction

The subaxial cervical spine is composed of the third through seventh vertebrae, of which the third through sixth exhibit relatively uniform anatomy. Bearing little weight, the cervical vertebral bodies are relatively small and thin compared to the size of their respective vertebral arches and vertebral foramina.

The spinal pedicle is located in the junction of vertebral body and the posterior vertebral arch. The most featured vertebral arteries transfer from the transverse foramina which perforate in the transverse processes. The pedicles get smaller caudal to C2, reaching a nadir around C3–C4.[1] Due to the differences in individual anatomy, there is significant disparity among the cervical pedicles. The height of the cervical pedicle ranges from 5.1 to 9.5 mm and their width ranges from 3 to 7.5 mm.[2,3] At C3–C4, 75% of pedicles have an average diameter less than 4 mm.[4]

Panjabi published a study on three-dimensional anatomy of the lower cervical spine in 1991.[5] This study demonstrated robust variation in cervical spine anatomy with little uniformity between patients and even within individual patients regarding the height and width, the axial projection points, and the axis angle of the cervical pedicles. In addition to the diminutive nature of the pedicles, cervical pedicles are bordered medially by the spinal canal/cord, laterally by the vertebral artery, and superiorly and inferiorly by the cervical nerve roots. This challenging anatomy makes accurate placement of pedicle screws even more critical. Screw misplacement may not only lead to inadequate fixation and stability, but also may lead to neurological, vascular, or visceral injury.

22.2 Computer-Assisted Navigation and Robotic Cervical Pedicle Screw Placement

Image-based computer-assisted navigation has been utilized in spine surgery to improve cervical pedicle screw insertion accuracy, making the procedure safer and more effective. Navigation allows the patient's anatomy to be revealed via intraoperative computer tomography (CT) registration so that the neighboring spinal cord, vertebral artery, nerve roots, and other important structures, normally not visualized, can be represented in surgery.

Although several recent studies have demonstrated improvement in pedicle screw placement in lower thoracic and lumbar spine,[6,7,8] the utility of pedicle screw placement in this setting is still debated.[9] Some critics claim that the navigation system distracts the surgeon's attention during the surgery and therefore the surgeon is unable to focus on the monitor. Additionally, although the trajectory may be more easily mapped, surgeon fatigue is not necessarily mitigated, and even with practice, the surgeon's force control, steadiness, repeatability, and durability may still be insufficient to face the challenge of complicated cervical spine surgery.

Robotics has recently been advocated as a tool to address precisely these issues. Coupled with navigation, the system allows an "eye" to reveal previously unseen structures and a "hand" to aid in steadiness and fatigue.[10,11]

The SpineAssist/Renaissance and the ROSA Spine robots have demonstrated promising results in clinical applications,[12,13] but neither has been studied in applications related to the cervical spine. Bertelsen et al described a new robotic system for atlantoaxial fixation in 2012, but its accuracy was not sufficient for clinical use (1.94-mm error in a cadaver trial).[10] The TIANJI robotic system (China) has been the most widely used device in China for cervical spinal surgery.

The TIANJI robot is a robot-assisted surgical navigation device based on 3D fluoroscopy,[14] and allows real-time navigation. The TIANJI robot has three main components: the robotic system, an optical tracking system, and a navigation system. The robotic arm has six degrees of freedom, and a universal tool base mounted at the end of the robot arm allows all instrumentation to be directly mounted. The optical tracking system is based on infrared reflection and consists of an infrared stereo camera and two reference frames. One reference frame is mounted on the patient's spinous process, and the other one is mounted on the universal tool base of the robotic arm. The infrared stereo camera captures the reflection from the two frames in real time and calculates their three-dimensional vector distance to allow the robotic arm to compensate for distance. The surgical planning and navigation system is based on the intraoperative 3D fluoroscopy images, and after registration, pedicle screw trajectories can be planned on the aligned images. The surgical planning and navigation system automatically calibrates to intraoperative positioning and can calculate the distance and angle between the real and planned trajectories and subsequently guide the movement of the robot arm. In this way, the robotic system can always maintain precise position within the predefined surgical trajectory.

In 2015, results of TIANJI system use were published, one report of robot-assisted anterior odontoid screw fixation and another of posterior C1–C2 transarticular screw fixation for atlantoaxial instability.[14,15] Currently, the system is in use in numerous hospitals in different provinces and cities in China serving more than 12 million people.

22.3 Indications

The indications for robotic subaxial cervical spine pedicle screw instrumentation include the following:
1. Cervical fracture or dislocation.
2. Cervical stenosis with instability.
3. Cervical stenosis with kyphosis.
4. Ossification of the posterior longitudinal ligament with stenosis.
5. Cervical postlaminectomy kyphosis.
6. Cervical spine instability caused by tumor.
7. Tuberculosis, rheumatoid, inflammation, and other factors with cervical instability.
8. Complex cervical deformity.

22.4 Techniques

We routinely place robot-assisted subaxial cervical spine pedicle screw instrumentation with the use of the TIANJI robotic system, previously described.
1. Preoperative X-ray, CT and MR images are essential to ensure the feasibility of the surgery and to plan preoperatively.
2. The patient is positioned prone with the head held using a Mayfield clamp, and shoulders and arms tucked at the side.
3. On a lateral fluoroscopic image, all potential screw trajectories should be adequately visualized and not obstructed by bone or soft tissue.
4. A posterior midline open approach or posterior percutaneous minimally invasive approach is used. The following steps are described using the percutaneous approach.
5. Fix the patient tracker firmly onto the Mayfield using a connector.
6. Connect the registrator to the arm of the robot and drag it into the scan area of the C-arm. Scan the operative area using the C-arm CT system (Arcadis Orbic 3D; Siemens Medical Solutions, Erlangen, Germany) and transfer the images into the robot system.
7. Plan the screws and decide the lengths and diameters using the reconstructed CT images.
8. After the screw trajectories are planned, bring the robotic arm into position which will allow accurate placement of the skin incision. Incise the skin and dilate in line with the robotic arm. Place soft tissue sleeve or retractors.
9. Locate the screw trajectory again using the robot. Insert the guide wire cannula through the robotic sleeve and make sure to put the tip of the cannula onto the bone cortex.
10. Place a 1.5-mm guide wire through the cannula and drill into bone, adjusting the amount of wire exposed in drill to limit the depth of penetration.
11. Remove the drill, the guide wire sleeve, the robot arm, and the retractors.
12. Repeat step 8 to 11 to insert all the guide wires.
13. Scan the operative area using the C-arm to verify the position of the guide wires.
14. Insert the cannulated screws and then rods and end caps
15. Once all hardware has been placed, close in a layered fashion per surgeon preference.

22.5 Notes

1. To do navigation or robot-assisted minimally invasive cervical surgery, the experience of open cervical surgery and the training of the computer-assisting equipment are essential.
2. During surgery, if there is any doubt as to the accuracy of the navigation or robot system, check the accuracy by locating several bone marks, such as the spinous process and the articular processes. Rescanning and re-registration is the key to restore the accuracy.
3. There are several factors that may affect the accuracy during surgery.
   a) Patient tracker movement. The patient tracker should be firmly placed onto the bone or the Mayfield clamp. Once the tracker is moved, or even touched, the accuracy and fidelity should be checked.
   b) Movement between cervical segments. Especially in cases of trauma or after manipulation, there may be motion between cervical segments, which can influence accuracy. Fix the patient tracker as near as possible to the target segments and operate gently to reduce the effect of segment movement. During the insertion of the guide wire, keep high rotation speed of the drill and low force toward the bone.
   c) Slipping of the guide wire on bone slope. Try to design the trajectory through a flatter bone surface if possible. Putting the cannula onto the bone surface can help get better control of the wire tip and reduce the chance of slipping and tip bend. Use a guided abrasive drill to make an entry hole if slipping persists.
   d) Cannula deflected by soft tissue. Adequate exposure or percutaneous approach can reduce the affect.
4. Since the maximum permissible error of a pedicle screw at the cervical and mid-thoracic spine is less than 1 mm,[16] any robot system whose accuracy does not meet this criteria should be evaluated with caution before the application in the cervical spine.

22.6 Learning Curve

Both the navigation and the robot systems require additional learning time for surgeons. However, the real-time multiplanar reconstruction of the surgical area provided by the systems can reduce the learning time compared to cervical spine surgery learned with fluoroscopic technique.

During the learning phase, these steps are recommended:
a) Operate first on the segment distant from the patient tracker.
b) Expose adequately to identify the entry points of the screws under direct vision and make sure they are consistent with the experience of traditional surgeries.
c) Check the accuracy using easily identified bone marks after each guide wire insertion. Do not hesitate to rescan

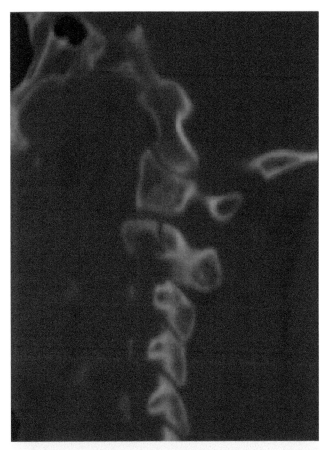

Fig. 22.1 The sagittal view CT shows cervical spine fracture, and the fracture line is close to the vertebral artery.

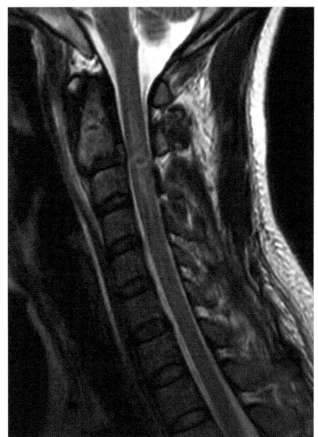

Fig. 22.2 The MRI shows edema signal in spinal cord.

whenever there is doubt about the accuracy, especially when the operative segment changes.

d) Use the depth scale to determine the final length of the screws and compare with the planning.

e) Use C-arm CT scan to verify the placement of the guide wires as well as the screws.

22.7 Case

Patient: LJRU, female, 46 years old.

Chief complaint: Movement and sensation disorders for 13 hours after car accident.

Present illness: Car accident 13 hours earlier, leading to neck pain, limb movement and sensation disorders, no dizziness, nausea, and vomiting. The patient visited local hospital, and CT shows cervical spine fracture in C2–C4. After rigid collar support, the patient was transported to our hospital.

Past history: Hypertension for 4 years and there was no relevant prior history.

Physical examination: Frankel C, muscle strength for upper and lower limbs is 0–II, neck hyperalgesia, and hypoesthesia below neck.

The CT shows cervical spine fracture in C2–C4 (▶ Fig. 22.1), and the MRI shows high signal in C2–C4 (▶ Fig. 22.2).

The patient underwent the TIANJI robot-assisted subaxial cervical spine pedicle screw instrumentation (▶ Fig. 22.3, ▶ Fig. 22.4); the surgery was successful and there were no intraoperative complications. The patient was discharged for rehabilitation on day 5.

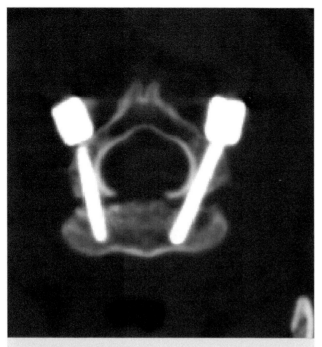

Fig. 22.3 The pedicle screws in C3.

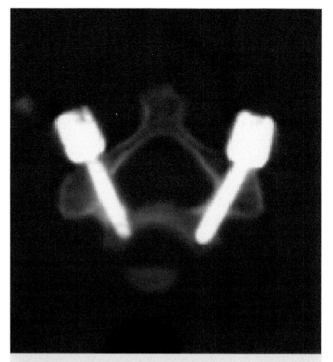

Fig. 22.4 The pedicle screws in C4.

References

[1] Sanelli PC, Tong S, Gonzalez RG, Eskey CJ. Normal variation of vertebral artery on CT angiography and its implications for diagnosis of acquired pathology. J Comput Assist Tomogr. 2002; 26(3):462–470

[2] An HS, Wise JJ, Xu R. Anatomy of the cervicothoracic junction: a study of cadaveric dissection, cryomicrotomy, and magnetic resonance imaging. J Spinal Disord. 1999; 12(6):519–525

[3] Ebraheim NA, Xu R, Knight T, Yeasting RA. Morphometric evaluation of lower cervical pedicle and its projection. Spine. 1997; 22(1):1–6

[4] Karaikovic EE, Daubs MD, Madsen RW, Gaines RW, Jr. Morphologic characteristics of human cervical pedicles. Spine. 1997; 22(5):493–500

[5] Panjabi MM, O'Holleran JD, Crisco JJ, III, Kothe R. Complexity of the thoracic spine pedicle anatomy. Eur Spine J. 1997; 6(1):19–24

[6] Tian W, Liu Y, Zheng S, Lv Y. Accuracy of lower cervical pedicle screw placement with assistance of distinct navigation systems: a human cadaveric study. Eur Spine J. 2013; 22(1):148–155

[7] Tian W, Lang Z. Placement of pedicle screws using three-dimensional fluoroscopy-based navigation in lumbar vertebrae with axial rotation. Eur Spine J. 2010; 19(11):1928–1935

[8] Wu H, Gao ZL, Wang JC, Li YP, Xia P, Jiang R. Pedicle screw placement in the thoracic spine: a randomized comparison study of computer-assisted navigation and conventional techniques. Chin J Traumatol. 2010; 13(4):201–205

[9] Verma R, Krishan S, Haendlmayer K, Mohsen A. Functional outcome of computer-assisted spinal pedicle screw placement: a systematic review and meta-analysis of 23 studies including 5,992 pedicle screws. Eur Spine J. 2010; 19(3):370–375

[10] Bertelsen A, Melo J, Sánchez E, Borro D. A review of surgical robots for spinal interventions. Int J Med Robot. 2013; 9(4):407–422

[11] Kim S, Chung J, Yi BJ, Kim YS. An assistive image-guided surgical robot system using O-arm fluoroscopy for pedicle screw insertion: preliminary and cadaveric study. Neurosurgery. 2010; 67(6):1757–1767, discussion 1767

[12] Chenin L, Peltier J, Lefranc M. Minimally invasive transforaminal lumbar interbody fusion with the ROSA(TM) spine robot and intraoperative flat-panel CT guidance. Acta Neurochir (Wien). 2016; 158(6):1125–1128

[13] Devito DP, Kaplan L, Dietl R, et al. Clinical acceptance and accuracy assessment of spinal implants guided with SpineAssist surgical robot: retrospective study. Spine. 2010; 35(24):2109–2115

[14] Tian W. Robot-assisted posterior C1–2 transarticular screw fixation for atlantoaxial instability: a case report. Spine. 2016; 41 Suppl 19:B2–B5

[15] Tian W, Wang H, Liu YJ. Robot-assisted anterior odontoid screw fixation: a case report. Orthop Surg. 2016; 8(3):400–404

[16] Rampersaud YR, Simon DA, Foley KT. Accuracy requirements for image-guided spinal pedicle screw placement. Spine. 2001; 26(4):352–359

23 Navigated and Robotic Anterior Odontoid Peg Fracture Fixation

Kartik Shenoy and Ali Bydon

Abstract:
Odontoid peg, or dens, fractures are being recognized more frequently due to the increasing use of computed tomography in the traumatically injured patient and consequently, there is an increased rate of operative intervention. Transverse or oblique fracture patterns are amenable to anterior fixation; however, precise placement of anterior odontoid screws is critical to achieving fracture union. Traditionally, biplanar fluoroscopy was used to place anterior odontoid screws, but the setup can be cumbersome and there is increased radiation exposure to the patient and surgeon. Navigation and robotics have allowed for more accurate placement of anterior odontoid screws while minimizing the amount of radiation, however the long-term clinical outcomes are still to be determined.

Keywords: anterior odontoid fixation, dens fracture, odontoid fracture, computer navigation, robotic spine surgery

23.1 Introduction

Odontoid fractures can be the result of spinal trauma and if missed can be life-threatening. Fractures of the odontoid peg, or dens, constitute 5 to 15% of all cervical spine injuries.[1] In 1928, Osgood and Lund reviewed 55 cases and found the mortality rate to be more than 50%.[2] Advances since then as described by Amyes and Anderson in a 1956 report of 63 cases had a mortality rate of 8% with a 5% rate of nonunion.[1] The high rate of mortality is largely a result of missed injuries, as the upper cervical spine is difficult to visualize on plain radiographs given the overlapping osseous structures. They are frequently missed due to the lack of clinical symptoms other than neck pain. With the advent of computed tomography (CT) and its application in the trauma setting, fractures are better identified and characterized.[3]

According to the Anderson-D'Alonzo classification, there are three types of odontoid peg fractures based on the fracture pattern from cephalad to caudal. Type I is a fracture of the tip usually due to an avulsion of the alar ligament. Type II is a more caudal fracture through the waist or base where the odontoid peg meets the body of the axis. The fracture line in a type III extends into the body and has a larger fracture bed surface area.[4] Type II fractures are typically treated operatively with either C1–C2 posterior fusion or anterior odontoid screw fixation. C1–C2 posterior fusion is performed most commonly with C1 lateral mass with C2 pedicle screws.[5,6,7] However, given that the C1–C2 articulation contributes greatly to cervical rotation, postfusion, the patient may lose up to 50% of neck rotation.

Anterior fixation with one or two odontoid screws is another treatment option; unlike a fusion, it offers the advantage of preserving rotation. In order to perform anterior fixation, the fracture pattern must be transverse or in the anterosuperior to posteroinferior orientation and reducible without significant comminution.[8] The surgeon must also be mindful of the patient's chest size, as insertion of the screw at the correct angle may be limited by a larger, barrel-shaped chest. When anterior fixation is appropriate, imaging using fluoroscopy or intraoperative CT is suggested for proper screw placement.

23.2 Traditional Surgical Technique

Anterior odontoid osteosynthesis can be performed using two biplanar fluoroscopy machines to obtain images of the odontoid peg in the true anteroposterior (AP) and lateral planes. Prior to incision, using halo traction, a Mayfield or manual reduction, reduction of the fracture should be attempted. With the patient in the supine position, the head is extended to facilitate reduction and screw insertion. Before making incision, a K-wire is placed along the neck in the intended direction and then confirmed on fluoroscopy to guide placement of a transverse, anteromedial incision. An anterior approach to C2–C3 is made via an incision at approximately the C5–C6 level. The platysma is divided and blunt dissection medial to the sternocleidomastoid is performed down to the prevertebral fascia. The fascia is then incised at the C2–C3 level and the disk space is identified. A partial removal of the anterosuperior edge of C3 body is performed to allow exposure of the inferior edge of C2 and the screw start point. A K-wire is then advanced under fluoroscopy and then a 4.5-mm cannulated cancellous screw is placed over the wire.[9]

23.3 Navigation

Navigation for anterior odontoid screw placement evolved through the need for more accurate screw placement and to minimize radiation exposure and complications. Although screws can be placed via fluoroscopy as described earlier, there are still complications such as screw cutout, vascular injury, or even neurological injury at a rate of 0.2 to 5%.[10,11] The need for accurate placement of screws led to the field of spinal navigation, and technology that was once used for precision pedicle screw placement is now used in anterior odontoid screw placement. There are a variety of navigation technologies available and they vary based on the imaging modality: fluoroscopy-based, three-dimensional fluoroscopy, and intraoperative CT.

23.3.1 Fluoroscopy-Based Computer Navigation

Fluoroscopy-based computer navigation, or virtual fluoroscopy, as described by Battaglia et al is a technique that employs the traditional two-dimensional C-arm images in conjunction with an optical tracking system and computer to allow real-time visual tracking of screw trajectory relative to preacquired images.[12] In this technique, standard AP and lateral fluoroscopic images are obtained and then instruments are calibrated and synchronized to a computer and a reference frame attached typically to a Mayfield frame. The software is then able to show predicted positions of instruments on the fluoroscopy screen in order to provide real-time feedback to the surgeon as instruments are positioned. According to Chibbaro et al, virtual fluoroscopy allows for surgeons to perform a high-risk surgery in a safer, easier, and faster way.[13] Although there is a learning curve, there is a significant reduction in fluoroscopy time which reduces radiation exposure to both the patient and the surgeon as a total of only four images are needed: AP and lateral pre- and postoperatively. These findings were also supported by Battaglia et al in which they directly compared traditional fluoroscopy to virtual fluoroscopy.[12]

23.3.2 Three-Dimensional Image-Based Navigation and Computed Tomography

The isocentric C-arm three-dimensional fluoroscopy is a form of intraoperative fluoroscopy and CT to provide standard fluoroscopic images as well as cross-sectional imaging in three planes allowing increased accuracy during surgery. A set of defined consecutive images are acquired in a 190-degree orbital plane and then multiplanar image reconstruction is performed to obtain real-time axial, sagittal, and coronal imaging of the cervical spine. Similar to the fluoroscopy technique detailed earlier, a reference frame is placed on a Mayfield or similar head clamp. After calibration, the trajectory of screws or instruments can be viewed in real time on the three-dimensional cross-sectional imaging. Summers et al reported a case series of nine patients who underwent anterior odontoid screw placement using isocentric C-arm three-dimensional fluoroscopy and found that all screws were accurately placed, and no additional operative time was needed.[14] Furthermore, using the three-

dimensional fluoroscopy, they were able to perform an immediate postoperative CT scan to ensure proper screw placement prior to leaving the operating room.

Many ensuing studies have investigated the role of three-dimensional fluoroscopy and found similar results.[15,16] Additional studies have directly compared three-dimensional fluoroscopy to the traditional technique and found a significantly less fluoroscopy time when using three-dimensional fluoroscopy without any difference in operating time, blood loss, or complications.[17] Martirosyan et al reported that total time in operating room was not statistically different in either group as the three-dimensional fluoroscopy group had shorter operative time but longer setup time, whereas the traditional fluoroscopy group had longer operative time but shorter preoperative setup.[18] In this study, they also reported on outcomes and found that patients in the three-dimensional fluoroscopy group had higher outcome scores and fusion rates without any difference in the rate of complications.

Intraoperative CT using an O-arm (Medtronic, Minneapolis, MN) can also be used with navigation-based placement of anterior odontoid screws.[19] In 2017, Pisapia et al presented the first report on using an O-arm for anterior odontoid screws in eight patients.[20] This technique also employs a reference point to be placed on the head clamp. After performing dissection, the O-arm is brought into the operating field and a full spin is performed to obtain cross-sectional imaging. A calibrated probe can be used to plan the start point and trajectory of the screw (▶ Fig. 23.1 and ▶ Fig. 23.2). Next, using a drill which is also registered to the system, the planned pathway is drilled (▶ Fig. 23.3). Real-time fluoroscopy can then be performed while drilling to ensure that the drill matches the planned path (▶ Fig. 23.4). The ability of the O-arm to capture AP and lateral fluoroscopic images while advancing the drill and screw is not a necessity but can be used to double check positioning. This is an advantage, as there is no movement of the O-arm when transitioning from an AP to lateral view as would be performed

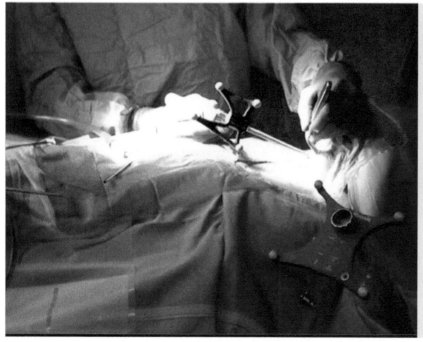

Fig. 23.1 After standard Smith Robinson approach to cervical spine, a calibrated probe is inserted at the start point to assess the trajectory of the planned odontoid screw.

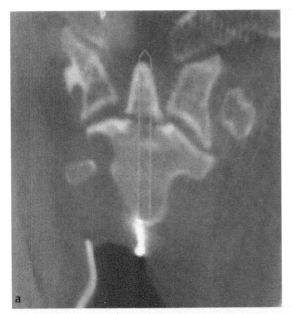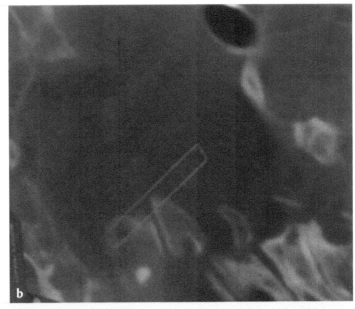

Fig. 23.2 Intraoperative proposed trajectory in coronal (**a**) and sagittal (**b**) planes determined from calibrated probe and navigation system.

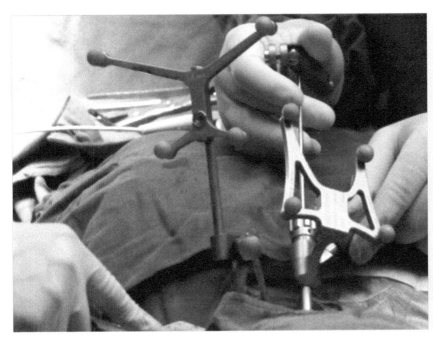

Fig. 23.3 Once the trajectory has been planned, a calibrated drill can be used to ensure that the same trajectory is maintained.

with traditional or three-dimensional fluoroscopy which could potentially get in the surgeon's way. Final intraoperative O-arm can confirm accurate screw placement (▶ Fig. 23.5). More studies utilizing the O-arm for anterior odontoid screw placement are needed and further studies comparing virtual fluoroscopy to three-dimensional fluoroscopy and O-arm with regard to outcomes and complications would allow for the safest, easiest, and most cost-effective technique to be identified.

23.4 Robotics

The use of robotics in spinal surgery was developed as early as 1992; however, the majority of advancements have been made in the last two decades.[21] Spinal surgical complications can be dire, given the presence of blood vessels, nerves, and the spinal cord all within a small operating field. Robots, unlike humans, do not suffer from fatigue and can be calibrated for greater accuracy. Although robots have been around for over 25 years, there has been a paucity of literature on robotic-assisted anterior odontoid fracture fixation. Tian et al described a robot-assisted anterior odontoid screw placement using the TiRobot system.[22] In this system, three-dimensional fluoroscopy is used to obtain cross-sectional imaging. Then using navigation, the software is calibrated, and the surgeon can then plan the start point and trajectory of the screw. This information is then transmitted to the robotic arm which guides the surgeon for screw placement based on reference frames on the patient and

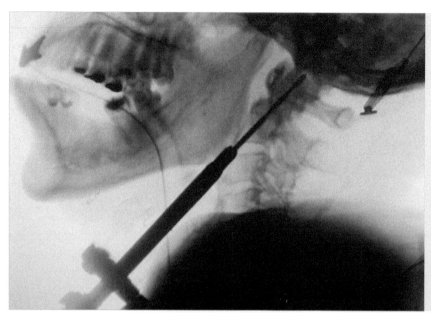

Fig. 23.4 Intraoperative fluoroscopy can confirm appropriate position of drill prior to actual screw placement.

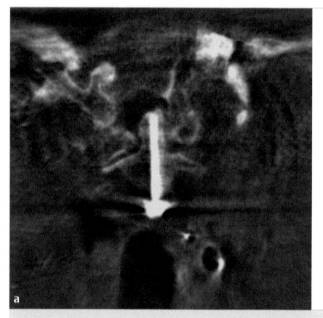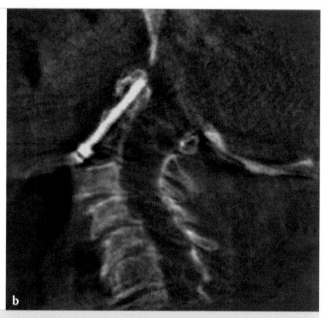

Fig. 23.5 Intraoperative O-arm confirms accurate screw placement in the coronal (**a**) and sagittal (**b**) planes.

on the robotic arm. The robotic arm ensures steadiness and reproducibility. In their case report, Tian et al reported successful placement of a single anterior odontoid screw within 0.9 mm of their planned position. The robot's ability to combine navigation for planning and accuracy for safety and predictability may prove superior in cases where a high level of precision is needed. However, like navigation, more research is needed, as currently there is only one published case report.

23.5 Outcomes Following Fixation

Odontoid fractures make up approximately 5 to 15% of all cervical spine injuries with a higher incidence in the elderly.[23]

C1–C2 posterior fusion is a suitable treatment option for type II fractures; however, when the fracture line is transverse or anterosuperior to posteroinferior, anterior fixation may be an acceptable alternative surgical option in select individuals. Anterior odontoid fixation has been reported to have a union rate of 95%.[9] Though, when adjusting for age, Platzer et al found a significantly higher rate of nonunion in patients over the age of 65 years.[24]

Some authors advocate for two anterior odontoid screws when the diameter of the dens is sufficient to accommodate two screws, as this construct theoretically offers more rotational stability, yet biomechanical studies have shown no significant difference in failure rates.[25,26] Moreover, when using two screws, the surface area of the fracture bed for healing is decreased potentially limiting the fusion rate; however, this has not been shown clinically.[27,28]

Opponents of anterior fixation argue that there is a high rate of screw failure and nonunion when performed in osteoporotic bone and a higher risk of perioperative complications due to approaches such as dysphagia and pneumonia.[29,30] With proper patient selection and surgical technique, complications can be minimized.

23.6 Future Directions

- Does the application of navigation and/or robotics increase the rate of union or decrease the rate of complications?
- Does an orthopaedic robot offer an advantage over navigation for anterior odontoid screw placement?
- Is there a difference in radiation exposure when using the O-arm compared to fluoroscopy?

23.7 Key Points

Navigation and robotics can be successfully and safely employed for anterior odontoid screw fixation. Although these technologies have been around for decades, they have only recently been applied to odontoid fracture fixation. These surgical techniques can be performed with no change in union or complication rate or surgical time and offer many advantages to increase surgical accuracy.

References

[1] Amyes EW, Anderson FM. Fracture of the odontoid process; report of sixty-three cases. AMA Arch Surg. 1956; 72(3):377–393

[2] Osgood RB, Lund CC. Fractures of odontoid process. N Engl J Med. 1928; 198:61–72

[3] Baumgarten M, Mouradian W, Boger D, Watkins R. Computed axial tomography in C1-C2 trauma. Spine. 1985; 10(3):187–192

[4] Anderson LD, D'Alonzo RT. Fractures of the odontoid process of the axis. J Bone Joint Surg Am. 1974; 56(8):1663–1674

[5] Elliott RE, Tanweer O, Boah A, et al. Outcome comparison of atlantoaxial fusion with transarticular screws and screw-rod constructs: meta-analysis and review of literature. J Spinal Disord Tech. 2014; 27(1):11–28

[6] Rajinda P, Towiwat S, Chirappapha P. Comparison of outcomes after atlantoaxial fusion with C1 lateral mass-C2 pedicle screws and C1-C2 transarticular screws. Eur Spine J. 2017; 26(4):1064–1072

[7] Sim HB, Lee JW, Park JT, Mindea SA, Lim J, Park J. Biomechanical evaluations of various c1-c2 posterior fixation techniques. Spine. 2011; 36(6):E401–E407

[8] Böhler J. Anterior stabilization for acute fractures and non-unions of the dens. J Bone Joint Surg Am. 1982; 64(1):18–27

[9] Eap C, Barresi L, Ohl X, et al. Odontoid fractures anterior screw fixation: a continuous series of 36 cases. Orthop Traumatol Surg Res. 2010; 96(7):748–752

[10] Zeidman SM, Ducker TB, Raycroft J. Trends and complications in cervical spine surgery: 1989–1993. J Spinal Disord. 1997; 10(6):523–526

[11] Graham JJ. Complications of cervical spine surgery. A five-year report on a survey of the membership of the Cervical Spine Research Society by the Morbidity and Mortality Committee. Spine. 1989; 14(10):1046–1050

[12] Battaglia TC, Tannoury T, Crowl AC, Chan DP, Anderson DG. A cadaveric study comparing standard fluoroscopy with fluoroscopy-based computer navigation for screw fixation of the odontoid. J Surg Orthop Adv. 2005; 14(4):175–180

[13] Chibbaro S, Benvenuti L, Carnesecchi S, Marsella M, Serino D, Gagliardi R. The use of virtual fluoroscopy in managing acute type II odontoid fracture with anterior single-screw fixation. A safe, effective, elegant and fast form of treatment. Acta Neurochir (Wien). 2005; 147(7):735–739, discussion 739

[14] Summers LE, Kouri JG, Yang M, Patrick Jacob R. Odontoid screw placement using Isocentric 3-dimensional C-arm fluoroscopy. J Spinal Disord Tech. 2008; 21(1):45–48

[15] Zou D, Zhang K, Ren Y, Wu Y, Yang Y, Li Y. Three-dimensional image navigation system-assisted anterior cervical screw fixation for treatment of acute odontoid fracture. Int J Clin Exp Med. 2014; 7(11):4332–4336

[16] Kantelhardt SR, Keric N, Giese A. Management of C2 fractures using Iso-C(3D) guidance: a single institution's experience. Acta Neurochir (Wien). 2012; 154(10):1781–1787

[17] Yang YL, Fu BS, Li RW, et al. Anterior single screw fixation of odontoid fracture with intraoperative Iso-C 3-dimensional imaging. Eur Spine J. 2011; 20(11):1899–1907

[18] Martirosyan NL, Kalb S, Cavalcanti DD, et al. Comparative analysis of isocentric 3-dimensional C-arm fluoroscopy and biplanar fluoroscopy for anterior screw fixation in odontoid fractures. J Spinal Disord Tech. 2013; 26(4):189–193

[19] Ailawadhi P, Agrawal D, Satyarthee GD, Gupta D, Sinha S, Mahapatra AK. Use of O-arm for spinal surgery in academic institution in India: experience from JPN apex trauma centre. Neurol India. 2011; 59(4):590–593

[20] Pisapia JM, Nayak NR, Salinas RD, et al. Navigated odontoid screw placement using the O-arm: technical note and case series. J Neurosurg Spine. 2017; 26(1):10–18

[21] Bertelsen A, Melo J, Sánchez E, Borro D. A review of surgical robots for spinal interventions. Int J Med Robot. 2013; 9(4):407–422

[22] Tian W, Wang H, Liu YJ. Robot-assisted anterior odontoid screw fixation: a case report. Orthop Surg. 2016; 8(3):400–404

[23] Platzer P, Thalhammer G, Oberleitner G, Schuster R, Vécsei V, Gaebler C. Surgical treatment of dens fractures in elderly patients. J Bone Joint Surg Am. 2007; 89(8):1716–1722

[24] Platzer P, Thalhammer G, Ostermann R, Wieland T, Vécsei V, Gaebler C. Anterior screw fixation of odontoid fractures comparing younger and elderly patients. Spine. 2007; 32(16):1714–1720

[25] Sasso R, Doherty BJ, Crawford MJ, Heggeness MH. Biomechanics of odontoid fracture fixation. Comparison of the one- and two-screw technique. Spine. 1993; 18(14):1950–1953

[26] Heller JG, Alson MD, Schaffler MB, Garfin SR. Quantitative internal dens morphology. Spine. 1992; 17(8):861–866

[27] Jenkins JD, Coric D, Branch CL, Jr. A clinical comparison of one- and two-screw odontoid fixation. J Neurosurg. 1998; 89(3):366–370

[28] ElSaghir H, Böhm H. Anderson type II fracture of the odontoid process: results of anterior screw fixation. J Spinal Disord. 2000; 13(6):527–530, discussion 531

[29] Vasudevan K, Grossberg JA, Spader HS, Torabi R, Oyelese AA. Age increases the risk of immediate postoperative dysphagia and pneumonia after odontoid screw fixation. Clin Neurol Neurosurg. 2014; 126:185–189

[30] Andersson S, Rodrigues M, Olerud C. Odontoid fractures: high complication rate associated with anterior screw fixation in the elderly. Eur Spine J. 2000; 9(1):56–59

24 Navigated and Robotic Posterior Atlantoaxial Fusion

Andrew H. Milby and James M. Schuster

Abstract:

The atlantoaxial articulation is a complex and challenging anatomic region for surgical dissection and instrumentation. Posterior atlantoaxial fusion is an important treatment modality for traumatic, degenerative, inflammatory, and developmental disorders. Transarticular and segmental C1–C2 screw fixation both remain useful instrumentation techniques for stabilization of this region to facilitate osseous fusion. Imaging of this region is difficult with conventional fluoroscopy, and intraoperative navigation has emerged as a useful method to improve the safety and accuracy of instrumentation placement. As clinical experience with the use of navigation has accumulated, additional benefits may include the potential for reductions in blood loss and radiation exposure to the surgical team. Limited clinical data exists regarding the use of robotic assistance for posterior C1–C2 fusion at this time. Future directions may involve the use of both modalities to facilitate reductions in the invasiveness and morbidity of posterior atlantoaxial fusion.

Keywords: atlas, axis, atlantoaxial, C1–C2, transarticular, Magerl, Goel, Harms

24.1 Introduction

The atlantoaxial articulation is a unique and highly stressed joint complex that supports and protects the craniocervical junction while permitting tremendous range of motion. While uncommon relative to other spinal disorders, acquired degeneration or instability of the C1–C2 articulation may result in severe disability due to pain or neurologic impairment. As such, fusion of this joint complex may be indicated for the relief of pain or prevention of neurologic deterioration in the setting of traumatic, degenerative, inflammatory, or other acquired atlantoaxial instability.

Historical methods for atlantoaxial fusion involved open decortication and bone grafting techniques but relied primarily upon external stabilization via collar, traction, or halo vest immobilization to achieve a biomechanical environment permissive of osseous fusion.[1,2] More sophisticated wiring techniques subsequently achieved additional construct stability when used in combination with structural autografts, but still necessitated prolonged external immobilization as an adjunct.[3,4] Additional posterior hook-and-clamp-based fixation systems have also been described.[5] The widespread adoption of screw fixation techniques in the subaxial cervical spine prompted investigation of additional screw fixation tracts within the atlantoaxial articulation. Magerl first described clinical experience with the C1–C2 transarticular screw trajectory for stabilization and fusion.[6,7] This elegant technique achieves excellent biomechanical stability but is technically demanding and dependent on the variable neurovascular anatomy of the atlantoaxial region. Indeed, it has been estimated that up to 23% of patients may have anatomy that is not permissive of safe bilateral transarticular screw passage.[8] Harms[9] and Goel[10] each

reported on their clinical experience with segmental C1–C2 fixation, leading to increased adoption of this technique for a variety of indications, including fractures, degenerative and inflammatory arthritis, and congenital malformations and/or instability. In particular, polyaxial locking screws have facilitated greater flexibility in screw trajectories to achieve fixation even in the setting of traumatically altered or congenitally aberrant anatomy. When combined with direct decortication of the C1–C2 joints and/or onlay interlaminar bone grafts, satisfactory clinical outcomes and high rates of osseous fusion have been observed following both transarticular and segmental fixation techniques.[11,12,13,14]

24.2 Background and Rationale

Frameless stereotactic navigation techniques have evolved in parallel for a variety of indications, notably intracranial and spinal procedures. The ability to recognize the spatial position and orientation of an instrument in real time when co-registered with a patient's specific three-dimensional cross-sectional imaging is of intuitive benefit to the surgeon. However, this data must ultimately be incorporated along with direct visual and tactile feedback to guide intraoperative decision-making. The anatomy of the C1–C2 articulation is particularly unforgiving with respect to dissection and instrumentation. The upper cervical spinal cord is in close proximity and is at risk of injury with medial deviation into the canal. The C2 nerves overlay the C1 pars screw starting point and C1–C2 joint, and are enveloped by a robust epidural venous plexus. The vertebral arteries course through the transverse foramina of C2 lateral and inferior to the C2 pedicle, and cranially over the arch of C1 in a highly variable fashion.[15,16,17] In addition, the occiput-C1 articulation is at risk with cranial deviation of the C1 pars screw trajectory. The relative lack of bone stock within the typical transarticular, C2 pedicle, and C1 pars screw trajectories leaves little room for error or re-drilling of cannulation attempts. These regions are also difficult to visualize with standard C-arm fluoroscopy due to the multiple superimposed bony contours from overlapping structures.

Regardless of the means of fixation employed, the posterior cervical approach involves significant morbidity in terms of muscular dissection, potential blood loss, and risk of infection. Rapid prototyping techniques have emerged to facilitate fabrication of custom patient-specific models or drill guides based upon preoperative imaging studies to potentially improve the consistency of instrumentation placement and decrease intraoperative radiation exposure.[18,19,20,21,22,23,24] However, use of such drill guides still necessitates an open surgical exposure with attendant soft tissue disruption and blood loss. Other surgeons have reported on less-invasive exposures and/or percutaneous techniques for decreasing the approach-related morbidity in C1–C2 fusion.[25,26,27,28,29,30] These techniques have relied heavily on the use of intraoperative fluoroscopic imaging. While the use of intraoperative navigation and robotic assistance has been investigated primarily as a means of increasing the safety and consistency of instrumentation placement in the C1–C2 region, it offers the potential to simultaneously facilitate less-invasive approaches and reduce surgical morbidity. These potential benefits must be weighed carefully against other factors, such as operative time, cost, and radiation exposure to the patient and surgical team when deciding whether or not to employ intraoperative navigation.

24.3 Surgical Technique

The senior author's specific technique and navigation system has been previously reported.[31] In general, the patient is positioned prone on a radiolucent table with the head fixed in a Mayfield clamp. Cervical alignment is assessed with cross-table lateral imaging and closed reduction maneuvers may be performed as indicated. If required by the navigation system, a fiducial array may be attached to the Mayfield adapter at the head of the bed. The room is set up with the navigation detector at the head of the bed and the display screen in the surgeon's line of sight (▶ Fig. 24.1). The patient is prepped and draped in a standard fashion, and a sterile fiducial array is attached to the adapter through the drape (▶ Fig. 24.2). A midline subperiosteal exposure of the C1–C2 region may be performed, or less-invasive approaches for percutaneous instrumentation may be considered. An intraoperative scan is then obtained using either fiducial registration or mapping of multiple points directly on the exposed osseous structures. The desired surgical instruments are then co-registered with the navigation scan. These may include a probe, drill guide, screwdriver, and/or burr at the surgeon's discretion. The navigated probe may be used to visualize the planned screw trajectories to aid determining the extent of exposure. The navigated burr may be used to notch the C1 lamina if desired to facilitate placement of instruments for C1 screw placement (▶ Fig. 24.3a). The navigated drill is used to verify the position and trajectory while drilling a starting point and recess for the navigated drill guide (▶ Fig. 24.3b,

c). The navigation tract is locked as surgical plan (▶ Fig. 24.4). Using the surgical plan the navigated drill guide then maintains a consistent trajectory during drilling of the screw tract and a new surgical plan is fixed (▶ Fig. 24.5, ▶ Fig. 24.6). A screw of appropriate length is selected to permit clearance of the C1 lamina (either fully threaded or with a smooth shaft to prevent C2 nerve irritation) and is then placed using the navigated screwdriver and the previous surgical plan. The process may be repeated for the desired C2 screw trajectory (pedicle, pars, or translaminar). Alternatively, the technique may also be used for C1–C2 transarticular screw placement. The construct is completed with rods, set screws, and/or cross links as indicated, and second intraoperative scan may be performed to confirm satisfactory appearance of the construct. Direct decortication of the C1–C2 joints may be performed prior to insertion of instrumentation and/or placement, and fixation of onlay grafts may be subsequently performed per the surgeon's preferred fusion technique.

24.4 Caveats and Potential Pitfalls

Navigation can be a useful adjunct for performing complex spinal surgery. It is especially useful in the setting of altered or aberrant anatomy, and especially at the craniocervical junction where there is little room for error. This includes cases of trauma, rheumatoid arthritis or other subluxating conditions, revisions, and cases with aberrant vertebral artery or bony anatomy. Additionally, for most systems, it allows confirmation of implant placement while still in the OR.

There are however some general and specific issues regarding utilizing navigation at the craniocervical junction that should be considered. First, we highly recommend that surgeons become working "experts" in all aspects of the navigation system, as nothing can be more frustrating than having scrub assistants and/or radiology technicians who are not familiar with these systems. In addition, having the image acquisition

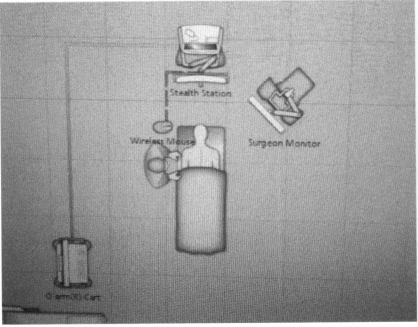

Fig. 24.1 Operating room setup for navigated posterior C1–C2 fusion.

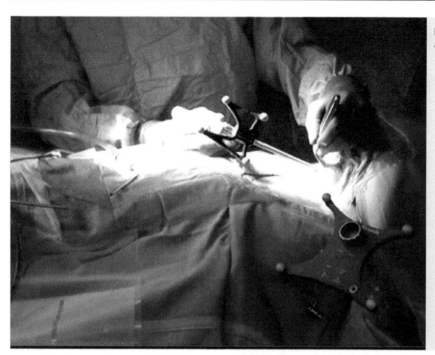

Fig. 24.2 Intraoperative image demonstrating attachment of sterile fiducial array.

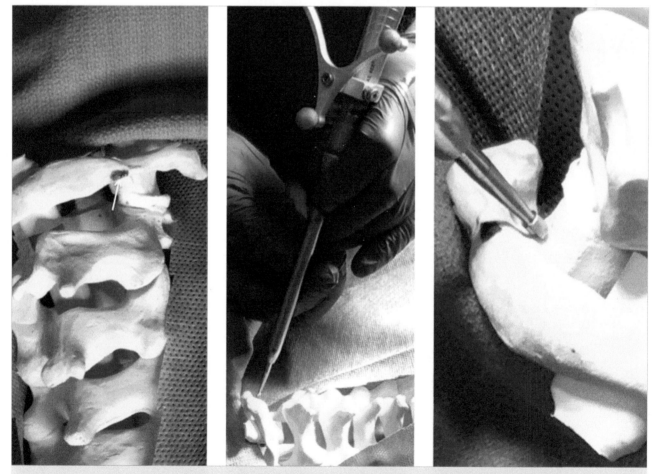

Fig. 24.3 Use of the navigated burr to notch the undersurface of the C1 lamina and create the lateral mass screw starting point.

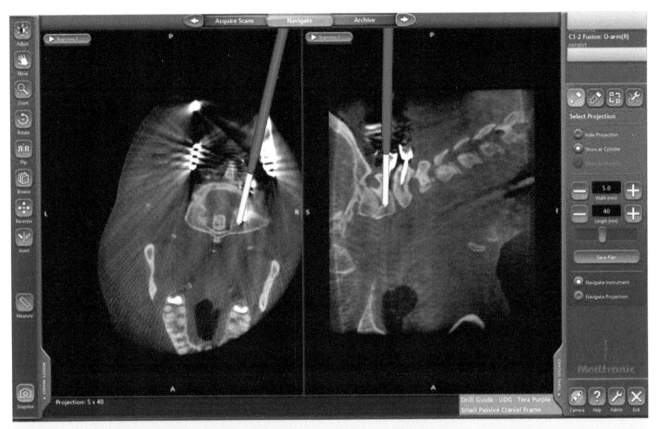

Fig. 24.4 Intraoperative image of navigation display with drill tract superimposed upon CT image.

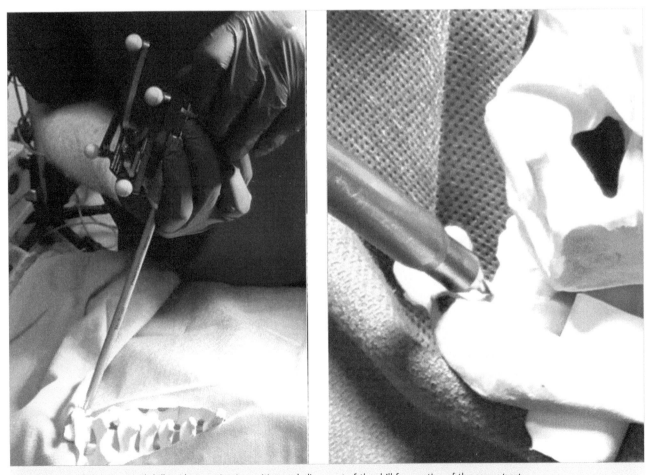

Fig. 24.5 Use of the navigated drill guide to maintain position and alignment of the drill for creation of the screw tract.

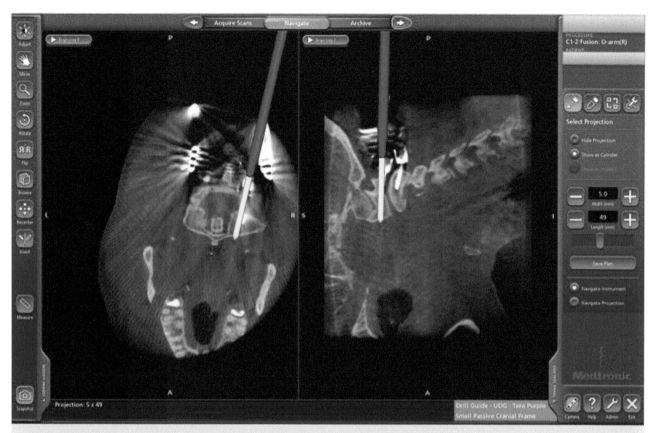

Fig. 24.6 Intraoperative image of navigation display with screwdriver and screw superimposed upon CT image.

system in the room and ready for operation in advance tremendously helps with workflow and avoids needless delays. We also feel that learning these techniques without the aid of navigation or using navigation as a confirmation is critical. This knowledge of appropriate starting points and trajectories helps the surgeon realize when the navigation may be "off." Additionally, if the system is not functioning properly during a case, the surgeon must rely on experience with anatomic and basic fluoroscopic techniques. Navigation is a virtual system, so it is important to periodically check the accuracy of the system by touching a specific anatomical structure such as the notch of the C2 spinous process. If there is any concern for accuracy, the practitioner should have a low threshold for reacquiring source images. Additionally, even under normal circumstances, there is more potential relative motion at the craniocervical junction when applying pressure with drill guides, drills, and screws, and especially in the setting of trauma. Because of this, there is some practitioner variability regarding the placement of the fiducial array. Some advocate attaching it to the Mayfield cranial clamp as described above. The advantage is that the array is out of the operative field. The disadvantage is the potential for relative motion between the clamp and the spine. The other option is to attach it to a structure in the operative field such as the C2 or C3 spinous process. The disadvantage is that it can be cumbersome to work around especially since the trajectory of the screws requires the detector for the system to be placed at the head of the bed. Additionally, because of the potential for relative motion with placement of retractors, generally we

recommend leaving the retractors in place for the image acquisition, where usually we would remove the retractors to avoid artifact with the spine. This increased mobility at C1–C2 is most likely a pitfall for robotic systems also.

Another way to utilize navigation is in a hybrid capacity in which navigation is used to determine starting points and plan trajectories, and then to use live fluoroscopy for drilling and screw placement. This can be done with standard fluoroscopy or by draping in image acquisition equipment and then using it in its fluoroscopic capacity. This is the technique we use for navigation assistant odontoid screw placement.[32]

24.5 Clinical Experience with Intraoperative Navigation for Atlantoaxial Fusion

24.5.1 Safety and Accuracy of Screw Placement

The primary focus of the use of intraoperative navigation for atlantoaxial fusion has been the safe and consistent placement of transarticular or segmental C1–C2 instrumentation (▶ Table 24.1). Two reports by Yang et al have compared screw placement accuracy between traditional fluoroscopy-based and navigation-assisted techniques for both transarticular[33] and segmental[34] screw placement. In the transarticular cohort, the

Table 24.1 Clinical series of intraoperative navigation for posterior atlantoaxial fusion

First author	Year	Total N	Treatment group N	Mean f/u (mo)	Mean age (yr)	Indication(s)	Primary outcome	Secondary outcome (s)	Notes	Level of evidence
Hitti[31]	2017	45	20	7.8	61.5	Traumatic and degenerative C1–C2 instability	Surgical blood loss	Operative time, rates of surgical complications	Reduction in EBL from 990 in fluoroscopy group to 438 in navigation group. Operative time longer in navigation group initially, but decreased over time	3
Smith[35]	2016	7	7	12	55.3	Traumatic, degenerative, and inflammatory atlantoaxial instability	Screw placement accuracy	Radiation dose, blood loss, fusion status	No screws required repositioning. Mean 39.0 mGy radiation dose. Mean 271 mL EBL. 100% fusion rate at 12 mos	4
Yang[33]	2015	42	18	18.4	45.1	Traumatic, degenerative, and inflammatory atlantoaxial instability	Screw placement accuracy	Radiation dose, blood loss, fusion status	97.2% screw accuracy in navigation group vs. 91.7% in fluoroscopy group; 236 vs. 308 mL EBL; 48 vs. 60 s fluoroscopy time	3
Yu[36]	2014	23	13	3	33.5	Craniovertebral junction malformation	Screw placement accuracy	Operative time, fusion status, Nurick grade	98.1% rate of accurate screw placement with 1.8 mm accuracy. 100% fusion rate over f/u period	4
Yang[34]	2013	24	12	10.8	46.0	Traumatic, degenerative, and inflammatory atlantoaxial instability	Screw placement accuracy	Radiation dose, blood loss, fusion status	95.8% screw accuracy in navigation group vs. 83.3% in fluoroscopy group; 304 mL vs. 463 mL EBL; 48 vs. 64 s fluoroscopy time	3
Uehara[37]	2012	20	20	33.75	57.9	Traumatic, degenerative, and inflammatory atlantoaxial instability	Screw placement accuracy	Radiographic parameters, JOA score, pain score	97.4% screw accuracy. One lateral perforation without clinical sequelae	4
Acosta[38]	2005	20	20	18	63.0	Traumatic, degenerative, inflammatory, malignant, and congenital atlantoaxial instability	Screw placement accuracy	Fusion status	92% accuracy in placing 36 screws in 20 patients. One nonunion in patient with malpositioned screw at 7 mo follow-up	4
Laherty[39]	2005	9	9	18	70.0	Traumatic, degenerative, inflammatory, and congenital atlantoaxial instability	Screw placement accuracy	Fusion status	100% accuracy in placement of 17 planned screws	4
Borm[40]	2004	17	14	9	60.0	Degenerative and inflammatory atlantoaxial instability	Screw placement accuracy	Analgesic intake postoperatively	Navigation used in conjunction with percutaneous transarticular screw placement via percutaneous cannulated technique. Two screw malpositions without clinical sequelae in setting of supplemental C1 claw fixation	4
Welch[41]	1997	10	4	6	46.4	Traumatic and degenerative atlantoaxial instability	Screw placement accuracy	Intraoperative complications	100% accuracy, no intraoperative complications, decreased intraoperative fluoroscopy	4

Abbreviation: EBL, estimated blood loss.

authors noted a 97.2% rate of accurate screw placement in the navigation group versus a 91.7% rate in the fluoroscopy group, though this difference was not statistically significant. One vertebral artery injury occurred in the fluoroscopy group that was successfully treated by endovascular occlusion. There were no neurologic complications in either group. Similar proportions were noted in the segmental instrumentation cohort, with a 95.8% rate in the navigation group that was significantly greater than the 83.3% in the fluoroscopy group (p=0.04). No vascular or neurologic complications occurred in either group. These retrospective cohort studies represent the highest level of evidence available regarding the comparative radiographic efficacy of screw placement for both the transarticular and segmental instrumentation constructs. The scarcity of serious adverse events with both techniques and small sample sizes preclude the formation of any conclusions regarding overall clinical superiority. Other retrospective clinical series are consistent with rates above, with reported screw placement accuracy with navigation ranging from 92 to 100%.[35,36,37,38,39,40,41]

24.5.2 Blood Loss

The robust epidural venous plexus surrounding the C2 nerve and overlying the C1–C2 joint space creates the potential for significant blood loss during surgical dissection. Navigation has been posited as a means of reducing the amount of dissection needed when compared to direct visualization of bony landmarks, therefore reducing surgical blood loss and its sequelae. Hitti et al reported a retrospective cohort study of 45 consecutive patients undergoing C1–C2 fusion with segmental instrumentation, assessing intraoperative blood loss and rates of transfusion.[31] Estimated blood loss (EBL) was significantly reduced in the navigation group (mean: 438 ± 104 mL) when compared with the fluoroscopy group (990 ± 199 mL; p = 0.02). No significant difference was seen in total volumes transfused between the groups. Yang et al also observed a significant reduction in mean EBL with the use of navigation (304 ± 48 mL) relative to fluoroscopy (463 ± 55 mL; p = 0.04).[34] These figures are also broadly consistent with the mean EBL of 271 ± 294 mL reported by Smith et al in their series of navigated C1–C2 fusions with segmental instrumentation.[35]

24.5.3 Radiation Exposure

Due to the utilization of an isocentric fluoroscopy–based navigation system, Yang et al were able to directly compare mean fluoroscopic times for both navigated and non-navigated transarticular and segmental C1–C2 fusion procedures. For transarticular screw placement, the mean fluoroscopic time in the navigated group (48.8 ± 1.1 seconds) was significantly reduced when compared to the conventional fluoroscopy group (60.3 ± 2.2 seconds; p < 0.001).[33] A similar reduction was also observed in the segmental instrumentation series (47.5 ± 1.5 vs. 64.0 ± 3.0 seconds; p < 0.001).[34] For computed tomography (CT)–based systems, direct comparison of radiation exposure is more challenging. Smith et al reported a mean patient radiation dose of 39.0 ± 13.7 mGy in their series,[35] compared to a historical mean of 6 mGy for conventional fluoroscopy.[42] However, the authors noted that this technique essentially eliminated radiation exposure for the surgical team. This is consistent with previous studies of CT-based navigation systems for instrumentation of the thoracolumbar spine.[43] Many surgeons routinely obtain postoperative CT scans to verify instrumentation following use of conventional intraoperative fluoroscopy. The potential for elimination of such scans with the use of CT-based intraoperative navigation may ultimately result in an equivalent total radiation dose to the patient in these circumstances.

24.5.4 Operative Time

The additional setup and complexity of navigation has been one barrier to its adoption. For the isocentric fluoroscopy-based navigation system, Yang et al reported a navigation-specific setup time ranging from 5 to 15 minutes in both their transarticular and segmental fixation cohorts, with equivalent total operative times.[33,34] Yu et al reported a similar 8 ± 1.5 minute setup time for a CT-based navigation system in their series.[36] Hitti et al reported that, following an initial learning curve, total operative times with CT-based navigation ultimately became equivalent to those with conventional fluoroscopy.[31]

24.6 Clinical Experience with Robotic Assistance for Atlantoaxial Fusion

Limited clinical experience to date has been accumulated regarding the use of robotic assistance for placement of atlantoaxial instrumentation. Indeed, a single case report by Tian from 2016 exists regarding the use of robotically assisted placement of a screw spanning C1–C2 in a trajectory not previously described due to aberrant anatomy of the craniocervical junction.[44] In addition to the robotic system physically placing the screw, the trajectory was also selected with assistance from surgical planning software. No safe trajectory could be identified on the right side, so a unilateral left-sided screw was placed. A postinstrumentation scan revealed a deviation of 0.9 mm from the planned trajectory with no breaches. A fusion from the occiput to C2 was subsequently performed. The author reported no complications attributable to this technique with the limitation of extremely short-term (5-day) follow-up and acknowledged that additional study is needed prior to further clinical adoption of this technique.

24.7 Conclusion

Posterior fusion of the atlantoaxial articulation remains an important means of restoring stability to this critical joint complex in the setting of degenerative, traumatic, inflammatory, or other acquired instability. Successful clinical outcomes and high fusion rates have been achieved with transarticular and segmental C1–C2 instrumentation techniques with use of anatomic landmarks and intraoperative fluoroscopy, though imaging of this region remains difficult and highly variable anatomy may place neurologic and vascular structures at risk with certain instrumentation trajectories. The use of intraoperative navigation has emerged as a means of increasing the safety and consistency of instrumentation placement in this region. Clinical reports to date suggest additional benefits in terms of reduced intraoperative blood loss and minimization of radiation exposure to the surgical team. Such benefits must be balanced against radiation exposure to the patient, cost, and increased complexity with potential effects on operative time. Limited data exists regarding the use of robotic assistance for atlantoaxial instrumentation placement. Further study will clarify the extent to which navigation and robotic techniques may facilitate reductions in the invasiveness and morbidity of posterior atlantoaxial fusion.

References

[1] Mixter SJ, Osgood RB. IV. Traumatic lesions of the atlas and axis. Ann Surg. 1910; 51(2):193–207

[2] Gallie WE. Skeletal traction in the treatment of fractures and dislocations of the cervical spine. Ann Surg. 1937; 106(4):770–776

[3] Brooks AL, Jenkins EB. Atlanto-axial arthrodesis by the wedge compression method. J Bone Joint Surg Am. 1978; 60(3):279–284

[4] Dickman CA, Sonntag VK, Papadopoulos SM, Hadley MN. The interspinous method of posterior atlantoaxial arthrodesis. J Neurosurg. 1991; 74(2):190–198

[5] Cybulski GR, Stone JL, Crowell RM, Rifai MH, Gandhi Y, Glick R. Use of Halifax interlaminar clamps for posterior C1-C2 arthrodesis. Neurosurgery. 1988; 22 (2):429–431

[6] Magerl F, Seemann PS. Stable posterior fusion of the atlas and axis by transarticular screw fixation, In: Kehr P, Weidner A, eds. Cervical Spine. New York, NY: Springer-Verlag; 1987:322–327

[7] Jeanneret B, Magerl F. Primary posterior fusion C1/2 in odontoid fractures: indications, technique, and results of transarticular screw fixation. J Spinal Disord. 1992; 5(4):464–475

[8] Paramore CG, Dickman CA, Sonntag VK. The anatomical suitability of the C1–2 complex for transarticular screw fixation. J Neurosurg. 1996; 85(2):221–224

[9] Harms J, Melcher RP. Posterior C1-C2 fusion with polyaxial screw and rod fixation. Spine. 2001; 26(22):2467–2471

[10] Goel A, Desai KI, Muzumdar DP. Atlantoaxial fixation using plate and screw method: a report of 160 treated patients. Neurosurgery. 2002; 51(6):1351–1356, discussion 1356–1357

[11] Coyne TJ, Fehlings MG, Wallace MC, Bernstein M, Tator CH. C1-C2 posterior cervical fusion: long-term evaluation of results and efficacy. Neurosurgery. 1995; 37(4):688–692, discussion 692–693

[12] Haid RW, Jr, Subach BR, McLaughlin MR, Rodts GE, Jr, Wahlig JB, Jr. C1-C2 transarticular screw fixation for atlantoaxial instability: a 6-year experience. Neurosurgery. 2001; 49(1):65–68, discussion 69–70

[13] Finn MA, Apfelbaum RI. Atlantoaxial transarticular screw fixation: update on technique and outcomes in 269 patients. Neurosurgery. 2010; 66(3) Suppl: 184–192

[14] Bourdillon P, Perrin G, Lucas F, Debarge R, Barrey C. C1-C2 stabilization by Harms arthrodesis: indications, technique, complications and outcomes in a prospective 26-case series. Orthop Traumatol Surg Res. 2014; 100(2):221–227

[15] Tokuda K, Miyasaka K, Abe H, et al. Anomalous atlantoaxial portions of vertebral and posterior inferior cerebellar arteries. Neuroradiology. 1985; 27(5): 410–413

[16] Hasan M, Shukla S, Siddiqui MS, Singh D. Posterolateral tunnels and ponticuli in human atlas vertebrae. J Anat. 2001; 199(Pt 3):339–343

[17] Young JP, Young PH, Ackermann MJ, Anderson PA, Riew KD. The ponticulus posticus: implications for screw insertion into the first cervical lateral mass. J Bone Joint Surg Am. 2005; 87(11):2495–2498

[18] Kawaguchi Y, Nakano M, Yasuda T, Seki S, Hori T, Kimura T. Development of a new technique for pedicle screw and Magerl screw insertion using a 3-dimensional image guide. Spine. 2012; 37(23):1983–1988

[19] Yang JC, Ma XY, Xia H, et al. Clinical application of computer-aided design-rapid prototyping in C1-C2 operation techniques for complex atlantoaxial instability. J Spinal Disord Tech. 2014; 27(4):E143–E150

[20] Hu Y, Yuan ZS, Kepler CK, et al. Deviation analysis of atlantoaxial pedicle screws assisted by a drill template. Orthopedics. 2014; 37(5):e420–e427

[21] Guo S, Lu T, Hu Q, Yang B, He X, Li H. Accuracy assessment of using rapid prototyping drill templates for atlantoaxial screw placement: a cadaver study. BioMed Res Int. 2016; 2016:5075879

[22] Pu X, Yin M, Ma J, et al. Design and application of a novel patient-specific 3D printed drill navigational guiding template in atlantoaxial pedicle screw placement. World Neurosurg. 2017

[23] Jiang L, Dong L, Tan M, Yang F, Yi P, Tang X. Accuracy assessment of atlantoaxial pedicle screws assisted by a novel drill guide template. Arch Orthop Trauma Surg. 2016; 136(11):1483–1490

[24] Jiang L, Dong L, Tan M, et al. A modified personalized image-based drill guide template for atlantoaxial pedicle screw placement: a clinical study. Med Sci Monit. 2017; 23:1325–1333

[25] Schmidt R, Richter M, Gleichsner F, Geiger P, Puhl W, Cakir B. Posterior atlantoaxial three-point fixation: comparison of intraoperative performance between open and percutaneous techniques. Arch Orthop Trauma Surg. 2006; 126(3):150–156

[26] Kaminski A, Gstrein A, Kälicke T, Muhr G, Müller EJ. Mini-open percutaneous transarticular screw fixation for acute and late atlantoaxial instability. Acta Orthop Belg. 2008; 74(1):102–108

[27] Holly LT, Isaacs RE, Frempong-Boadu AK. Minimally invasive atlantoaxial fusion. Neurosurgery. 2010; 66(3) Suppl:193–197

[28] Taghva A, Attenello FJ, Zada G, Khalessi AA, Hsieh PC. Minimally invasive posterior atlantoaxial fusion: a cadaveric and clinical feasibility study. World Neurosurg. 2013; 80(3–4):414–421

[29] Srikantha U, Khanapure KS, Jagannatha AT, Joshi KC, Varma RG, Hegde AS. Minimally invasive atlantoaxial fusion: cadaveric study and report of 5 clinical cases. J Neurosurg Spine. 2016; 25(6):675–680

[30] Alhashash M, Shousha M, Gendy H, Barakat AS, Boehm H. Percutaneous posterior trans-articular atlantoaxial fixation for the treatment of odontoid fractures in the elderly: a prospective study. Spine. 2017

[31] Hitti FL, Hudgins ED, Chen HI, Malhotra NR, Zager EL, Schuster JM. Intraoperative navigation is associated with reduced blood loss during C1-C2 posterior cervical fixation. World Neurosurg. 2017; 107:574–578

[32] Pisapia JM, Nayak NR, Salinas RD, et al. Navigated odontoid screw placement using the O-arm: technical note and case series. J Neurosurg Spine. 2017; 26 (1):10–18

[33] Yang Y, Wang F, Han S, et al. Isocentric C-arm three-dimensional navigation versus conventional C-arm assisted C1-C2 transarticular screw fixation for atlantoaxial instability. Arch Orthop Trauma Surg. 2015; 135(8):1083–1092

[34] Yang YL, Zhou DS, He JL. Comparison of isocentric C-arm 3-dimensional navigation and conventional fluoroscopy for C1 lateral mass and C2 pedicle screw placement for atlantoaxial instability. J Spinal Disord Tech. 2013; 26(3):127–134

[35] Smith JD, Jack MM, Harn NR, Bertsch JR, Arnold PM. Screw placement accuracy and outcomes following O-arm-navigated atlantoaxial fusion: a feasibility study. Global Spine J. 2016; 6(4):344–349

[36] Yu X, Li L, Wang P, Yin Y, Bu B, Zhou D. Intraoperative computed tomography with an integrated navigation system in stabilization surgery for complex craniovertebral junction malformation. J Spinal Disord Tech. 2014; 27(5): 245–252

[37] Uehara M, Takahashi J, Hirabayashi H, et al. Computer-assisted C1-C2 transarticular screw fixation "Magerl Technique" for atlantoaxial instability. Asian Spine J. 2012; 6(3):168–177

[38] Acosta FL, Jr, Quinones-Hinojosa A, Gadkary CA, et al. Frameless stereotactic image-guided C1-C2 transarticular screw fixation for atlantoaxial instability: review of 20 patients. J Spinal Disord Tech. 2005; 18(5):385–391

[39] Laherty RW, Kahler RJ, Walker DG, Tomlinson FH. Stereotactic atlantoaxial transarticular screw fixation. J Clin Neurosci. 2005; 12(1):62–65

[40] Börm W, König RW, Albrecht A, Richter HP, Kast E. Percutaneous transarticular atlantoaxial screw fixation using a cannulated screw system and image guidance. Minim Invasive Neurosurg. 2004; 47(2):111–114

[41] Welch WC, Subach BR, Pollack IF, Jacobs GB. Frameless stereotactic guidance for surgery of the upper cervical spine. Neurosurgery. 1997; 40(5):958–963, discussion 963–964

[42] Bandela JR, Jacob RP, Arreola M, Griglock TM, Bova F, Yang M. Use of CT-based intraoperative spinal navigation: management of radiation exposure to operator, staff, and patients. World Neurosurg. 2013; 79(2):390–394

[43] Tabaraee E, Gibson AG, Karahalios DG, Potts EA, Mobasser JP, Burch S. Intraoperative cone beam-computed tomography with navigation (O-ARM) versus conventional fluoroscopy (C-ARM): a cadaveric study comparing accuracy, efficiency, and safety for spinal instrumentation. Spine. 2013; 38(22):1953–1958

[44] Tian W. Robot-assisted posterior C1–2 transarticular screw fixation for atlantoaxial instability: a case report. Spine. 2016; 41 Suppl 19:B2–B5

25 Robotic Posterior Thoracic Pedicle Screw Placement

Marco C. Mendoza, R. Alden Milam IV, and Eric B. Laxer

Abstract

This chapter describes robotic-assisted thoracic pedicle screw placement using the Renaissance System (MAZOR Robotics, Ltd., Israel), which enables the surgeon to accurately plan and insert pedicle screws based on a preoperative CT. Potential benefits of this navigation technique include decreased radiation exposure as well as increased accuracy and safety, particularly in revision and/or deformity cases. Here, we will describe the method of preoperative planning followed by the assembly of various frame constructs and the registration process. Lastly, we will discuss the screw insertion technique and technical pearls to avoid screw malposition.

Keywords: navigation, pedicle screw, thoracic, robotics, CT, Mazor, computer

25.1 Introduction

Pedicle screw constructs are a widely accepted modality for deformity correction and spinal stabilization. Implantation can be technically challenging particularly in patients with severe deformity, osteoporosis, or malignancy. Misplaced screws may lead to devastating neurologic and vascular complications. Pedicle screw–related complications have been reported to range from 1 to 6%.[1,2,3,4,5,6] This has led to the development of new techniques to improve safety and accuracy. One such advancement involves a computer-assisted robotic device that guides pedicle screw placement based on a preoperatively planned trajectory (MAZOR Robotics, Ltd., Israel).[7,8] This chapter will focus on the surgical technique of the Renaissance System, which is composed of two main components, the Renaissance Workstation and the RBT device (▶ Fig. 25.1).

The technique can be divided into four steps: (1) Planning; (2) Frame construct; (3) Registration; and (4) Screw insertion. All four steps will be discussed below, followed by a section on additional pearls. Use of the robotic system is possible for open or percutaneous techniques.

25.2 Planning

The patient undergoes a preoperative computed tomographic (CT) scan of the thoracic spine following Mazor's Renaissance low-dose protocol (~150–200 mA) with continuous, 1-mm cuts. This can be done using any CT scanner. Using a flash drive or DVD, the CT scan is then transferred to any computer that has been loaded with Mazor's Renaissance software. The surgeon is then able to evaluate the patient's anatomy, and plan all aspects of screw decision-making such as screw size, location, starting point, and trajectory. Screw accuracy is confirmed in axial, sagittal, and coronal planes. This allows for ideal screw position in each pedicle. Once all the screws have been planned, rods are virtually added, allowing the surgeon to view the planned construct in multiple planes. This is an extremely helpful step as screw adjustments can be made as needed to allow for better alignment of the entire construct. The plan is then transferred

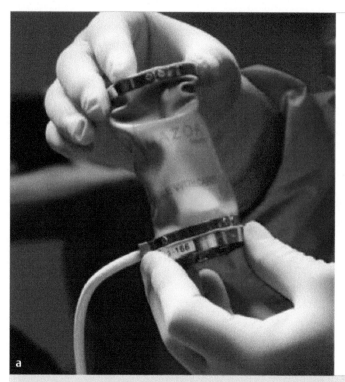
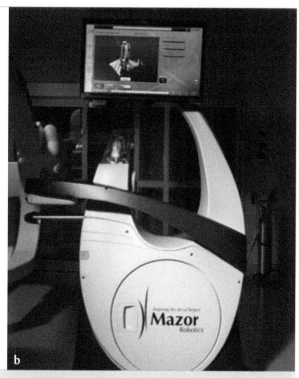

Fig. 25.1 The robotic guidance system (**a**) is a cylindrical 250-g device that can move in 6 degrees of freedom and is controlled by the workstation (**b**) that runs an interface software which facilitates preoperative planning, and intraoperative image acquisition and registration.

via flash drive to Mazor's intraoperative workstation, available for the day of surgery, and can be further edited directly on the workstation at any time if needed. Another option, if available, is to perform an intraoperative CT scan after the patient has been placed under anesthesia and positioned for surgery, then directly transfer the CT images to the Mazor workstation and construct the plan directly on the workstation in the OR.

25.3 Frame Construct

There are four mounting options for the Mazor robotic system depending on the clinical indication and preference: a clamp mount, a multidirectional bridge mount, a bed mount, and a Hover T mount. All mounting options are rigidly attached to the patient's spine to ensure maximum accuracy of screw placement. When instrumenting the thoracic spine, the Hover T is a popular option due to its bony fixation to the patient. It may be utilized in open and MIS procedures. Typically for thoracic pedicle screws, side block assemblies will be mounted on the cross bar so that the ball-and-socket joints face the feet of the patient. The side blocks are fixed to the patient using 4-mm Schantz pins. Afterward, the bridge is inserted through the cross bar and stabilized cranially using a 2.5-mm head pin inserted into the spinous process (▶ Fig. 25.2). The spinous process selected should be two levels above the planned vertebra to be instrumented. The bridge should hover freely without any external pressure but be placed as close as possible to the skin.

In open procedures, the clamp is a commonly utilized option and is attached to the spinous process centered over the area of interest. After performing a bilateral paraspinal exposure, the clamp mount may be attached. Next, a bridge is connected and fixed on each end with a K-wire inserted into the adjacent spinous processes maximizing stability (▶ Fig. 25.3). This technique is typically utilized for scoliosis and similar deformity cases. However, it may be utilized in MIS cases as well. At the minimum, a 3-cm incision is required in order to seat the clamp.

The multidirectional bridge is another mounting option that provides maximum stability. Prior to draping, bed adapters are attached to the bed rail on each side of the patient. These are typically placed just caudal to the planned incision. After draping, the bed adapters may then be fixed to the bed rail via an adapter that is underneath the drapes. The bed adapters should be positioned across from each other. The adapters should be maximally tightened because failure to do so may lead to wobbling of the bridge and inaccurate screw placement. A 2.5-mm head pin is then inserted directly into a spinous process above the planned instrumentation. It is essential that the pin has good purchase in the spinous process to maximize stability of the bridge. The multidirectional bridge is then attached so that it hovers directly over the patient. There should be minimal contact between the bridge and the patient as this can result in undue pressure on the bridge leading to screw malposition. The bridge may now translate laterally in either direction parallel to the patient's spinal column.

25.4 Registration

The Renaissance Spine Image Adaptor is attached to the C-arm. The C-arm console will then be connected directly to the Mazor workstation through a video cable. Next, an image is taken in the vertical position. The C-arm must be calibrated correctly to operate with the Renaissance Workstation. The C-arm image intensifier is affected by surrounding electromagnetic fields, which results in slight deformations of the images. This calibration process enables the software to compensate for such deformities, thereby improving accuracy.

After the selected mount is in proper position, the 3D marker is attached to the bridge at the level of interest. The position of the marker on the bridge should be entered into the workstation. To ensure proper orientation, there is an icon on the marker that should match the position of the patient. The C-arm is brought into the field and AP and 60-degree oblique images are obtained. It is imperative that all beads of the 3D marker be visible in the image to ensure proper registration. These images are then matched to the preoperative 3D CT scan. This enables the workstation to coordinate the preoperative CT

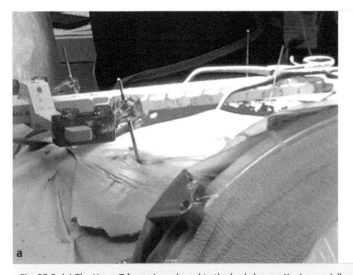
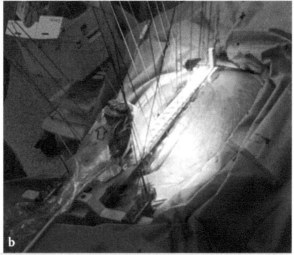

Fig. 25.2 (a) The Hover T frame is anchored to the body by one K-wire cranially and two Steinmann pins into each of the posterior superior iliac spines. **(b)** Guidewires are then inserted accordingly based on preoperative templating. These procedures can be performed with limited use of fluoroscopy. Note the robot in image **(b)** just next to the open blue arrow.

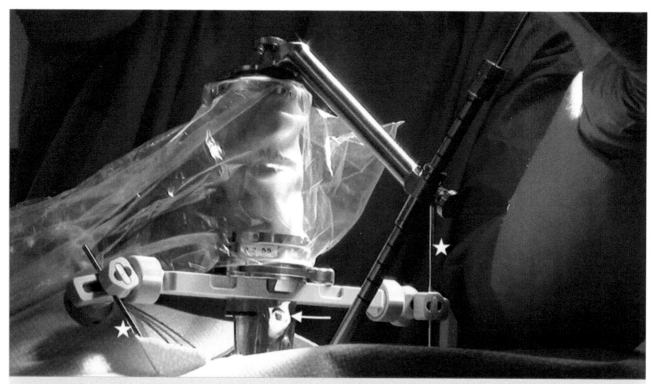

Fig. 25.3 Depiction of spinous process clamp mount. A specifically designed bridge is mounted on the clamp (*white arrow*) which allows access to three vertebrae (two motion segments). Note the fixation pins at each end of the bridge (*stars*).

images with the updated location of the platform and the vertebra. The 3D sync process registers and synchronizes the preoperative CT scan with the patient's spine and mounting platform. Each vertebra is registered separately independent of anatomic landmarks so that deformities and prior operations or disk space changes do not alter accuracy or performance.

25.5 Screw Insertion

After the registration procedure, a target vertebra is selected from the preoperative plan. The RBT may be activated and aligned to the planned trajectory. The software will then show the surgeon where the RBT device is to be mounted onto the platform. The device should be brought in from the foot of the bed and locked in place using the latch. It is imperative that the RBT device is handled only at the top and bottom end plates. The workstation will also instruct the surgeon which arms and tools to use for the planned trajectory. If screws are placed percutaneously, then an 11 blade on the scalpel holder may be used to incise the skin and then fascia. If screws are to be inserted through an open approach then the prior step may be skipped and the appropriate length cannula will then be inserted through the aiming arm followed by a blunt trochar. The blunt trochar should be pushed and rotated down to bone to clear a soft tissue path for the cannula. Using direct visualization and/or tactile feel, the trochar should contact the bony start point without any displacement or skiving. Hypertrophic facets in degenerative cases may lead to skiving laterally. The facet may be burred down to ensure that the drill bit is not

deflected from the planned starting point. Before removing the trochar, the cannula is pulled back approximately 5 mm as contact between the bone and the cannula can also lead to skiving and inaccurate screw paths. The blunt trochar is then exchanged for the drill guide. The drill guide does have sharp teeth at its tip to aid docking. It should impact in place to avoid any inaccuracy; however, one hand should be used to stabilize the cannula at all times. The appropriate drill bit is then inserted through the cannula. The depth is preset based on the preoperative plan so the drill may be buried until it is fully seated on the back of the cannula. If there is more than 3 cm between the drill guide and the stopper, then the inappropriate drill bit is being used. The surgeon should feel an endpoint throughout the length of the drill path otherwise the screw trajectory may be inaccurate. Next, a reduction tube and guidewire are inserted through the drill guide (▶ Fig. 25.4). A bony endpoint should be appreciated and the guidewire may be gently impacted into the bone. The aiming arm is removed, followed by the RBT while ensuring the guidewire remains seated. The surgeon may now complete screw insertion over the guidewire. The RBT may now be sent for the next screw trajectory.

It is at the surgeon's discretion whether or not to insert all wires first followed by screws or to instrument each level sequentially. The robotic system is designed to be accurate to 1 mm and potentially decreases radiation exposure. However, if at any point the screw purchase or trajectory appears incorrect, then fluoroscopy may be utilized to confirm screw position. In open procedures, it is imperative that the cannula should be docked onto the spine without any deflection from the surrounding soft tissue. If needed, retract the paraspinal

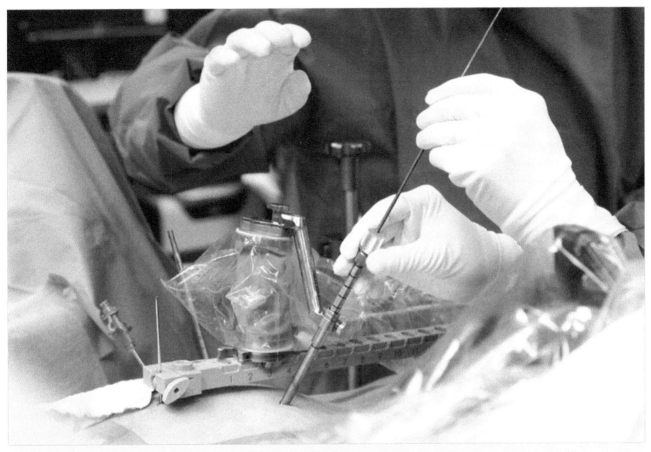

Fig. 25.4 Intraoperative photograph demonstrating percutaneous screw preparation. The reduction tube is inserted through the drill guide. Notice that one hand is utilized to stable the drill guide to maintain proper trajectory and accuracy.

musculature to avoid undue pressure on the cannula, which may lead to screw malposition. If a screw is malpositioned, then a new trajectory may be formulated using the workstation or the screw may be redirected and inserted using a freehand technique. Prior studies have reported robotic-assisted screws to be 87 to 93% accurate.[9,10,11] The most common reason for screw malposition is skiving off the side of the facet.

Robotic-assisted screw placement is still relatively new technology; therefore, efficacy and accuracy are still unproven compared to traditional techniques. There is additionally also a learning curve and such a technique may increase operative time and use of fluoroscopy initially. However, with time, speed and safety of a case will be elevated particularly in the setting of complex deformity or revision cases where normal bony landmarks are lost.

25.6 Technical Pearls

- Regardless of which mount is utilized, rigid fixation to the bed and/or bone should be achieved as subtle, inadvertent motion may lead to screw malposition.
- The blunt trochar should contact the bone without skiving. If needed, burr down the facet to create a stable entry point.

- Before removing the trochar, retract the cannula approximately 5 mm as the cannula can easily be diverted off its planned trajectory.
- There should always be an endpoint throughout the drill path, otherwise the trajectory is incorrect. Check that the RBT was docked appropriately and that the appropriate tools were used. Also, verify there is no soft tissue deflecting the cannula.

References

[1] Jutte PC, Castelein RM. Complications of pedicle screws in lumbar and lumbosacral fusions in 105 consecutive primary operations. Eur Spine J. 2002; 11 (6):594–598
[2] Kosmopoulos V, Schizas C. Pedicle screw placement accuracy: a meta-analysis. Spine. 2007; 32(3):E111–E120
[3] Kotani Y, Abumi K, Ito M, Minami A. Improved accuracy of computer-assisted cervical pedicle screw insertion. J Neurosurg. 2003; 99(3) Suppl:257–263
[4] Podolsky DJ, Martin AR, Whyne CM, Massicotte EM, Hardisty MR, Ginsberg HJ. Exploring the role of 3-dimensional simulation in surgical training: feedback from a pilot study. J Spinal Disord Tech. 2010; 23(8):e70–e74
[5] Rajasekaran S, Vidyadhara S, Ramesh P, Shetty AP. Randomized clinical study to compare the accuracy of navigated and non-navigated thoracic pedicle screws in deformity correction surgeries. Spine. 2007; 32(2):E56–E64
[6] Tian NF, Huang QS, Zhou P, et al. Pedicle screw insertion accuracy with different assisted methods: a systematic review and meta-analysis of comparative studies. Eur Spine J. 2011; 20(6):846–859

[7] Lieberman IH, Togawa D, Kayanja MM, et al. Bone-mounted miniature robotic guidance for pedicle screw and translaminar facet screw placement: Part I—Technical development and a test case result. Neurosurgery. 2006; 59(3): 641–650, discussion 641–650

[8] Togawa D, Kayanja MM, Reinhardt MK, et al. Bone-mounted miniature robotic guidance for pedicle screw and translaminar facet screw placement: Part 2—Evaluation of system accuracy. Neurosurgery. 2007; 60(2) Suppl 1: ONS129–ONS139, discussion ONS139

[9] Hu X, Ohnmeiss DD, Lieberman IH. Robotic-assisted pedicle screw placement: lessons learned from the first 102 patients. Eur Spine J. 2013; 22(3):661–666

[10] Molliqaj G, Schatlo B, Alaid A, et al. Accuracy of robot-guided versus freehand fluoroscopy-assisted pedicle screw insertion in thoracolumbar spinal surgery. Neurosurg Focus. 2017; 42(5):E14

[11] Schatlo B, Molliqaj G, Cuvinciuc V, Kotowski M, Schaller K, Tessitore E. Safety and accuracy of robot-assisted versus fluoroscopy-guided pedicle screw insertion for degenerative diseases of the lumbar spine: a matched cohort comparison. J Neurosurg Spine. 2014; 20(6):636–643

26 Robotic Minimally Invasive Transforaminal Lumbar Interbody Fusion

Alfred J. Pisano and Donald F. Colantonio III

Abstract:

The introduction of robot-assisted devices in spine surgery offers another tool in the surgeon's armamentarium for use in transforaminal lumbar interbody fusion (TLIF). This chapter summarizes the technical aspects, challenges and benefits, of robotically assisted minimally invasive TLIF and presents an overview of recent outcomes.

Keywords: transforaminal lumbar interbody fusion, robot, ROSA, SpineAssist, minimally invasive

26.1 Background

The transforaminal lumbar interbody fusion (TLIF) was first described by Harms and Jeszensky in 1998 and has since been widely utilized in the treatment of degenerative lumbar spine conditions.[1] The technique was developed as an alternative to posterior lumbar interbody fusion (PLIF) for lumbar interbody arthrodesis through a posterior approach. TLIF enables access to the disk space via a unilateral facetectomy and therefore reduces the amount of nerve root retraction required compared to PLIF. The decreased nerve retraction reduces the risk of neurologic injury while achieving similar fusion rates.[2]

The minimally invasive approach to the spine was developed in order to prevent the muscle and soft-tissue damage associated with traditional open spinal surgeries. Minimally invasive TLIF has been demonstrated to achieve similar outcomes to open TLIF with decreased perioperative pain and decreased paraspinal muscle injury. Although minimally invasive TLIF has become increasingly more utilized to treat degenerative lumbar spine disease, it remains technically challenging. Limited line of sight while operating through cannulas requires surgeons to rely on imaging and navigation systems to perform the procedure safely and efficiently.[3] Robot-guided systems have been utilized to further assist surgeons when performing minimally invasive spine procedures.

The most commonly utilized devices in robot-assisted TLIF surgeries are the SpineAssist (MAZOR Surgical Technologies, Israel), the ROSA Spine (Medtech, France), and the Globus Excelsius system. The devices are designed to assist the surgeon with pedicle screw placement and can assist in interbody placement. The systems can be used with either percutaneous or open approach. There are many aspects of robot-assisted TLIF that are common to both machines, although each has unique features as well.

26.2 Technique

Robot-assisted TLIF, whether performed through a minimally invasive or standard open approach, is dependent on several key factors in order to be conducted safely and effectively. Preoperative imaging and planning, positioning of both the patient and the robot, and approach and preparation of pedicles are all key elements to performing a successful robot-assisted TLIF.

26.2.1 ROSA Spine

The ROSA Spine device is a robotic arm with tracking capabilities and a navigation system. Its platform includes the robotic arm attached to a base coupled with a haptic sensor and a touch screen surgical workstation as well as an optical navigation camera.

The patient is positioned prone on a radiolucent operating table and the surgical site is prepped in sterile fashion. The O-arm (Medtronic) is covered with a sterile drape and positioned opposite the surgeon and slightly to his or her left in order to obtain intraoperative imaging. The ROSA Spine robot is covered with a sterile drape and positioned adjacent to the table and with the base perpendicular to the patient. The optical navigation camera is positioned at the foot of the bed and angled to face the operative site.[4,5]

A percutaneous reference pin is placed at the iliac wing. The robot's position is then coregistered to the patient reference using the optical camera. Next, the fiducial box attached to the robot arm is positioned using the robot's haptic properties. The fiducial box should be placed just over the skin at the operating site. CT imaging is obtained using the O-arm in breath-hold mode and subsequently transferred to the ROSA Spine surgical workstation. The utilization of breath-hold mode allows the robot to track movements of the spine induced by respiration. Recording of 3D images is conducted with automatic recognition by the fiducial box.[4,5]

Following image registration, the surgeon begins surgical planning. The first step is planning the trajectory for bilateral pedicle screw placement at the targeted levels to be fused. The surgeon choses his or her desired entry point and target point for the trajectory of each screw and then determines the length and diameter of each screw. During the planning process, the surgeon has access to the axial, sagittal, and coronal views on the robot's workstation and can also look along or perpendicular to the planned trajectory.

The robot arm is positioned along the trajectory and the movement tracking function is activated. Movement of the patient's body is tracked and accounted for with the robot's real-time navigation capability which allows instruments to remain along the planned trajectory throughout the procedure. Dilators are attached to the robot arm and positioned just above the skin at the first level to be instrumented. A small skin incision is made and the dilators are placed through the skin and muscle to access the entry point on the pedicle. A drill with a 3-mm bit is inserted through the dilator and an entry hole is drilled into the pedicle. The drill bit and all other instruments are tracked using real-time navigation. It is recommended to drill 20 mm through the bone and perform back-and-forth drill movements until no resistance is met in order to avoid a "ripping effect" between the drill and the bone. The back-and-forth movement serves to widen the entry point.[5]

A guide tube needle is placed through the dilator and then through the pedicle into the posterior vertebral body and a guide wire is inserted. The guide wire and all instruments are tracked with computer-aided navigation utilizing one of the percutaneous ancillary systems compatible with the ROSA Spine (Sextant, Longitude, or Socore) and monitored in real time. If the position of an instrument displayed by the navigation system differs from the planned trajectory, the true position can be confirmed using intraoperative fluoroscopy. The guide-tube needle is removed and dilators are placed through the muscles over the guide wire. The pedicles are then tapped and screws are placed percutaneously via the guide wire. The two percutaneous incisions are then joined in order to place a minimally invasive retractor and expose the articular facet. Next, a unilateral facetectomy is performed and the nerve root is released and retracted. TLIF may be performed according to each surgeon's preference. Thorough diskectomy is performed and ultimately a TLIF cage is placed with the option to use real-time navigation during diskectomy and cage insertion to minimize use of fluoroscopy.[4,5]

The procedure is conducted in a similar fashion for an open approach. The steps for intraoperative imaging and pedicle screw planning are the same as for a minimally invasive approach. When the lamina and articular facets of the vertebral bodies to be fused are exposed, the robot arm is positioned and the pedicles are drilled with robotic assistance. Pedicle screws are placed similarly with robot assistance.

Following arthrodesis, a CT scan is performed to verify final positioning. Once acceptable placement of hardware has been confirmed, the wound is closed in standard fashion.

26.2.2 SpineAssist Robot

The SpineAssist robot is a parallel manipulator device that utilizes a semiactive mode in positioning surgical instruments. The main components of the system are the robot itself and the SpineAssist workstation. The robot uses three outrigger arms which are designed to accommodate a drill guide sleeve. There are also two mounting options for the robot: the spinous process clamp and the Hover-T Minimally Invasive Frame (MAZOR). The spinous process clamp is used to attach the robot directly to a single spinous process near the target levels through a small incision. The spinous process clamp allows access to two motion segments with the robot attached to a specially designed bridge that has three accommodations for the robot. The Hover-T Minimally Invasive Frame is used to secure the robot to a frame attached to the patient with a K-wire and two Steinmann pins. The frame has a central bar that is aligned along the spine with a base that allows the robot to be attached in one of 19 different positions.[6]

The first step in utilizing the SpineAssist platform involves preoperative imaging and planning. A CT scan is obtained using the SpineAssist protocol. The CT must use 0.4- to 1-mm slices all in parallel and all in the same dimensions without compression. The images are then transferred to the SpineAssist workstation or to the surgeon's personal computer. The SpineAssist software is then able to generate 3D virtual images of each vertebra of interest to be used for surgical planning. The surgeon uses the reconstructed 3D images to plan the optimal entry point, trajectory, length, and diameter of pedicle screws. If the surgeon uses a computer other than the SpineAssist workstation, that device must be present in the operating room or the plan must be transferred via portable storage to the SpineAssist workstation.[6]

Several steps must take place in the operating room prior to the initiation of the procedure, and these should ideally occur prior to the patient being in the room. First, the accuracy of the SpineAssist system must be verified. The device is mounted on a jig with three-hole positions that are recognized by the software. The verification process is initiated and the software positions the robot according to the holes in the jig. A K-wire is placed through the drill sleeve and into one hole at a time to verify the starting point and trajectory.[6]

Another important step that can take place at the same time as system accuracy verification is the calibration of intraoperative fluoroscopy. The system utilizes a specifically designed phantom that is attached onto the image intensifier of C-arm. The phantom has two surfaces that contain metal beads which are recognized by the software and used to calibrate C-arm images and control for distortions caused by surrounding electronic fields in the operating room. Once the phantom is attached, the C-arm is aligned with the orientation of the patient and an anteroposterior (AP) and lateral X-ray without any objects in the field of view for calibration. Four additional images are required once the patient is in position to complete calibration.[6]

The patient is positioned prone on a radiolucent operating table and prepped and draped in sterile fashion. At this point, either the spinous process clamp or the Hover-T Minimally Invasive Frame is attached to the patient. To affix the spinous process clamp, the target level is identified and an approximately 4-cm incision is made over the spinous process. The clamp is attached to the spinous process and the bridge is attached to the clamp. This can be done with or without fluoroscopic guidance. To attach the Hover-T Minimally Invasive Frame, a K-wire is placed through the frame into one of the spinous processes and two Steinmann pins are then placed through the frame into the posterior-superior iliac spine (PSIS) on either side. Pin placement can be performed with or without fluoroscopic guidance.[6]

Once the preferred mounting platform is anchored to the patient, four X-rays are taken to complete the image registration process. First, an AP and lateral X-rays are taken without the targeting device in place. Then the targeting device is attached to the mounting platform and another set of AP and lateral X-rays is taken. At this point, the image registration process is complete and no further imaging is required throughout the operation. The software automatically registers the four intraoperative images to the preoperative CT images and planned screw trajectories. The surgeon then uses the workstation to verify that the synchronized images are matched appropriately (the software also independently evaluates the accuracy of the image match). Imaging should be repeated if the fluoroscopic images are not well matched to the preoperative CT. The surgeon's plan is displayed as an overlay on the synchronized images once accurate image registration is achieved.[6]

The SpineAssist system is now ready for pedicle screw placement. The surgeon selects a vertebral body to instrument and the software determines the appropriate position to attach the SpineAssist robot based on which mounting platform is used.

The software also determines which arm to use. If the Hover-T Frame is used, the software displays all combinations of robot positions and arms that the surgeon may select. The robot is secured in the chosen position and the software moves the robot to achieve the planned entry point and trajectory. Next, the arm is attached to the robot's top plate and a cannulated drill guide is placed into the guide sleeve. A drill bit is then introduced into the cannulated drill guide. A small skin incision is made to introduce an obturator and bluntly dissect through soft tissues to bone along the trajectory of the drill. The drill is advanced along the trajectory to the entry point and a hole is made through the cortex. A K-wire is then placed in the hole and advanced into the vertebral body. Next a screw hole is drilled and the pedicle is probed to check for any breach followed by insertion of the pedicle screw. This process is repeated at each level until all screws are placed.[6]

Once pedicle screws are in place, dilators can be placed in order to perform a facetectomy. The nerve root is released and retracted and the surgeon conducts a thorough diskectomy. TLIF cages are then placed and positioning is confirmed with fluoroscopy.

26.2.3 Excelsius GPS Robot

The Excelsius GPS robot contains a navigation platform married to a robotic arm and is currently utilized in spine surgery for pedicle screw placement. Preoperative imaging may be used to plan pedicle screws preoperatively and then merged with intraoperative imaging or an entirely intraoperative process may be employed. Our preference is to obtain a preoperative CT scan with 1 mm thin or less slices and preoperatively plan our pedicle screw trajectories. We then utilize intraoperative fluoroscopy to obtain perfect AP and lateral images and merge the intraoperative data with our preoperative scans. Alternatively, an O-arm (Medtronic) can be used to obtain an intraoperative scan from which to plan screws and subsequently reference for robotic pedicle screw placement.

26.2.4 Intraoperative Workflow

Two reference pins are placed, one into each PSIS, and serve as fiducials (▶ Fig. 26.1). Initially, a small incision is made over the right PSIS, and soft-tissue dissection is performed to place the Excelsius GPS standard Quattro spike directly into the PSIS. The Quattro spike provides a point of rigid fixation for the system's dynamic reference frame. A second incision is then made over the contralateral PSIS to place the surveillance marker into rigid bony anatomy to track the relative distance to the dynamic reference base (DRB) to identify unwanted shifts in the DRB during the procedure, tracked by the camera throughout the procedure. The fiducials are detected automatically in the intraoperative scan and are used to register the patient's anatomy during the scan to the DRB.

After placement of the reference markers, the C-arm is brought into the field with the fluoroscopy registration fixture attached to the image intensifier, acquiring one true AP and one true lateral intraoperative fluoroscopic image for each planned level, noting that the same image may be used for multiple levels (▶ Fig. 26.2). Levels are appropriately labeled utilizing a centroid marker.

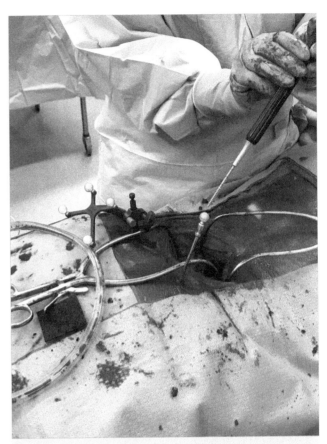

Fig. 26.1 Globus Quattro spike inserted into right posterior superior iliac spine (PSIS) and Globus surveillance marker with attached reference clamp at left PSIS.

Once all images are captured and identified, the software performs a seeded merge between the preoperative CT scans, DRR file, and the intraoperative fluoroscopy images (▶ Fig. 26.3). This merge is checked manually to ensure bony landmarks are matched, ensuring navigational integrity (▶ Fig. 26.4).

The robotic system is then brought into the sterile field. The base station is then docked after assurance that all of the previously planned screw trajectories are reachable by the end effector.

Starting with the screw trajectory farthest from the dynamic reference base, the desired screw plan is selected and the robotic arm precisely aligns into the desired trajectory. The GPS instruments are displayed as they are advanced through the end effector. For multiple-level fusions, we bring the robotic arm in for each level and mark the location of planned skin penetration. We then make a single skin incision in a "best fit" line (i.e., averaging a straight line between the medial to lateral lineup of the planned screw trajectories), which minimizes the chance of skin or fascia deflecting the instrumentation leading to possible screw misplacement.

After skin incision, we dissect through the subcutaneous tissue to the level of the fascia, which is then widely incised in line with the skin incision. The robotic arm is then brought into the field for each of the planned pedicle screw trajectories. The real-time instrument/implant trajectory is displayed on the patient images along with the planned screw allowing confirmation of the

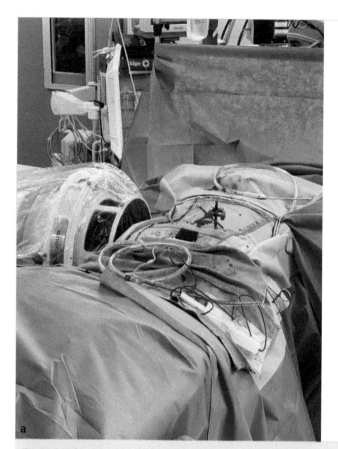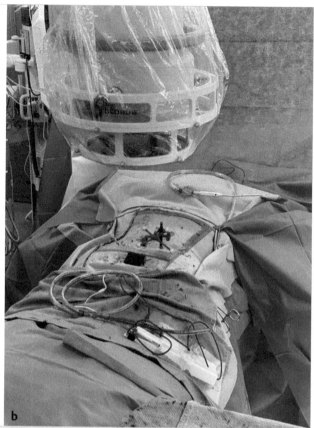

Fig. 26.2 (a,b) Perfect anteroposterior and lateral fluoroscopic images must be obtained with fluoroscopy registration fixture attached to the image intensifier and images then merged with preoperative CT.

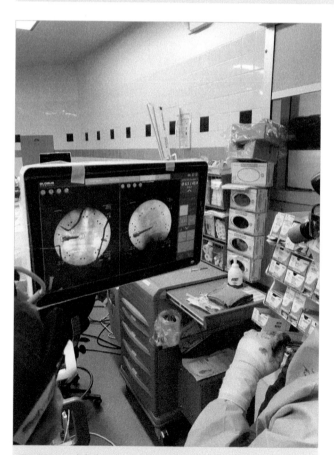

Fig. 26.3 In all fluoroscopic technique, screws can be planned based on fluoroscopic imaging using pedicle shadows on anteroposterior and lateral projections.

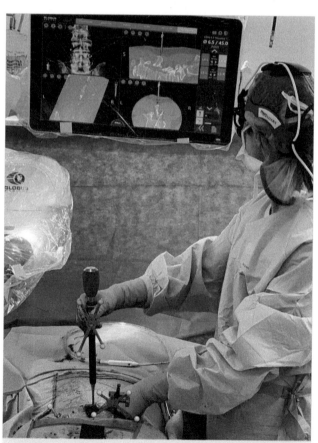

Fig. 26.4 Identifiable bony landmarks are checked with intraoperative navigation to ensure integrity of the planned screw trajectories. Here, the surgeon is placing the probe on the spinous process and confirming its localization on the navigation platform.

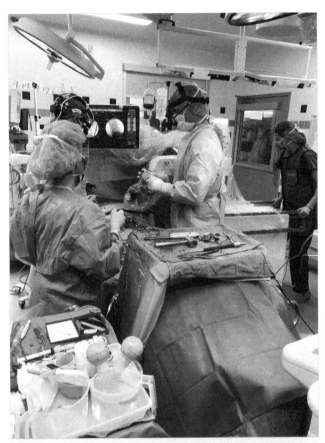

Fig. 26.5 The robotic arm is automatically brought into the field in the correct location for planned pedicle screw placement.

desired trajectory. Observation is made periodically between the monitor and surgical site to ensure consistency between tactile and navigation feedback.

We prefer to use a blunt tip side cutting drill (3.5 × 30 mm side-cutting, high-speed/low-torque drill) to make the pedicle screw holes as we find this drill the least likely to skive and cause screw misplacement. After drilling the screw trajectory in the robotic arm, screws are then placed through the arm of the preplanned width and diameter (▶ Fig. 26.5). Once all implants have been successfully placed, rods are placed and secured with end caps and locked into final position. Prior to breaking screw tabs, we obtain an AP and lateral fluoroscopic image to ensure that the screws appear appropriately positioned. Once, screws have been placed, TLIF may proceed as per surgeon's protocol. The Quattro spikes and surveillance marker are then removed and the wounds are closed in a standard layered fashion (▶ Fig. 26.6).

26.3 Outcomes

In assessing the efficacy of robotic TLIF, pedicle screw accuracy is paramount. Evaluation of surgical parameters such as radiation administered is likewise essential in judging the practicality of robotic TLIF. As robotic TLIF is a novel technology, data evaluating these characteristics are somewhat limited.

However, here we will evaluate the available data in regard to screw accuracy and surgical outcomes with an understanding that as these technologies evolve and surgeons become more adept in their use, these data may change.

26.3.1 Pedicle Screw Accuracy

Numerous studies have evaluated the accuracy of the SpineAssist robot in vivo in comparison to freehand technique. A systematic review and meta-analysis identified five early studies that compared pedicle screw accuracy between the SpineAssist robot (both percutaneous and open) and freehand technique. Their analysis included 600 robotic pedicle screws and 400 freehand screws. They did not find a difference between the rate of Gertzbein-Robbins Grade A pedicle screws (RR: 1.08, $p = 0.52$.) or Grade B pedicle screws (RR: 1.02, $p = 0.93$).[7] Furthermore, neither percutaneous nor open robotic assist demonstrated a difference in accuracy when compared to freehand technique.[8]

Numerous subsequent case series have validated these early findings with reported accuracy rates of 90 to 100%.[9] The largest case series to date evaluated 3,271 pedicle screws with the SpineAssist robot and found a GRS Grade A or B rate of 98.3%.[10] Interestingly, one study demonstrated a difference in screw accuracy between robotic pedicle screws and freehand technique. In the study by Ringel et al, robot-assisted screws were less accurate overall (93 vs. 85%) and tended to veer laterally.[11] The authors theorized that the bed mount platform for the robot may not have provided enough stability for accurate screw placement. A study by van Dijk et al demonstrated that aberrant screws breached the pedicle laterally 68% of the time, while 35% of breaches occurred medially.[12]

Several techniques have been employed to mitigate screw aberrancy. Kuo et al evaluated a novel technique with the SpineAssist robot. Using secondary registration, they were able to increase pedicle screw accuracy. By first placing k-wires and evaluating trajectory prior to screw implantation, they noted a 6% error rate with K-wires deviating greater than 3 mm. They repositioned the errant K-wires and were able to achieve a final accuracy of 98.7%.[13] In addition to secondary registration, the Peteron technique theoretically reduces the risk of lateral breach by flattening the entry point with a drill. This serves to mitigate robotic arm slippage on the lateral face of the facet. Furthermore, selection of the most lateral to medial screw trajectory available for each pedicle may reduce the incidence of lateral slippage as well. Interestingly, Macke et al found an improved accuracy rate when patients received a prone CT preoperatively (97.6 vs. 92.4% accuracy).[14]

One study has demonstrated improved efficacy of robotic technique over navigation assistance. Roser et al compared pedicle screw accuracy between a freehand group, robotic group, and navigation group and found GRS Grade A rates of 97.5, 99, and 92%, respectively.[15]

The majority of available data pertains to the SpineAssist robot. However, one study by Lonjon et al evaluated screw accuracy with the ROSA robot compared to the freehand technique. They found an accuracy rate of 97.2% with the robot compared to 92% with a freehand technique.[16] While this technology is promising, additional studies are needed to further validate its performance.

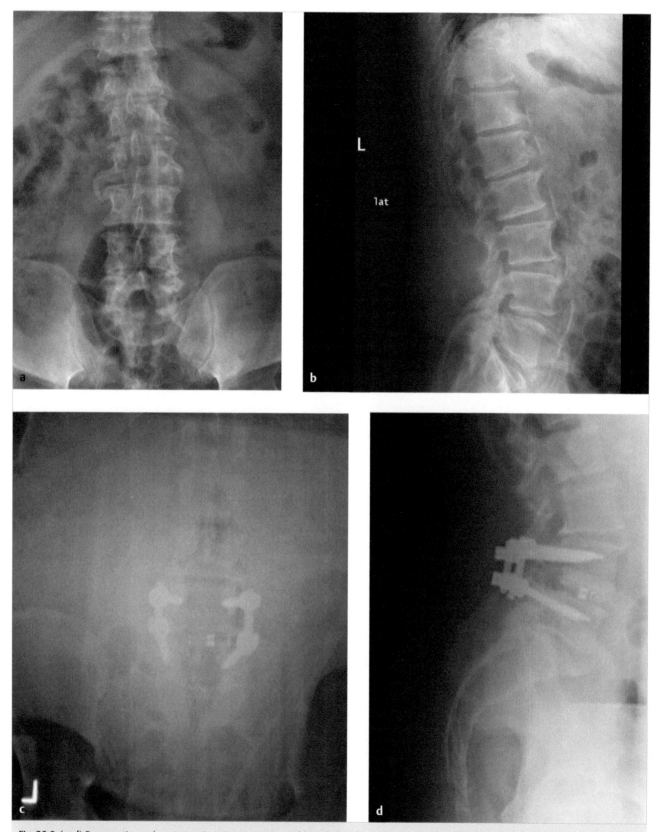

Fig. 26.6 (a–d) Preoperative and postoperative anteroposterior and lateral plain film imaging of robotically placed pedicle screw and transforaminal lumbar interbody fusion case.

26.3.2 Radiation Exposure

Decrease in radiation exposure is one of the proposed benefits of robotically assisted screw placement. Several studies have compared radiation dosage administered using robotic assistance versus freehand screw placement. These studies generally demonstrate a significant reduction or equivalent administration of intraoperative radiation when using the SpineAssist robot. Hyun et al found that fluoroscopy time with the robot was 3.5 seconds per screw compared to 13.3 seconds for the freehand technique.[17] Similarly, Kantelhardt et al found a decrease in fluoroscopy time with the SpineAssist robotic technique (34 vs. 77 seconds per screw).[8] The one available study evaluating radiation exposure with the ROSA robot demonstrated an increase in fluoroscopy time compared to freehand technique (25 vs. 10 seconds per screw).[16]

These studies do not account for radiation administered preoperatively needed for templating. However, one study utilized low-dose CT preoperatively and was able to reduce radiation exposure to the patient and was still able to use the images for preoperative templating.[18] However, more studies are needed to evaluate this technique as this study did not comment on screw accuracy.

26.4 Complications

Minimally invasive TLIF is a technically challenging procedure and robotic assistance devices have been incorporated into this technique with the goal of minimizing common complications. Pedicle screw malposition, durotomy, nerve root injury, pseudoarthrosis, and hardware failure remain concerns of minimally invasive TLIF even with the use of robotic assistance. Introducing a robotic device to the procedure, however, also generates a new set of potential complications due to reliance on a nonhuman element. The primary adverse outcome reported due to robot failure is screw malposition which has been attributed to several factors. Soft-tissue pressure on the guiding arm,[11,19] inability to surgically obtain the target angle for screw placement as determined by software,[9] difficulty in keeping the drill guide positioned on the slope of the facet,[11,13,20] and conducting preoperative CT in the standard supine position rather than prone[14] have been shown to contribute to screw malpositioning. Additionally, several studies describe aborting the robotic procedure due to software registration failure or inability to obtain adequate fluoroscopic imaging prior to robot utilization.[9]

26.5 Conclusion

Robotic TLIF is a novel technology with promising outcomes. Two commercially available robots, the SpineAssist by MAZOR and the ROSA by Medtech, seek to improve pedicle screw accuracy through trajectory planning and tool positioning. While further research is needed in regard to clinical outcomes, numerous studies have demonstrated their efficacy and safety.

References

[1] Harms JG, Jeszenszky D. Die posteriore, lumbale, interkorporelle Fusion in unilateraler transforaminaler Technik. Oper Orthop Traumatol. 1998; 10(2): 90–102

[2] Humphreys SC, Hodges SD, Patwardhan AG, Eck JC, Murphy RB, Covington LA. Comparison of posterior and transforaminal approaches to lumbar interbody fusion. Spine. 2001; 26(5):567–571

[3] Schröder ML, Staartjes VE. Revisions for screw malposition and clinical outcomes after robot-guided lumbar fusion for spondylolisthesis. Neurosurg Focus. 2017; 42(5):E12

[4] Chenin L, Peltier J, Lefranc M. Minimally invasive transforaminal lumbar interbody fusion with the ROSA(TM) Spine robot and intraoperative flat-panel CT guidance. Acta Neurochir (Wien). 2016; 158(6):1125–1128

[5] Lefranc M, Peltier J. Evaluation of the ROSA™ Spine robot for minimally invasive surgical procedures. Expert Rev Med Devices. 2016; 13(10):899–906

[6] Lieberman IH, Togawa D, Kayanja MM, et al. Bone-mounted miniature robotic guidance for pedicle screw and translaminar facet screw placement: Part I–Technical development and a test case result. Neurosurgery. 2006; 59(3): 641–650, discussion 641–650

[7] Liu H, Chen W, Wang Z, Lin J, Meng B, Yang H. Comparison of the accuracy between robot-assisted and conventional freehand pedicle screw placement: a systematic review and meta-analysis. Int J CARS. 2016; 11 (12):2273–2281

[8] Kantelhardt SR, Martinez R, Baerwinkel S, Burger R, Giese A, Rohde V. Perioperative course and accuracy of screw positioning in conventional, open robotic-guided and percutaneous robotic-guided, pedicle screw placement. Eur Spine J. 2011; 20(6):860–868

[9] Joseph JR, Smith BW, Liu X, Park P. Current applications of robotics in spine surgery: a systematic review of the literature. Neurosurg Focus. 2017; 42(5): E2

[10] Devito DP, Kaplan L, Dietl R, et al. Clinical acceptance and accuracy assessment of spinal implants guided with SpineAssist surgical robot: retrospective study. Spine. 2010; 35(24):2109–2115

[11] Ringel F, Stüer C, Reinke A, et al. Accuracy of robot-assisted placement of lumbar and sacral pedicle screws: a prospective randomized comparison to conventional freehand screw implantation. Spine. 2012; 37(8):E496–E501

[12] van Dijk JD, van den Ende RPJ, Stramigioli S, Köchling M, Höss N. Clinical pedicle screw accuracy and deviation from planning in robot-guided spine surgery: robot-guided pedicle screw accuracy. Spine. 2015; 40(17):E986–E991

[13] Kuo KL, Su YF, Wu CH, et al. Assessing the intraoperative accuracy of pedicle screw placement by using a bone-mounted miniature robot system through secondary registration. PLoS One. 2016; 11(4):e0153235

[14] Macke JJ, Woo R, Varich L. Accuracy of robot-assisted pedicle screw placement for adolescent idiopathic scoliosis in the pediatric population. J Robot Surg. 2016; 10(2):145–150

[15] Roser F, Tatagiba M, Maier G. Spinal robotics: current applications and future perspectives. Neurosurgery. 2013; 72 Suppl 1:12–18

[16] Lonjon N, Chan-Seng E, Costalat V, Bonnafoux B, Vassal M, Boetto J. Robot-assisted spine surgery: feasibility study through a prospective case-matched analysis. Eur Spine J. 2016; 25(3):947–955

[17] Hyun SJ, Kim KJ, Jahng TA, Kim HJ. Minimally invasive robotic versus open fluoroscopic-guided spinal instrumented fusions. Spine. 2017; 42(6):353–358

[18] Sensakovic WF, O'Dell MC, Agha A, Woo R, Varich L. CT radiation dose reduction in robot-assisted pediatric spinal surgery. Spine. 2017; 42(7):E417–E424

[19] Barzilay Y, Liebergall M, Fridlander A, Knoller N. Miniature robotic guidance for spine surgery–introduction of a novel system and analysis of challenges encountered during the clinical development phase at two spine centres. Int J Med Robot. 2006; 2(2):146–153

[20] Schatlo B, Molliqaj G, Cuvinciuc V, Kotowski M, Schaller K, Tessitore E. Safety and accuracy of robot-assisted versus fluoroscopy-guided pedicle screw insertion for degenerative diseases of the lumbar spine: a matched cohort comparison. J Neurosurg Spine. 2014; 20(6):636–643

27 Robotic Anterior Lumbar Interbody Fusion

Patricia Zadnik Sullivan, Tristan Blase Fried, and William C. Welch

Abstract:

Robotic anterior lumbar interbody fusion (ALIF) is an innovative technique combining the advantages of laparoscopic technology and robotic surgical systems. Anterior approaches to lumbar spinal fusion are indicated for patients with lumbar instability and radiographic evidence of decreased lumbar lordosis or loss of interbody disk height. Historically, a large abdominal incision is made to allow an access surgeon to approach the anterior lumbar spine, then a neurosurgeon or an orthopaedic surgeon removes a disk and places an interbody cage. The use of a combined laparoscopic and robotic surgical system allows the surgeon to maintain manual dexterity and a wide view of the surgical field despite smaller incisions. One limitation of this technique is its reliance on multiple surgical teams, and poorly described federal and local regulations for its use. This chapter will review the technical aspects of robotic-assisted ALIF and discuss the advantages and limitations of this technique.

Keywords: robotic surgery, laparoscopy, anterior lumbar interbody fusion, anterior lumbar spine

27.1 Introduction

Robotic surgical systems provide surgeons with increased dexterity and improve the operative view while eliminating the need for a surgical assistant to manipulate the endoscope. The surgeon is seated at a console in the operating room, controlling the wristed instruments at the end of the robotic arms. One of the most popular robotic systems, the da Vinci Surgical Robot, was developed by Intuitive Surgical and has been described in porcine, human cadaver, and human patient models of robotic anterior lumbar interbody fusion (R-ALIF).[1,2,3,4] This robotic system utilizes arms that can be fitted with scalpels, graspers, and electrocautery; however, no bone-cutting or rongeur instruments have been developed for use. The da Vinci robot has been approved by the United States Food and Drug Administration (FDA) for general surgery procedures involving laparoscopy, as well as urological, gynecological, and a subset of cardiac procedures.[5] To date, the FDA has not approved the use of robotic surgical systems in ALIF procedures.

Early technical notes for the use of the R-ALIF described proof of principle on living pigs and human cadavers.[4,6] These studies describe the use of the robot for the entirety of the procedure; and allow the neurosurgeon, orthopaedic surgeon, or neurosurgical researcher to complete all stages of the procedure. Unfortunately, most neurosurgeons and orthopaedic surgeons are not familiar with the laparoscope or credentialed to utilize the robotic surgical system from the start to the end of the case; thus, nonhuman and human cadaver models are the only technical descriptions of purely robotic techniques. Federal, vendor-specific, and hospital regulations restrict the use of the surgical robots for placement of instrumentation in human patients, and further large-scale studies will be needed before the widespread adoption of this technique. Furthermore, as orthopaedic and neurosurgical subspecialties continue to modify resident education, it is unclear if endoscopic and robot-assisted surgery will be incorporated into surgical training.

27.2 Technical Description

27.2.1 Animal Model

The proof of principle robot-assisted ALIF is described in a pig model.[3,4,6] Both the transperitoneal and retroperitoneal approaches are described in the pig model; however, the retroperitoneal approach will be described for illustration. The pig is placed in a right lateral decubitus position and a flank incision is made for a blunt tip balloon trocar for insufflation. Multiple incisions are made including a camera port, two robotic arm insertion ports, and assist port located above the camera. The robotic surgical system is docked and the surgeon takes a seat at the robotic console, directing the robotic arms using the device. The psoas muscle is identified and retracted to visualize the lateral aspect of the lumbar interbody disk space. The annulus is incised and disk material removed. An additional incision is made for the cage insertion port. An endoscope and expandable cage instruments are used to prepare the end plate. Finally, an expandable cage is inserted. A radiograph of the porcine lumbar spine is taken to confirm successful interbody placement. Technical difficulties complicated this approach, with the robot repeatedly freezing, requiring repositioning of the robotic arms and increasing the overall operative time to 6 hours.[6]

27.2.2 Patient Case Reports

In the technical description of robotic-assisted laparoscopic ALIF in human patients,[1,2,4] the patient is positioned supine on a radiolucent table and prepped and draped in the usual fashion. A modified lithotomy position is used to provide internal retraction of pelvic viscera. Preoperative fluoroscopy provides localization for the level of interest. An access surgeon, specifically a urological or general surgeon with experience in the surgical robot, introduces the needle into the umbilicus for insufflation. A camera port is then introduced via the umbilicus. A 30-degree endoscope is used to enter the abdomen to visualize safe entry of an assistant port, as well as two or three additional instrument ports. The robot may then be docked to the camera port and instruments introduced to the abdominal cavity for transperitoneal dissection of the lumbar disk space of interest (▶ Fig. 27.1). Red rubber catheters may be used for intermittent, atraumatic retraction of the great vessels depending on the level of interest. The presacral plexus is identified and retracted, and the sacral artery and vein may be ligated or clipped.

When the anterior disk space is fully exposed, fluoroscopy is used to confirm the correct level. Due to federal regulations, the robot may not be used for placement of spinal instrumentation; therefore, technical approaches for the robotic ALIF proceed using standard laparoscopy techniques. Specifically, a 2-cm

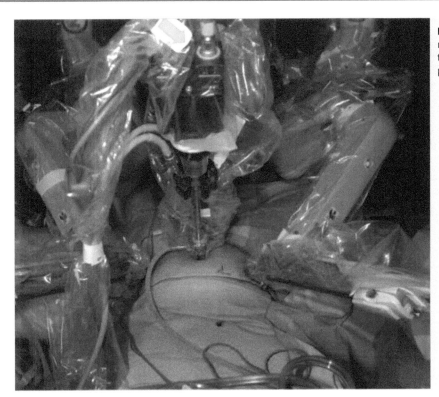

Fig. 27.1 Intraoperative photograph surgical robot docked to patient. The patient is supine in the lithotomy position. (Reproduced with permission from Lee et al.[1])

incision is made approximately 5 cm superior to the pubic symphysis and a gel port is introduced to maintain pneumoperitoneum and allow passage of spinal instrumentation. This incision should reflect the angle necessary to approach the disk space of interest, and take into consideration the patient's specific anatomy as well as the size of the implantable cage. The disk annulus is then incised, and the disk material and the end plates prepared for cage placement. A spacer is placed to confirm proper restoration of disk height and lordosis, and the final cage is packed with bone morphogenetic protein or other osteoinductive material, and placement is confirmed via intraoperative fluoroscopy.

27.3 Comparison to Open Anterior Lumbar Interbody Fusion

Anterior lumbar interbody fusion is advantageous for patients with lumbar instability who require restoration of disk height and stabilization. The anterior approach allows the surgeon to restore disk height and introduce lumbar lordosis, and may be used alone or in combination with posterior laminectomy and fusion. A clear view of the anatomy is necessary for safe cage placement, as the lumbosacral plexus overlies the anterior lumbar vertebral bodies, and the iliac vein and artery bifurcate anterior to L4. During dissection, damage to the lumbosacral plexus may result in decreased sensation in the legs or retrograde ejaculation in male patients.[7,8,9,10,11,12] Unfortunately, in patients who have undergone multiple prior abdominal surgeries, including common procedures such as hysterectomies, inguinal hernia repairs, and cesarean sections, the traditional open anterior approach may be limited by postsurgical adhesions which restrict dissection to the anterior lumbar spine.

Other limitations of the open anterior approach include increased abdominal muscle tone in an unparalyzed, anesthetized patient, if neuromonitoring is used during the case. Abdominal contractility can displace abdominal retractors, obstructing the view of the anterior disk space. Finally, in obese patients, standard abdominal retractors may be unable to meet the length required to access the anterior lumbar spine.

To combat these limitations, laparoscopic-assisted ALIF affords surgeons a better view of the anterior disk space. In multiple general surgical studies, laparoscopic surgeries reduce the length of surgical incisions, decrease postoperative pain, and decrease length of stay.[13,14] Lysis of adhesions may be performed concomitantly, allowing the surgeon to have unobstructed access to the anterior lumbar vertebral body. However, in contrast to open ALIF which can be completed via a retroperitoneal approach, laparoscopic ALIF is generally transperitoneal. Retroperitoneal approaches are thought to reduce the risk of retrograde ejaculation due to decreased manipulation of the lumbosacral plexus. Although retroperitoneal laparoscopic approaches are described for other general surgical procedures including adrenalectomy, there have been no case reports of retroperitoneal laparoscopic robot-assisted ALIF in human patients. For these reasons, although laparoscopic approaches for ALIF reduce scar size and generate a better view for the surgeon, there are data suggesting that transperitoneal ALIF increases the risk of retrograde ejaculation.[15]

One additional limitation of laparoscopy is the need for long handles on the instrument, reducing or eliminating much-needed tactile feedback. The learning curve for endoscopic approaches is higher when compared to open approaches, because the surgeon must adjust to following her hands on a television screen while attempting to manipulate the distal tip of instruments that are more than a foot away. To combat this difficulty, the surgical robot utilizes hand tools to increase surgical dexterity. Compared with laparoscopic surgeries, the use of the surgical robot can also help reduce surgeon fatigue due to the lack of a fulcrum effect. Although there are advantages to the robot, the lack of rongeur and bone cutting instruments has limited its adoption in orthopaedic and neurosurgery.

27.3.1 Limitations of Robotic Techniques

In the adoption of this new technology, operative time and measures of surgical quality must be monitored to ensure patient safety. In one report of transperitoneal ALIF, the entire procedure from incision to closure took only 175 minutes and a 25-mL blood loss was reported.[4] The authors report that the patient was discharged on postoperative day 1. Of note, this patient was a healthy 52-year-old woman with a body mass index (BMI) of 27. In a series of 11 patients undergoing robotic-assisted ALIF, operative time varied by surgical level.[2] For L5–S1 fusions ($n = 5$ patients), the average time per operation was 187.4 minutes; the average blood loss was 65 mL; and the average hospital stay was 4 days. Among patients with L4–L5 fusions ($n = 2$ patients), the average time per operation was 220 minutes; the average blood loss was 50 mL; and the average hospital stay was 3.5 days. The final group was the two-level fusion of L4–L5 and L5–S1 ($n = 4$ patients). The average time was 275.5 minutes; the average blood loss was 75 mL; and the average hospital stay was 6 days. There were no reported cases of postoperative ileus or intraoperative vascular injury. Patients were all relatively young (35–60 years old) with low BMI (20–34).[2]

The surgical case cohorts reflect the mean patient age and BMI reported in large cohort studies. In a study using National Surgical Quality Improvement Program (NSQIP) data for open ALIF patients, average age was 52 years and BMI was 29.[16] Unlike the R-ALIF data, cohort studies of open ALIF patients report more complications, including vascular injuries and retrograde ejaculation.[8,11,12,16,17,18,19,20,21] In these studies, the role of an access surgeon was variable. In contrast, given the federal regulations and current training environment, an access surgeon is required in robotic laparoscopic-assisted ALIF surgery. In one systemic meta-analysis of open ALIF, role of an access surgeon was associated with a significantly increased rate of postoperative retrograde ejaculation and ileus, as well as a higher rate of intraoperative vascular injury.[15] The role of an access surgeon was also associated with significantly decreased neurological injury, decreased peritoneal injury, and a statistically significant lower rate of overall postoperative complications.[15]

27.4 Conclusion

Robot-assisted laparoscopic ALIF is technically feasible as an alternative to standard open ALIF approaches with lower reported complication rates in small cohort studies compared to open ALIF. Regulatory limitations and constraints on surgical training may prohibit the widespread adoption of this method, and currently an access surgeon trained in the use of the surgical robot is required for all procedures.

References

[1] Lee JY, Bhowmick DA, Eun DD, Welch WC. Minimally invasive, robot-assisted, anterior lumbar interbody fusion: a technical note. J Neurol Surg A Cent Eur Neurosurg. 2013; 74(4):258–261

[2] Lee Z, Lee JY, Welch WC, Eun D. Technique and surgical outcomes of robot-assisted anterior lumbar interbody fusion. J Robot Surg. 2013; 7(2):177–185

[3] Kim MJ, Ha Y, Yang MS, et al. Robot-assisted anterior lumbar interbody fusion (ALIF) using retroperitoneal approach. Acta Neurochir (Wien). 2010; 152(4):675–679

[4] Beutler WJ, Peppelman WC, Jr, DiMarco LA. The da Vinci robotic surgical assisted anterior lumbar interbody fusion: technical development and case report. Spine. 2013; 38(4):356–363

[5] United States Food and Drug Administration. Surgical Specialties - Regulatory Clearance. Web Archive. Intuitive Surgical; 2013

[6] Yang MS, Yoon DH, Kim KN, et al. Robot-assisted anterior lumbar interbody fusion in a Swine model in vivo test of the da Vinci surgical-assisted spinal surgery system. Spine. 2011; 36(2):E139–E143

[7] Carragee EJ, Mitsunaga KA, Hurwitz EL, Scuderi GJ. Retrograde ejaculation after anterior lumbar interbody fusion using rhBMP-2: a cohort controlled study. Spine J. 2011; 11(6):511–516

[8] Comer GC, Smith MW, Hurwitz EL, Mitsunaga KA, Kessler R, Carragee EJ. Retrograde ejaculation after anterior lumbar interbody fusion with and without bone morphogenetic protein-2 augmentation: a 10-year cohort controlled study. Spine J. 2012; 12(10):881–890

[9] Lindley EM, McBeth ZL, Henry SE, et al. Retrograde ejaculation after anterior lumbar spine surgery. Spine. 2012; 37(20):1785–1789

[10] Mobbs RJ, Phan K, Daly D, Rao PJ, Lennox A. Approach-related complications of anterior lumbar interbody fusion: results of a combined spine and vascular surgical team. Global Spine J. 2016; 6(2):147–154

[11] Tepper G, Rabbani R, Yousefzadeh M, Prince D. Quantitative assessment of retrograde ejaculation using semen analysis, comparison with a standardized qualitative questionnaire, and investigating the impact of rhBMP-2. Spine. 2013; 38(10):841–845

[12] Than KD, Wang AC, Rahman SU, et al. Complication avoidance and management in anterior lumbar interbody fusion. Neurosurg Focus. 2011; 31(4):E6

[13] Anadol ZA, Ersoy E, Taneri F, Tekin E. Outcome and cost comparison of laparoscopic transabdominal preperitoneal hernia repair versus Open Lichtenstein technique. J Laparoendosc Adv Surg Tech A. 2004; 14(3):159–163

[14] Ge B, Wu M, Chen Q, et al. A prospective randomized controlled trial of laparoscopic repair versus open repair for perforated peptic ulcers. Surgery. 2016; 159(2):451–458

[15] Phan K, Xu J, Scherman DB, Rao PJ, Mobbs RJ. Anterior lumbar interbody fusion with and without an "access surgeon": a systematic review and meta-analysis. Spine. 2017; 42(10):E592–E601

[16] Abt NB, De la Garza-Ramos R, Olorundare IO, et al. Thirty day postoperative outcomes following anterior lumbar interbody fusion using the National Surgical Quality Improvement Program database. Clin Neurol Neurosurg. 2016; 143:126–131

[17] Garcia RM, Choy W, DiDomenico JD, et al. Thirty-day readmission rate and risk factors for patients undergoing single level elective anterior lumbar interbody fusion (ALIF). J Clin Neurosci. 2016; 32:104–108

[18] Choy W, Barrington N, Garcia RM, et al. Risk factors for medical and surgical complications following single-level ALIF. Global Spine J. 2017; 7(2):141–147

[19] Asha MJ, Choksey MS, Shad A, Roberts P, Imray C. The role of the vascular surgeon in anterior lumbar spine surgery. Br J Neurosurg. 2012; 26(4):499–503

[20] Hrabalek L, Sternbersky J, Adamus M. Risk of sympathectomy after anterior and lateral lumbar interbody fusion procedures. Biomed Pap Med Fac Univ Palacky Olomouc Czech Repub. 2015; 159(2):318–326

[21] Rothenfluh DA, Koenig M, Stokes OM, Behrbalk E, Boszczyk BM. Access-related complications in anterior lumbar surgery in patients over 60 years of age. Eur Spine J. 2014; 23 Suppl 1:S86–S92

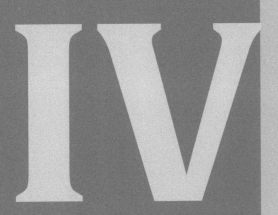

Part IV
Techniques Using Alternative Modalities for Complex Spine Pathology

IV

28 Intraoperative Ultrasound-Guided Intradural Tumor Resection

Yamaan S. Saadeh, Jay K. Nathan, and Mark E. Oppenlander

Abstract:

Ultrasound is a cost-effective, practical, and efficient imaging modality used during spinal intradural tumor operations to supplement surgical planning, enhance resection, and limit potential complications. Intraoperative ultrasound use has increased over the past several decades for intradural tumor resections, and the technology is widely available and approaching use as a standard of care. In this chapter, we describe the history of ultrasound use in intradural tumor surgery, multiple techniques for intraoperative utilization, limitations of ultrasound, and a summary of current literature. Additionally, our chapter explores the emerging applications for intraoperative ultrasound, such as integration with neuronavigation technology and the use of existing ultrasound contrast agents to enhance intraoperative imaging and resection of spinal intradural tumors.

Keywords: intraoperative imaging, ultrasound, intradural tumor

28.1 Introduction

Intradural spinal tumors represent a minority of all tumors involving the spinal canal, though they present unique challenges for the surgeon. One of these is visibility: Due to their location deep to the dura mater, they are not readily apparent following laminectomy, as opposed to epidural tumors, which often are (▶ Fig. 28.1). Intramedullary lesions can be even more challenging to visualize, requiring significant myelotomy for exposure. Risks of operating on intradural lesions include incomplete resection and spinal cord injury. Careful planning with preoperative imaging is essential (▶ Fig. 28.2), though intraoperative image guidance can help mitigate risk by providing real-time information to the surgeon to guide dural opening, refine goals of surgery, and estimate extent of resection. Ultrasound represents a rapid, readily accessible, reliable, and cost-effective imaging modality to serve this intraoperative role.

28.2 Background

Ultrasound technology relies on sound waves that, by definition, have a frequency exceeding what is audible to the human ear. These waves are emitted from a transducer, travel through space, and generate a signal when they are reflected back toward the transducer by an object. The majority of medical applications of ultrasound utilize frequencies in the range of 3 to 18 MHz.[1]

The earliest patents for ultrasonic devices were filed in 1912; however, the use of ultrasound for medical diagnosis was not documented until 1942 by Karl Dussik, an Australian neurologist who published a case report of ultrasound use for detecting an intracranial lesion. The routine use of medical ultrasound did not occur until the 1960s, when ultrasound devices became

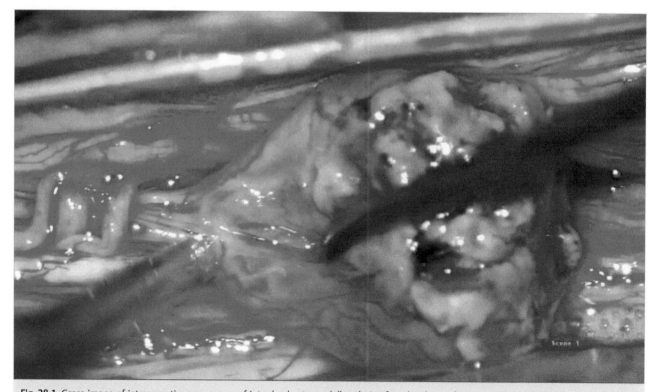

Fig. 28.1 Gross image of intraoperative appearance of intradural extramedullary lesion found to be a schwannoma on pathology.

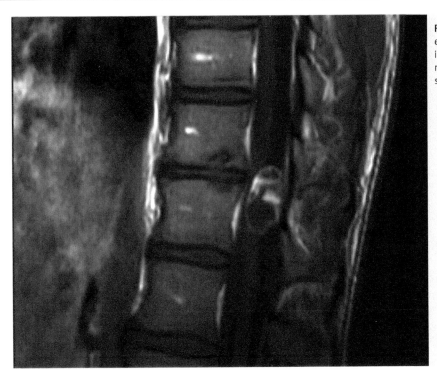

Fig. 28.2 Preoperative sagittal MRI with contrast enhancement demonstrating a cystic septated intradural extramedullary lesion in the lower region of the thoracic spine compressing the spinal cord.

increasingly commercially available.[2] Multiple case reports and case series from this decade describe ultrasound use for intracranial lesions.[3,4,5] The first documented use of ultrasound for visualizing a spinal intradural lesion was in 1978 by Reid.[6] Within the literature, there is evidence of increasing interest in the use of ultrasound for cases of spinal intradural tumors as the utility of ultrasound is better understood and as ultrasound technology becomes more ubiquitous within the operating room.

There are multiple commercially available medical ultrasound machines which have documented use for neurosurgical cases. At our institution, we utilize the Hitachi ProSound Alpha 7 machine with the Hitachi "hockey-stick" transducer probe for spinal intradural lesions. Other ultrasound manufacturers include GE, Philips, Siemens, and Toshiba (▶ Fig. 28.3).

The most commonly known and utilized mode of ultrasound imaging is B-mode imaging, which uses a linear array of transducers to generate a two-dimensional image of a plane through the body. The brightness of different areas on the image depends on the ability of various tissues to reflect sound waves, referred to as echogenicity. Brighter areas represent tissue that reflects more of the incident ultrasound wave and are therefore termed hyperechoic. Darker areas on the image represent weak ultrasonic reflection and are termed hypoechoic. High-density lesions include many solid tumors and are generally hyperechoic (bright) on ultrasound imaging, while fluid-filled areas such as intracranial ventricles and tumor cysts reflect ultrasound waves poorly and are hypoechoic. Doppler or duplex ultrasound is another commonly used mode to visualize blood flow magnitude and direction.

28.3 Uses

Various uses of intraoperative ultrasound during the resection of intradural tumors have been described, including real-time operative planning, diagnosis, and evaluation of resection.

28.3.1 Evaluation of Exposure

Intraoperative ultrasound can be used initially at the time of dural exposure to verify correct localization over the tumor. Evaluation of the extent of bony exposure bilaterally as well as superiorly and inferiorly is prudent to avoid a narrow working corridor during tumor resection. Ultrasound can be used to verify exposure of dura both above and below the level of the lesion, as well as laterally to the margins of the spinal canal. If inadequate exposure is found, appropriate widening of the exposure prior to dural opening should be performed to minimize the potential for bone fragments and blood to enter the thecal sac (▶ Fig. 28.4).

28.3.2 Differential Diagnosis

Imaging characteristics of different lesions on ultrasound may provide some indication regarding the diagnosis of an intradural lesion.[7] Astrocytomas and gangliogliomas tend to be isoechoic to the spinal cord parenchyma, though the cord is often expanded secondary to the lesion. Ependymomas are generally hyperechoic compared to the spinal cord, and the contrast between spinal cord and lesion tends to be greater.[8] Hypoechoic intratumoral cysts are also more often associated with astrocytomas. Hemangioblastomas are visualized as nodular hyperechoic areas often surrounded by an anechoic cyst.[9]

Extramedullary tumors also frequently have ultrasound characteristics that may suggest a diagnosis. Meningiomas tend to be hyperechoic and are infrequently associated with cysts, while schwannomas are generally hypoechoic and associated with cysts.[10] Neurofibromas have ultrasonic characteristics similar to schwannomas, and differentiating them based on ultrasound is not reliable.[11]

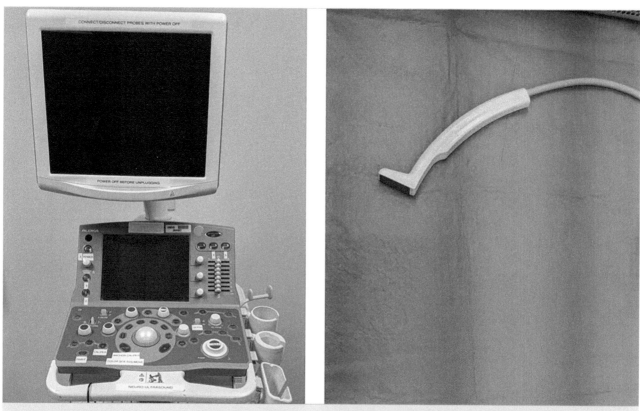

Fig. 28.3 The Hitachi ProSound Alpha 7 machine with "hockey-stick" transducer probe, our preferred probe for use in intradural spine cases.

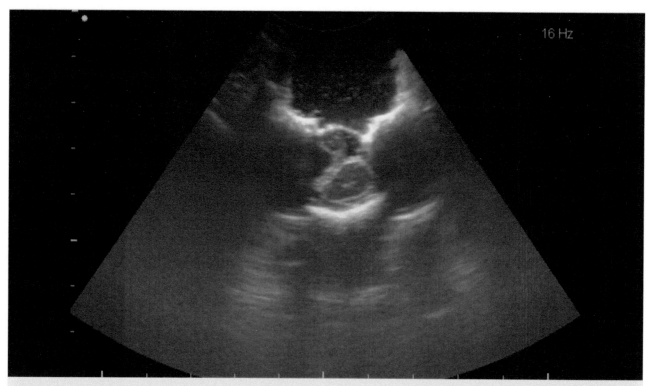

Fig. 28.4 An axial oriented intraoperative ultrasound image demonstrating use of ultrasound in the fluid-filled surgical bed. The laminectomy defect is visible and exposes the full extent of the spinal canal. The spinal cord is visible ventrally with tumor present dorsally.

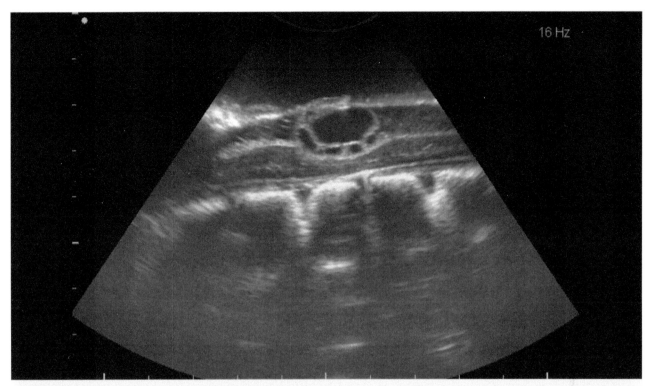

Fig. 28.5 A sagittal oriented intraoperative ultrasound image demonstrating the craniocaudal extent of the intradural extramedullary lesion with CSF visible above and below the level of the lesion. The cord is ventral to the lesion.

28.3.3 Durotomy Planning

Determining the cranial and caudal extents of an intradural lesion allows planning an appropriate length durotomy that traverses the entire extent of the lesion. Durotomy should initially be made slightly above or below the lesion, at an area with sufficient cerebrospinal fluid (CSF) between the dura and neural elements to safely access the subarachnoid space. The durotomy can then be extended until it traverses the extent of the lesion (▸ Fig. 28.5).

28.3.4 Myelotomy Planning

Surgical resection of intramedullary tumors generally requires myelotomy, unless the tumor extends to the pia at the spinal cord surface. Intraoperative ultrasound can be used to determine the length of myelotomy necessary to expose the extent of the lesion. The location of myelotomy can also be guided by ultrasound based on where the lesion comes closest to the spinal cord surface.

28.3.5 Extent of Resection

Intraoperative ultrasound can also add utility in cases that lack a clear visual delineation or dissection plane between lesional and nonlesional tissue. Sequential images in real time allow frequent intraoperative feedback on the progress of resection, allowing for identification of residual tumor tissue, cysts, or calcifications. Intraoperative ultrasound can be useful even in

cases where an infiltrative lesion may be isoechoic to the spinal cord. Real-time images can be compared to pre-resection images to assess progress as well as the caliber of the remaining spinal cord.

28.3.6 Evaluating Vasculature and Contrast-Enhanced Ultrasound Imaging

The Doppler mode can be used on intraoperative ultrasound to assess the angioarchitecture of the arterial and venous system of the spinal cord. For hypervasculature tumors, such as hemangioblastomas, Doppler mode ultrasound may help identify vascular pedicles that supply the tumor and assist in planning the approach.[9]

Contrast-enhanced ultrasound is an emerging technique in the United States that has had relatively widespread use within Europe and Asia for more than a decade. Contrast-enhanced ultrasound relies on the intravenous injection of microbubbles measuring 2 to 20 μm (similar to the size of red blood cells) which remain intravascular and thus are able to avoid sequestration in the lungs. These microbubbles result in increased signal from areas of high vascularity and superior assessment of the microvasculature.[12] Additionally, unlike magnetic resonance imaging (MRI) and computed tomography (CT) contrast agents, these microbubbles do not enter the interstitial space outside the vasculature. Rather, they remain trapped in the vasculature for several minutes until they are cleared from the circulation. This allows for repeated use of the ultrasound contrast agent without loss of image contrast, as can occur with repeated use of CT or MRI contrast agents as they diffuse into the interstitial space.

Historically, contrast-enhanced ultrasound has been used for cardiac and liver studies, though there are a number of case series reporting the ability of contrast-enhanced ultrasound to show lesional tissue in intra-axial brain tumors.[13,14,15] Several case reports also detail the use of contrast-enhanced ultrasound to enhance the imaging of lesional tissue for intradural spine tumors.[9,16] This emerging technology appears to be a promising method to improve real-time assessment of residual lesional tissue in spinal intramedullary tumor resection.

28.4 Limitations

As with all imaging modalities, ultrasound is not without limitations. Perhaps the most characteristic limitation of ultrasound is that its quality relies heavily on the skill and experience of the user. While CT and MRI utilize standard, reproducible protocols, myriad settings for the ultrasound machine can be manipulated at the time of each acquisition, and it is incumbent on the user to understand how this impacts image quality and diagnostic accuracy. Probe selection, position, and angulation are just some of these important factors. For surgeons and support staff less accustomed to intraoperative ultrasound use, this customizability can add time and frustration to an operation, creating an initial barrier to adoption.

Even in the hands of a user experienced with optimized imaging settings, physical limitations affect image quality. Hyperechoic tissues reduce transmission of ultrasound waves to structures farther from the probe. Similar to opaque materials casting visible shadows from light, this ultrasonic shadowing reduces the ability to discriminate echogenicity of deeper structures. Thus, resolution is impaired and so too is the clinical meaning of the image. Hemostatic agents are a common hyperechoic culprit. Signal strength and imaging depth adjustments are machine settings that can help improve imaging in this circumstance.

Direct risk to the patient from ultrasound imaging is typically considered very low. While there is energy transfer to imaged tissues from incident sound waves, producing heat, this is typically below a threshold needed to cause clinically significant effects when ultrasound is used for diagnostic purposes.

28.5 Outcomes

Intraoperative ultrasound use during the resection of intradural tumors has increased over the past two decades. Although there are no direct comparison studies of patients undergoing resection of intradural spinal tumors with and without the use of ultrasound, multiple reports document its utility and safety. Prada et al described a series of 34 patients in whom intraoperative ultrasound was able to identify anatomical landmarks, including dural and arachnoid membranes, dentate ligaments, anterior and posterior rootlets, and the spinal cord vasculature.[17] The central canal is also readily visible.[18]

Epstein et al described their experience with 186 cases of intramedullary spinal cord lesions, reporting that the use of intraoperative ultrasonography greatly facilitated radical resection.[8] In a series of 10 patients with a variety of pathologies,

including intradural tumors, intraoperative ultrasound improved localization ability for biopsies and assessment of decompression of the cord in the setting of spinal cord cysts.[18] Maiuri et al reported on the use of intraoperative ultrasound in 20 patients to guide the extent of exposure and assist with resection.[19] In a series of 78 patients who underwent resection of intradural tumors with use of intraoperative sonography, surgeons reported increased ability to verify extent of exposure and guidance of myelotomy, and 76% of patients experienced neurological improvement.[20]

28.6 Future Directions

As surgical teams become more accustomed to using intraoperative ultrasound, new roles will be identified, and barriers to adoption related to unfamiliarity will be reduced. An application to transform a smartphone into a "virtual ultrasound probe" aids in training, simulation, and preoperative rehearsal.[21] For intradural tumor resection cases requiring corpectomy and/or spinal instrumentation for stabilization, ultrasound has shown promise in evaluating corpectomy width and cord expansion after decompression,[22] pedicle screw holes prior to screw placement,[23] and anterior spinal artery flow as spinal alignment is manipulated.[24] Because of its ability to provide real-time updates of intraoperative anatomy, ultrasound coupled with automated image analysis could be used to refine stereotactic guidance systems, to account for patient or reference frame movement after image acquisition or spinal cord drift following dural opening.[25] Robotic arms could hold and reposition ultrasound probes for the surgeon. To obviate the need to look away from the surgical field at an ultrasound display, the ultrasound image could be viewed within augmented reality glasses or within a microscope viewer, superimposed on the patient's visible anatomy.

There are also promising reports of integrating existing technology into neurosurgical applications of ultrasound. Ultrasound contrast agents are a potentially cost-effective, rapid, and easy-to-use supplement to intraoperative ultrasound that may enhance the capability to differentiate lesional from nonlesional tissue.[15] There is also discussion of integrating current three-dimensional (3D) ultrasound technology intraoperatively to construct 3D images of real-time surgical anatomy and assist with assessment of resection.[26] This technique may also be incorporated into neuronavigation, which is ubiquitously used for localization and assessment of resection. A major limitation of neuronavigation is the loss of accuracy that occurs intraoperatively with CSF egress and the changes in local anatomy that occur throughout resection. Incorporation of 3D ultrasound with neuronavigation has the potential to provide real-time neuronavigation updates to correct for the limitations in existing technology.[27]

References

[1] Carovac A, Smajlovic F, Junuzovic D. Application of ultrasound in medicine. Acta Inform Med. 2011; 19(3):168–171
[2] Shampo MA, Kyle RA. Karl Theodore Dussik: pioneer in ultrasound. Mayo Clin Proc. 1995; 70(12):1136
[3] Dyck P, Kurze T, Barrows HS. Intra-operative ultrasonic encephalography of cerebral mass lesions. Bull Los Angeles Neurol Soc. 1966; 31(3):114–124

[4] Schlagenhauff R, Glasauer F. The use of intraoperative echoencephalography. In: Rand E, ed. Recent Advances in Diagnostic Ultrasound. Springfield, IL: Charles C Thomas; 1971:74–86

[5] Sugar O, Uematsu S. The use of ultrasound in the diagnosis of intracranial lesions. Surg Clin North Am. 1964; 44:55–64

[6] Dohrmann GJ, Rubin JM. History of intraoperative ultrasound in neurosurgery. Neurosurg Clin N Am. 2001; 12(1):155–166, ix

[7] Jallo GI, Freed D, Epstein F. Intramedullary spinal cord tumors in children. Childs Nerv Syst. 2003; 19(9):641–649

[8] Epstein FJ, Farmer JP, Schneider SJ. Intraoperative ultrasonography: an important surgical adjunct for intramedullary tumors. J Neurosurg. 1991; 74(5): 729–733

[9] Vetrano IG, Prada F, Nataloni IF, Bene MD, Dimeco F, Valentini LG. Discrete or diffuse intramedullary tumor? Contrast-enhanced intraoperative ultrasound in a case of intramedullary cervicothoracic hemangioblastomas mimicking a diffuse infiltrative glioma: technical note and case report. Neurosurg Focus. 2015; 39(2):E17

[10] Matsuzaki H, Tokuhashi Y, Wakabayashi K, Ishihara K, Iwahashi M. Differences on intraoperative ultrasonography between meningioma and neurilemmoma. Neuroradiology. 1998; 40(1):40–44

[11] Reynolds DL, Jr, Jacobson JA, Inampudi P, Jamadar DA, Ebrahim FS, Hayes CW. Sonographic characteristics of peripheral nerve sheath tumors. AJR Am J Roentgenol. 2004; 182(3):741–744

[12] Wilson SR, Greenbaum LD, Goldberg BB. Contrast-enhanced ultrasound: what is the evidence and what are the obstacles? AJR Am J Roentgenol. 2009; 193(1):55–60

[13] Lekht I, Brauner N, Bakhsheshian J, et al. Versatile utilization of real-time intraoperative contrast-enhanced ultrasound in cranial neurosurgery: technical note and retrospective case series. Neurosurg Focus. 2016; 40(3):E6

[14] Prada F, Mattei L, Del Bene M, et al. Intraoperative cerebral glioma characterization with contrast enhanced ultrasound. BioMed Res Int. 2014; 2014: 484261

[15] Prada F, Perin A, Martegani A, et al. Intraoperative contrast-enhanced ultrasound for brain tumor surgery. Neurosurgery. 2014; 74(5):542–552, discussion 552

[16] Vetrano IG, Prada F, Erbetta A, DiMeco F. Intraoperative ultrasound and contrast-enhanced ultrasound (CEUS) features in a case of intradural extramedullary dorsal schwannoma mimicking an intramedullary lesion. Ultraschall Med. 2015; 36(4):307–310

[17] Prada F, Vetrano IG, Filippini A, et al. Intraoperative ultrasound in spinal tumor surgery. J Ultrasound. 2014; 17(3):195–202

[18] Dohrmann GJ, Rubin JM. Intraoperative ultrasound imaging of the spinal cord: syringomyelia, cysts, and tumors—a preliminary report. Surg Neurol. 1982; 18(6):395–399

[19] Maiuri F, Iaconetta G, de Divitiis O. The role of intraoperative sonography in reducing invasiveness during surgery for spinal tumors. Minim Invasive Neurosurg. 1997; 40(1):8–12

[20] Regelsberger J, Fritzsche E, Langer N, Westphal M. Intraoperative sonography of intra- and extramedullary tumors. Ultrasound Med Biol. 2005; 31(5):593–598

[21] Perin A, Prada FU, Moraldo M, et al. USim: a new device and app for case-specific, intraoperative ultrasound simulation and rehearsal in neurosurgery. A preliminary study. Oper Neurosurg (Hagerstown). 2017(Jun):29

[22] Moses V, Daniel RT, Chacko AG. The value of intraoperative ultrasound in oblique corpectomy for cervical spondylotic myelopathy and ossified posterior longitudinal ligament. Br J Neurosurg. 2010; 24(5):518–525

[23] Kantelhardt SR, Bock CH, Larsen J, et al. Intraosseous ultrasound in the placement of pedicle screws in the lumbar spine. Spine. 2009; 34(4):400–407

[24] Degreif J, Wenda K. Ultrasound-guided spinal fracture repositioning. Surg Endosc. 1998; 12(2):164–169

[25] Dekomien C, Roeschies B, Winter S. System architecture for intraoperative ultrasound registration in image-based medical navigation. Biomed Tech (Berl). 2012; 57(4):229–237

[26] Unsgaard G, Rygh OM, Selbekk T, et al. Intra-operative 3D ultrasound in neurosurgery. Acta Neurochir (Wien). 2006; 148(3):235–253, discussion 253

[27] Rasmussen IA, Jr, Lindseth F, Rygh OM, et al. Functional neuronavigation combined with intra-operative 3D ultrasound: initial experiences during surgical resections close to eloquent brain areas and future directions in automatic brain shift compensation of preoperative data. Acta Neurochir (Wien). 2007; 149(4):365–378

29 Stereotactic Radiosurgery for Treatment of Primary and Metastatic Spinal Tumors

Ori Barzilai, Adam M. Schmitt, Mark H. Bilsky, and Ilya Laufer

Abstract

Spinal tumors are a frequent occurrence and the improvement in available cancer therapy is leading to longer survival. The biggest advancement in oncological treatment of spinal tumors has been the development and integration of spine stereotactic radiosurgery (SRS) which has dramatically improved the ability to provide safe and durable control of spine tumors. For treatment of metastatic spinal disease, an abundance of data show that radiosurgery provides high rates of local-tumor control with limited treatment-associated morbidity. Surgery continues to play an important role in the treatment of spinal metastases, but the integration of SRS has changed both the indications and surgical techniques. Radiosensitive tumors can be effectively treated with conventional external beam radiation therapy, while radioresistant tumors without significant epidural extension can be effectively treated with upfront SRS. In the setting of high-grade epidural spinal cord compression, dose constraints prohibit the delivery of an optimal radiation dose to the entire tumor volume without risking radiation-induced myelitis: thus, surgery is often required not only to decompress the spinal cord but also to provide a margin for the safe delivery of SRS. The role for SRS in the treatment of primary spinal tumors continues to evolve, but there is mounting clinical evidence that chordoma is radioresponsive to SRS. As radiosurgical technologies have become accessible worldwide, utilization of radiosurgery for the treatment of spinal pathology has grown. Spine surgeons must be familiar with radiosurgical concepts including simulation, contouring, and treatment planning to optimize decision making.

Keywords: spine, stereotactic radiosurgery, stereotactic body radiotherapy, tumor, metastases, sarcoma

29.1 Introduction

Spinal tumors are classified as either primary or metastatic depending on the site of origin. Metastatic spinal cord tumors are far more frequent than primary tumors, as it is known that approximately 40% of all people with cancer develop spinal metastases and postmortem studies suggest that up to 90% of cancer patients may have microscopic evidence of spinal metastases.[1,2] Almost 20% of patients diagnosed with spinal metastases progress to symptomatic cord compression.[3,4,5]

Treatment goals for patients with spine tumors include durable local tumor control, preservation or restoration of neurological function, maintenance of spinal stability, and palliation of pain. The goals of treatment among patients with spinal metastases are palliative. However, some patients with primary tumors, especially benign or low-grade malignant primary spine tumors, may be cured. Historically, treatment responses for osseous tumors to systemic therapy were limited and thus conventional external beam radiation therapy (cEBRT) was the mainstay of treatment for spinal tumors.[6,7,8] In current practice, the integration of medical and technological advancements has led to complex multimodality therapy strategy. The biggest advancement in the oncological treatment of spinal tumors has been the development and integration of spine stereotactic radiosurgery (SSRS) which has dramatically improved the ability to provide meaningful, durable control of spine tumors. This is particularly important and necessary in the current era of extended survivals seen with modern systemic therapy.

As radiosurgical technologies have become accessible worldwide, utilization of radiosurgery for the treatment of spinal pathology has rapidly growing. Spine surgeons must familiarize with radiosurgical concepts to optimize decision making. This chapter will discuss the basic concepts of radiosurgery for primary and metastatic tumors.

29.2 Terminology

Stereotactic body radiotherapy (SBRT) is an umbrella term describing single fraction or hypofractionated image-guided delivery of focused high-dose radiotherapy to targets throughout the body. The fractionation schedule generally varies between one and five fractions, with single-fraction SBRT occasionally being referred to as stereotactic radiosurgery (SRS; ▶ Table 29.1). Once radiosurgery has been selected as the treatment of choice, whether in a primary setting or in the postoperative setting, the treatment process consists of several stages.

First, a *simulation* is performed. This is the process of obtaining up-to-date imaging, for accurate delineation of tumor and organs at risk (OARs), with patients placed in an immobilization frame that would provide reproducible positioning during therapy planning and delivery. Delivery precision is confirmed through reproducible immobilization, intraprocedural target location confirmation using on-board imaging, active motion detection, and corrections during treatment delivery.[9,10,11]

Next, *contouring* of the treatment target and OARs is performed on a designated software platform. Optimal imaging translates into optimal contouring and hence often, particularly in the postoperative setting where hardware-related artifacts are common, a computed tomography (CT) myelography is performed during simulation in order to clearly delineate the position of the spinal cord. Alternatively, noncontrast CT can be performed and fused with a contrast-enhanced MRI. Three main volumes are contoured: the *gross tumor volume (GTV)*, *clinical target volume (CTV)*, and *planning target volume (PTV)*.[12] The GTV represents the actual tumor seen on imaging. The CTV is the area of potential microscopic spread of tumor cells that includes the GTV and adjacent bone marrow spaces. The PTV is a geometric expansion around the CTV with a 2- to 3-mm margin to ensure that the CTV receives the planned dose. This margin accounts for factors that are challenging to control precisely such as physical errors of the treatment delivery, uncertainty of patient positioning and motion during treatment, and organ

Table 29.1 Spine radiosurgery glossary

SRS—stereotactic radiosurgery	Spine radiosurgery treatment delivered in a single fraction
SBRT—spine body radiation therapy	Hypofractionated image-guided delivery of focused high-dose radiotherapy to target throughout the body
GTV—gross tumor volume	Palpable disease at surgery or gross tumor seen on imaging
CTV—clinical target volume	Region of potential microscopic spread of tumor cells that includes the GTV
PTV—planning target volume	Geometric construct that encompasses the CTV and adds an additional margin of tissue to ensure that the CTV receives the intended dose
OAR—organ at risk	Organs near or within the proposed treatment field. Most important OAR for spine radiosurgery is the spinal cord
Simulation	The process of obtaining up-to-date imaging, for accurate delineation of tumor and OARs, with patients placed in an immobilization frame that would provide reproducible positioning during therapy planning and delivery
Contouring	The process of outlining the GTV, CTV, PTV, and OARs on a designated treatment planning software
Planning	Optimally applying the desired/prescribed dose while accounting for the allowable dose to surrounding normal structures

motion during treatment. Guidelines exist for contouring in both the primary[13] (▶ Fig. 29.1) and postoperative setting[14,15] (▶ Fig. 29.2) and spine surgeons should familiarize with them. In the postoperative setting, the full preoperative tumor volume is used for the GTV delineation, with respective expansions also made around the preoperative tumor.

Lastly, treatment *planning* is performed. The plan is generated based on the prescribed radiation dose and the tolerable dose to the surrounding OARs. Due to the complexity of decision making involved in these cases, it is preferable for treatment plans to be generated in a multidisciplinary fashion composed of radiation oncology, medical physics, and neurosurgery teams.

29.3 Radiobiology of Stereotactic Radiosurgery

Conventional external beam radiation therapy results in mitotic or cytotoxic cell death via breakage of double-stranded DNA within a tumor and may subsequently decompress the spinal cord.[8,16,17] Using cEBRT, radiation is typically delivered through one to four beams to a treatment field that spreads beyond the tumor margins. Hence, the dose of radiation is limited since vital OARs that surround the tumor receive doses of radiation similar to the doses prescribed to the tumor.[18] Healthy tissues are able to repair most of the damage from this radiation, while tumor cells generally have impaired DNA repair mechanisms and can succumb to these fractionated doses of radiation. Treatment response rates to cEBRT are variable, likely due to the limitations in radiation-dose delivery to the tumor. Historically,

tumors have been classified as either radiosensitive or radioresistant based on the response to cEBRT. Lymphoma, myeloma, and seminoma are considered radiosensitive histologies, as are solid tumors such as breast and prostate.[19,20] Renal cell carcinoma (RCC), colon, non-small cell lung carcinomas (NSCLC), sarcomas, melanoma, thyroid, and hepatocellular carcinoma represent radioresistant tumors.[7,8,19,20]

Patients with radiosensitive tumors can be treated effectively with cEBRT, irrespective of the degree of epidural spinal cord compression (ESCC).[6,8] Furthermore, patients with radiosensitive tumors are more likely to maintain ambulation and remain ambulatory longer than patients with unfavorable histologies after cEBRT.[8,20,21,22]

The integration of SSRS has revolutionized the treatment of spinal metastases. Radiosurgery provides high-dose per fraction and uses intensity-modulated radiotherapy consisting of numerous beam angles (typically nine or more) to create conformal radiation contoured to optimize the dose delivered to the target while minimizing injury dose to OARs. Technological advancements in treatment planning and delivery including patient and tumor immobilization, image guidance, and intensity-modulated radiation delivery through multi-leaf collimators have made spinal SBRT safe and effective.[23,24] Ultimately, the ability to deliver high-dose per fraction of conformal radiation enables delivery of cytotoxic tumoral doses, which, in turn, overcomes the radioresistance of most tumors to cEBRT.[25] In experimental models, different radiobiologic responses have been shown between low-dose and high-dose per fraction radiation.[26,27] High-dose per fraction (i.e., > 10 Gy per fraction radiation) kills tumor cells via breakage of double-stranded DNA but additionally elicits tumor control through effects on the tumor vasculature.[28] One theory is that SRS induces the sphingomyelinase pathway, which, in turn, results in microvascular endothelial dysfunction and apoptosis, subsequent hypoperfusion of tumor tissue and ultimately tumor cell destruction.[29] The vascular damage then causes ischemic or indirect/secondary tumor cell death within a few days after radiation exposure. Moreover, the extensive tumor cell death secondary to both the radiation and the vascular damage may lead to the release of tumor-associated antigens and various proinflammatory cytokines, thereby triggering an antitumor immune response.[30,31] Ultimately, by all these pathways, SRS offers improved tumor cell death with limited side effects.

SSRS yields a clinical benefit regardless of tumor histology, providing a durable symptomatic response and high local-control rates, but these responses appear to be dose dependent.[32,33,34] Recent evidence[35] shows excellent outcomes with SSRS for traditionally radioresistant histologies such as RCC,[36,37,38] sarcoma,[39] and melanoma.[40]

29.4 Toxicity and Limitations

Dose constraints have been established for all major OARs[41,42] with the spinal cord considered the most critical OAR for SSRS. Multiple studies report low risk of toxicity after spinal SRS. Exceedingly rare cases of radiation myelopathy have been attributed to single-fraction spinal radiation, confirming that this is a highly infrequent complication of spinal radiation.[42] To our knowledge, hypofractionated treatment of the spine has not been reported to result in Grade 3 or 4 neurologic toxicity.

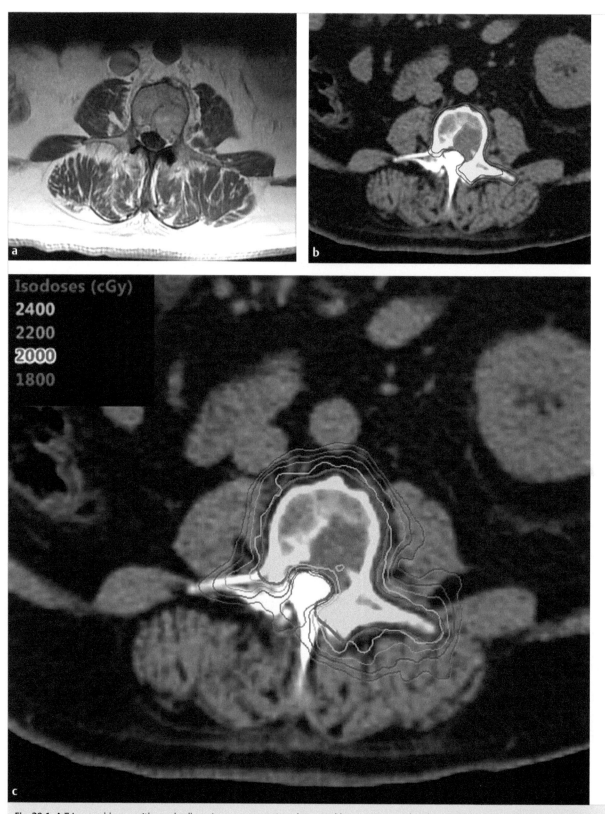

Fig. 29.1 A 74-year-old man with renal cell carcinoma metastatic to lungs and bones. Presented with general fatigue and stiffness and mid back pain and was neurologically intact at presentation. MRI of the spine revealed a vertebral body lesion in L3 with no epidural extension. He underwent SSRS, 24 Gy in a single fraction with well-controlled disease at 18-month follow-up. (a) Contrast-enhanced axial MRI demonstrating the tumor with no epidural involvement. (b) Contouring: the GTV is outlined in green, CTV in blue, and PTV in red. (c) Treatment plan with dosimetry map. CTV, clinical target volume; GTV, gross tumor volume; PTV, planning target volume; SSRS, spine stereotactic radiosurgery.

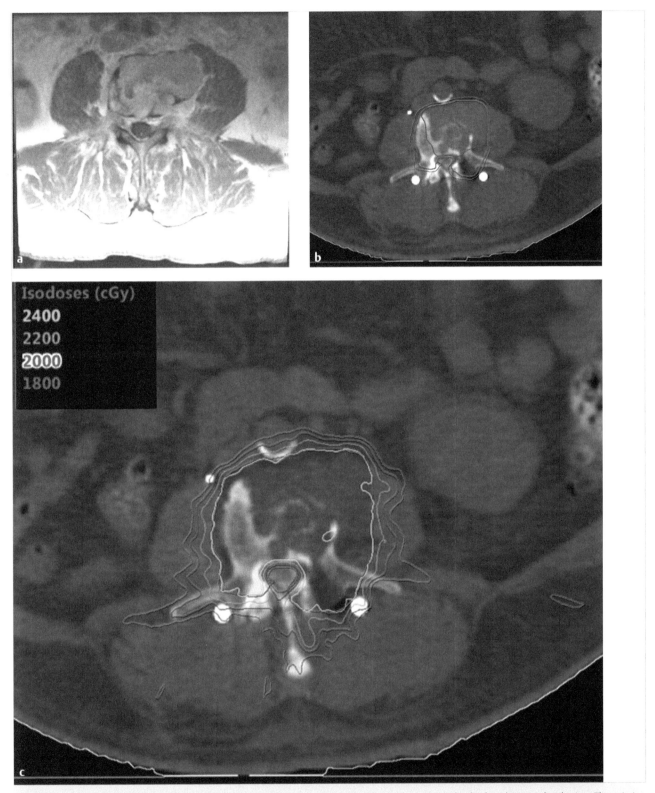

Fig. 29.2 A 67-year-old man s/p with metastatic renal cell carcinoma. Presented with severe mechanical radiculopathy in L4 distribution. The pain is primarily localized to the lower back, worst with positional change and radiates down the lateral aspect of the left lower extremity. MRI demonstrated an L4 burst fracture with severe left-side foraminal stenosis secondary to tumor infiltration. Following embolization of the tumor, he underwent percutaneous stabilization and minimal access facetectomy and foraminal decompression. Following surgery, he underwent SSRS, 24 Gy in a single fraction. (a) Contrast-enhanced axial MRI demonstrating the tumor with severe left-side foraminal stenosis. (b) Contouring: the GTV is outlined in green, CTV in blue, and PTV in red. (c) Treatment plan with dosimetry map. CTV, clinical target volume; GTV, gross tumor volume; PTV, planning target volume; SSRS, spine stereotactic radiosurgery.

Most adverse events are mild and involve Grade 1 or 2 skin and esophageal toxicity,[43] but mucositis, dysphagia, diarrhea, paresthesias, transient laryngitis, and radiculitis[43,44,45,46,47,48] have also been described. Single cases of Grade 3 vomiting, diarrhea, costochondritis, and dysphagia have been reported after hypofractionated treatment.[49,50]

Vertebral compression fractures (VCF) following SSRS have been described in up to 40% of treatments compared to a minimal (< 5%) risk following cEBRT.[51] Risk factors identified are older age, a lytic session, higher radiation doses, vertebral misalignment, or the presence of a preexisting VCF, and therefore some advocate pretreatment kyphoplasty in select patients.[51,52,53,54,55] However, the quoted fracture rate of 40% refers to radiographic fractures, but the symptomatic fracture rate requiring an intervention is much smaller and our previous study demonstrated only 7% risk of symptomatic fracture at 5-year follow-up.[56]

29.5 Stereotactic Radiosurgery in Metastatic Spine Disease

Treatment goals for patients with spinal metastases are palliative and include preservation of neurologic function, restoration and maintenance of spinal stability, and pain management.[57]

Multiple authors have reported excellent outcomes in treatment of spinal metastases with spine radiosurgery for traditionally radioresistant histologies in patients with minimal or no spinal cord compression.[58,59] Local control (LC) rates of 88% in the noncervical spine have been shown prospectively[58] and a multi-institutional retrospective analysis of 387 cases demonstrated LC of 84% at 2 years when using SBRT.[59] Other series have demonstrated comparable results.[60,61] Recently, we presented a case series of 811 lesions treated in 657 patients with a single-fraction SRS in which dose was analyzed as a continuous variable ranging from 18 to 26 Gy.[32] Local failure rates for the low-dose and high-dose groups were 5 versus 0.41% at 12 months, 15 versus 1.6% at 24 months, and 20 versus 2.1% at 48 months, respectively. In this study, 82% of the tumors were traditionally radioresistant and 50% had failed prior cEBRT, but tumor responses were found to be independent of tumor histology and prior radiation for the high-dose cohorts.[32]

The rationale for surgery in patients with metastatic spine tumors is largely predicated on the study by Patchell et al, in which patients randomized to direct surgical decompression followed by cEBRT had longer overall survival (OS), improved maintenance or recovery of ambulation, better preservation of bowel and bladder function, and decreased narcotic requirements compared to cEBRT alone.[62] This study provides class I evidence in support of direct surgical decompression for patients with solid tumor metastases resulting in high-grade ESCC and/or myelopathy.[62] The integration of SSRS as a postoperative adjuvant has transformed the goals of surgery and significantly decreased the associated morbidity compared to techniques traditionally employed with cEBRT. The need to deliver high-dose per fraction radiation to the entire tumor, including the epidural extension, with a safe margin from OARs, particularly the spinal cord, requires a small distance between the spinal cord and the tumor. Currently, only patients with high-grade ESCC from radioresistant tumors require spinal cord decompression for neurologic salvage and instrumented fusions for spinal stabilization. Using SSRS, the surgical goal is to create a target for the safe delivery of SSRS rather than resecting tumor for wide margins or cytoreduction. The term "separation surgery" describes a posterolateral epidural decompression with posterior instrumented fusion that focused on reconstitution of spinal fluid space to create a margin between the tumor and spinal cord. A retrospective review of 186 patients found this strategy to be both safe and effective for establishing durable local tumor control with the combination of separation surgery and high-dose SBRT providing LC above 90% at 1-year follow-up.[63] The LC was achieved regardless of tumor histology or prior radiation history. Others have since demonstrated similar results.[64,65]

29.6 Stereotactic Radiosurgery in Primary Spine Tumors

Unlike metastatic disease, for primary benign or malignant spinal column tumors, oncologic resection with wide margins for a curative goal is still considered the primary treatment modality. Unfortunately, in many of these cases, wide or "en-bloc" resections are not feasible or are associated with significant morbidity. Consequently, adjuvant therapies to enhance LC are needed. As these tumors are considered radioresistant to cEBRT, the role of both photon- and proton-based high-dose radiations for primary spinal column tumors is currently being explored. Delaney et al showed promising results using a combination of photon and proton (median dosage: 70.2 Gy relative biological effectiveness [RBE]) radiation, demonstrating a 5-year LC rate as high as 94% for primary spine sarcomas.[66] A neoadjuvant high-dose radiation followed by surgery followed by high-dose postoperative radiation has likewise demonstrated excellent results in the treatment of spinal sarcomas, showing 5-year OS, LC, locoregional control (LRC), and distant control (DC) of 81, 62, 60, and 77%, respectively.[67] Carbon ion therapy, a heavy particle radiation, is known to have a biological advantage compared to photons and protons secondary to increased RBE.[68,69] Improved LC rates for chordomas have been reported in retrospective single-center studies using this technology.[70]

Yamada et al published preliminary results using photon-based single-fraction SSRS for the treatment of spinal chordomas. In this cohort of 24 patients, 23 (95%) demonstrated stable or reduced tumor burden based on serial MRI in a median follow-up of 24 months.[71] A systematic literature review on the safety and LC of radiation therapy for spinal chordomas concluded that the use of pre- and/or postoperative photon image-guided radiotherapy (IGRT) or proton or carbon ion therapy should be considered for patients undergoing surgery for the treatment of primary and recurrent chordomas in the mobile spine and sacrum, since these RT modalities may improve LC.[72]

Taken together, though still considered experimental, promising initial results demonstrate value in the incorporation of high-dose radiation for primary spinal tumors. Future studies will determine the role of radiosurgery in this treatment paradigm.

29.7 Intradural Spinal Tumors

Surgery remains the first choice treatment for spinal intradural tumors.[73] Gerszten et al reported on the use of radiosurgery for the treatment of benign intradural extramedullary tumors, as they observed no subacute or long-term spinal cord toxicity in 41 patients treated for these pathologies.[74] Sachdev et al have since reported on 103 benign intradural tumors treated with radiosurgery with only one tumor progression during the mean follow-up period of 33 months.[75] Moreover, for intramedullary spinal cord tumors, a systematic literature review on SRS concluded that the technique is safe and effective in selected cases.[76] Despite these promising results, long-term data of the safety of this treatment are lacking. The concern for long-term toxicity and malignant transformation of these benign tumors currently precludes large-scale treatment and anticipation is growing for long-term outcomes from treatment in experimental settings.

29.8 Conclusion

The integration of radiosurgery for the treatment of spinal tumors has been transformative. For the treatment of metastatic spinal disease, radiosurgery provides high rates of local tumor control with limited treatment-associated morbidity. In the setting of high-grade epidural tumor extension, dose constraints prohibit the delivery of optimal radiation doses without risk to the spinal cord and hence, separation surgery is still indicated for circumferential decompression and restoration of the thecal sac. The role for radiosurgery in the treatment of primary spinal tumors is still in evolution; yet, promising results in experimental settings exist and it is likely that radiosurgery will play a more significant role in their treatment in the near future.

References

[1] Cobb CA, III, Leavens ME, Eckles N. Indications for nonoperative treatment of spinal cord compression due to breast cancer. J Neurosurg. 1977; 47(5):653–658

[2] Wong DA, Fornasier VL, MacNab I. Spinal metastases: the obvious, the occult, and the impostors. Spine. 1990; 15(1):1–4

[3] Klimo P, Jr, Schmidt MH. Surgical management of spinal metastases. Oncologist. 2004; 9(2):188–196

[4] North RB, LaRocca VR, Schwartz J, et al. Surgical management of spinal metastases: analysis of prognostic factors during a 10-year experience. J Neurosurg Spine. 2005; 2(5):564–573

[5] Sinson GP, Zager EL. Metastases and spinal cord compression. N Engl J Med. 1992; 327(27):1953–1954, author reply 1954–1955

[6] Gerszten PC, Mendel E, Yamada Y. Radiotherapy and radiosurgery for metastatic spine disease: what are the options, indications, and outcomes? Spine. 2009; 34(22) Suppl:S78–S92

[7] Mizumoto M, Harada H, Asakura H, et al. Radiotherapy for patients with metastases to the spinal column: a review of 603 patients at Shizuoka Cancer Center Hospital. Int J Radiat Oncol Biol Phys. 2011; 79(1):208–213

[8] Maranzano E, Latini P. Effectiveness of radiation therapy without surgery in metastatic spinal cord compression: final results from a prospective trial. Int J Radiat Oncol Biol Phys. 1995; 32(4):959–967

[9] Lo SS, Fakiris AJ, Chang EL, et al. Stereotactic body radiation therapy: a novel treatment modality. Nat Rev Clin Oncol. 2010; 7(1):44–54

[10] Foote M, Bailey M, Smith L, et al. Guidelines for safe practice of stereotactic body (ablative) radiation therapy. J Med Imaging Radiat Oncol. 2015; 59(5):646–653

[11] Li W, Sahgal A, Foote M, Millar BA, Jaffray DA, Letourneau D. Impact of immobilization on intrafraction motion for spine stereotactic body radiotherapy using cone beam computed tomography. Int J Radiat Oncol Biol Phys. 2012; 84(2):520–526

[12] Barzilai O, Laufer I, Robin A, Xu R, Yamada Y, Bilsky M. Hybrid therapy for metastatic epidural spinal cord compression: technique for separation surgery and spine radiosurgery. Operative Neurosurg. 201 9; 16(3):310–318

[13] Cox BW, Spratt DE, Lovelock M, et al. International Spine Radiosurgery Consortium consensus guidelines for target volume definition in spinal stereotactic radiosurgery. Int J Radiat Oncol Biol Phys. 2012; 83(5):e597–e605

[14] Redmond KJ, Robertson S, Lo SS, et al. Consensus contouring guidelines for postoperative stereotactic body radiation therapy for metastatic solid tumor malignancies to the spine. Int J Radiat Oncol Biol Phys. 2017; 97(1):64–74

[15] Redmond KJ, Lo SS, Soltys SG, et al. Consensus guidelines for postoperative stereotactic body radiation therapy for spinal metastases: results of an international survey. J Neurosurg Spine. 2017; 26(3):299–306

[16] Bilsky MH, Lis E, Raizer J, Lee H, Boland P. The diagnosis and treatment of metastatic spinal tumor. Oncologist. 1999; 4(6):459–469

[17] Vignard J, Mirey G, Salles B. Ionizing-radiation induced DNA double-strand breaks: a direct and indirect lighting up. Radiother Oncol. 2013; 108(3):362–369

[18] Lovelock DM, Zhang Z, Jackson A, et al. Correlation of local failure with measures of dose insufficiency in the high-dose single-fraction treatment of bony metastases. Int J Radiat Oncol Biol Phys. 2010; 77(4):1282–1287

[19] Rades D, Fehlauer F, Stalpers LJ, et al. A prospective evaluation of two radiotherapy schedules with 10 versus 20 fractions for the treatment of metastatic spinal cord compression: final results of a multicenter study. Cancer. 2004; 101(11):2687–2692

[20] Rades D, Fehlauer F, Schulte R, et al. Prognostic factors for local control and survival after radiotherapy of metastatic spinal cord compression. J Clin Oncol. 2006; 24(21):3388–3393

[21] Gilbert RW, Kim JH, Posner JB. Epidural spinal cord compression from metastatic tumor: diagnosis and treatment. Ann Neurol. 1978; 3(1):40–51

[22] Katagiri H, Takahashi M, Inagaki J, et al. Clinical results of nonsurgical treatment for spinal metastases. Int J Radiat Oncol Biol Phys. 1998; 42(5):1127–1132

[23] Alongi F, Arcangeli S, Filippi AR, Ricardi U, Scorsetti M. Review and uses of stereotactic body radiation therapy for oligometastases. Oncologist. 2012; 17 (8):1100–1107

[24] Chang BK, Timmerman RD. Stereotactic body radiation therapy: a comprehensive review. Am J Clin Oncol. 2007; 30(6):637–644

[25] Chan NK, Abdullah KG, Lubelski D, et al. Stereotactic radiosurgery for metastatic spine tumors. J Neurosurg Sci. 2014; 58(1):37–44

[26] Zhang B, Bowerman NA, Salama JK, et al. Induced sensitization of tumor stroma leads to eradication of established cancer by T cells. J Exp Med. 2007; 204(1):49–55

[27] Fuks Z, Kolesnick R. Engaging the vascular component of the tumor response. Cancer Cell. 2005; 8(2):89–91

[28] Song CW, Kim MS, Cho LC, Dusenbery K, Sperduto PW. Radiobiological basis of SBRT and SRS. Int J Clin Oncol. 2014; 19(4):570–578

[29] Garcia-Barros M, Paris F, Cordon-Cardo C, et al. Tumor response to radiotherapy regulated by endothelial cell apoptosis. Science. 2003; 300(5622):1155–1159

[30] Lee Y, Auh SL, Wang Y, et al. Therapeutic effects of ablative radiation on local tumor require CD8 + T cells: changing strategies for cancer treatment. Blood. 2009; 114(3):589–595

[31] Kaur P, Asea A. Radiation-induced effects and the immune system in cancer. Front Oncol. 2012; 2:191

[32] Yamada Y, Katsoulakis E, Laufer I, et al. The impact of histology and delivered dose on local control of spinal metastases treated with stereotactic radiosurgery. Neurosurg Focus. 2017; 42(1):E6

[33] Yamada Y, Lovelock DM, Yenice KM, et al. Multifractionated image-guided and stereotactic intensity-modulated radiotherapy of paraspinal tumors: a preliminary report. Int J Radiat Oncol Biol Phys. 2005; 62(1):53–61

[34] Gerszten PC, Burton SA, Ozhasoglu C, Welch WC. Radiosurgery for spinal metastases: clinical experience in 500 cases from a single institution. Spine. 2007; 32(2):193–199

[35] Barzilai O, Fisher CG, Bilsky MH. State of the art treatment of spinal metastatic disease. Neurosurgery. 2018; 82(6):757–769

[36] Ghia AJ, Chang EL, Bishop AJ, et al. Single-fraction versus multifraction spinal stereotactic radiosurgery for spinal metastases from renal cell carcinoma: secondary analysis of Phase I/II trials. J Neurosurg Spine. 2016; 24(5):829–836

[37] Gerszten PC, Burton SA, Ozhasoglu C, et al. Stereotactic radiosurgery for spinal metastases from renal cell carcinoma. J Neurosurg Spine. 2005; 3 (4):288–295

[38] Zelefsky MJ, Greco C, Motzer R, et al. Tumor control outcomes after hypofractionated and single-dose stereotactic image-guided intensity-modulated radiotherapy for extracranial metastases from renal cell carcinoma. Int J Radiat Oncol Biol Phys. 2012; 82(5):1744–1748

[39] Chang UK, Cho WI, Lee DH, et al. Stereotactic radiosurgery for primary and metastatic sarcomas involving the spine. J Neurooncol. 2012; 107(3):551–557

[40] Gerszten PC, Burton SA, Quinn AE, Agarwala SS, Kirkwood JM. Radiosurgery for the treatment of spinal melanoma metastases. Stereotact Funct Neurosurg. 2005; 83(5–6):213–221

[41] Schipani S, Wen W, Jin JY, Kim JK, Ryu S. Spine radiosurgery: a dosimetric analysis in 124 patients who received 18 Gy. Int J Radiat Oncol Biol Phys. 2012; 84(5):e571–e576

[42] Sahgal A, Weinberg V, Ma L, et al. Probabilities of radiation myelopathy specific to stereotactic body radiation therapy to guide safe practice. Int J Radiat Oncol Biol Phys. 2013; 85(2):341–347

[43] Yamada Y, Bilsky MH, Lovelock DM, et al. High-dose, single-fraction image-guided intensity-modulated radiotherapy for metastatic spinal lesions. Int J Radiat Oncol Biol Phys. 2008; 71(2):484–490

[44] Benzil DL, Saboori M, Mogilner AY, Rocchio R, Moorthy CR. Safety and efficacy of stereotactic radiosurgery for tumors of the spine. J Neurosurg. 2004; 101 Suppl 3:413–418

[45] Degen JW, Gagnon GJ, Voyadzis JM, et al. CyberKnife stereotactic radiosurgical treatment of spinal tumors for pain control and quality of life. J Neurosurg Spine. 2005; 2(5):540–549

[46] Chang EL, Shiu AS, Mendel E, et al. Phase I/II study of stereotactic body radiotherapy for spinal metastasis and its pattern of failure. J Neurosurg Spine. 2007; 7(2):151–160

[47] Hamilton AJ, Lulu BA. A prototype device for linear accelerator-based extracranial radiosurgery. Acta Neurochir Suppl (Wien). 1995; 63:40–43

[48] Cox BW, Jackson A, Hunt M, Bilsky M, Yamada Y. Esophageal toxicity from high-dose, single-fraction paraspinal stereotactic radiosurgery. Int J Radiat Oncol Biol Phys. 2012; 83(5):e661–e667

[49] Wang XS, Rhines LD, Shiu AS, et al. Stereotactic body radiation therapy for management of spinal metastases in patients without spinal cord compression: a phase 1–2 trial. Lancet Oncol. 2012; 13(4):395–402

[50] Terezakis SA, Lovelock DM, Bilsky MH, Hunt MA, Zatcky J, Yamada Y. Image-guided intensity-modulated photon radiotherapy using multifractioned regimen to paraspinal chordomas and rare sarcomas. Int J Radiat Oncol Biol Phys. 2007; 69(5):1502–1508

[51] Sahgal A, Whyne CM, Ma L, Larson DA, Fehlings MG. Vertebral compression fracture after stereotactic body radiotherapy for spinal metastases. Lancet Oncol. 2013; 14(8):e310–e320

[52] Boehling NS, Grosshans DR, Allen PK, et al. Vertebral compression fracture risk after stereotactic body radiotherapy for spinal metastases. J Neurosurg Spine. 2012; 16(4):379–386

[53] Cunha MV, Al-Omair A, Atenafu EG, et al. Vertebral compression fracture (VCF) after spine stereotactic body radiation therapy (SBRT): analysis of predictive factors. Int J Radiat Oncol Biol Phys. 2012; 84(3):e343–e349

[54] Jawad MS, Fahim DK, Gerszten PC, et al. on behalf of the Elekta Spine Radiosurgery Research Consortium. Vertebral compression fractures after stereotactic body radiation therapy: a large, multi-institutional, multinational evaluation. J Neurosurg Spine. 2016; 24(6):928–936

[55] Sahgal A, Atenafu EG, Chao S, et al. Vertebral compression fracture after spine stereotactic body radiotherapy: a multi-institutional analysis with a focus on radiation dose and the spinal instability neoplastic score. J Clin Oncol. 2013; 31(27):3426–3431

[56] Virk MS, Han JE, Reiner AS, et al. Frequency of symptomatic vertebral body compression fractures requiring intervention following single-fraction stereotactic radiosurgery for spinal metastases. Neurosurg Focus. 2017; 42(1):E8

[57] Barzilai O, Laufer I, Yamada Y, et al. Integrating evidence-based medicine for treatment of spinal metastases into a decision framework: neurologic, oncologic, mechanicals stability, and systemic disease. J Clin Oncol. 2017; 35(21):2419–2427

[58] Garg AK, Shiu AS, Yang J, et al. Phase 1/2 trial of single-session stereotactic body radiotherapy for previously unirradiated spinal metastases. Cancer. 2012; 118(20):5069–5077

[59] Guckenberger M, Mantel F, Gerszten PC, et al. Safety and efficacy of stereotactic body radiotherapy as primary treatment for vertebral metastases: a multi-institutional analysis. Radiat Oncol. 2014; 9:226

[60] Harel R, Pfeffer R, Levin D, et al. Spine radiosurgery: lessons learned from the first 100 treatment sessions. Neurosurg Focus. 2017; 42(1):E3

[61] Miller JA, Balagamwala EH, Angelov L, et al. Stereotactic radiosurgery for the treatment of primary and metastatic spinal sarcomas. Technol Cancer Res Treat. 2016

[62] Patchell RA, Tibbs PA, Regine WF, et al. Direct decompressive surgical resection in the treatment of spinal cord compression caused by metastatic cancer: a randomised trial. Lancet. 2005; 366(9486):643–648

[63] Laufer I, Iorgulescu JB, Chapman T, et al. Local disease control for spinal metastases following "separation surgery" and adjuvant hypofractionated or high-dose single-fraction stereotactic radiosurgery: outcome analysis in 186 patients. J Neurosurg Spine. 2013; 18(3):207–214

[64] Rock JP, Ryu S, Shukairy MS, et al. Postoperative radiosurgery for malignant spinal tumors. Neurosurgery. 2006; 58(5):891–898, discussion 891–898

[65] Bate BG, Khan NR, Kimball BY, Gabrick K, Weaver J. Stereotactic radiosurgery for spinal metastases with or without separation surgery. J Neurosurg Spine. 2015; 22(4):409–415

[66] DeLaney TF, Liebsch NJ, Pedlow FX, et al. Long-term results of Phase II study of high dose photon/proton radiotherapy in the management of spine chordomas, chondrosarcomas, and other sarcomas. J Surg Oncol. 2014; 110(2):115–122

[67] Rotondo RL, Folkert W, Liebsch NJ, et al. High-dose proton-based radiation therapy in the management of spine chordomas: outcomes and clinicopathological prognostic factors. J Neurosurg Spine. 2015; 23(6):788–797

[68] Krämer M, Weyrather WK, Scholz M. The increased biological effectiveness of heavy charged particles: from radiobiology to treatment planning. Technol Cancer Res Treat. 2003; 2(5):427–436

[69] Dea N, Gokaslan Z, Choi D, Fisher C. Spine oncology - primary spine tumors. Neurosurgery. 2017; 80 3S:S124–S130

[70] Uhl M, Welzel T, Jensen A, et al. Carbon ion beam treatment in patients with primary and recurrent sacrococcygeal chordoma. Strahlenther Onkol. 2015; 191(7):597–603

[71] Yamada Y, Laufer I, Cox BW, et al. Preliminary results of high-dose single-fraction radiotherapy for the management of chordomas of the spine and sacrum. Neurosurgery. 2013; 73(4):673–680, discussion 680

[72] Pennicooke B, Laufer I, Sahgal A, et al. Safety and local control of radiation therapy for chordoma of the spine and sacrum: a systematic review. Spine. 2016; 41 Suppl 20:S186–S192

[73] Ottenhausen M, Ntoulias G, Bodhinayake I, et al. Intradural spinal tumors in adults-update on management and outcome. Neurosurg Rev. 2018; 42(2):371–388

[74] Gerszten PC, Burton SA, Ozhasoglu C, McCue KJ, Quinn AE. Radiosurgery for benign intradural spinal tumors. Neurosurgery. 2008; 62(4):887–895, discussion 895–896

[75] Sachdev S, Dodd RL, Chang SD, et al. Stereotactic radiosurgery yields long-term control for benign intradural, extramedullary spinal tumors. Neurosurgery. 2011; 69(3):533–539, discussion 539

[76] Hernández-Durán S, Hanft S, Komotar RJ, Manzano GR. The role of stereotactic radiosurgery in the treatment of intramedullary spinal cord neoplasms: a systematic literature review. Neurosurg Rev. 2016; 39(2):175–183, discussion 183

Part V
Easing the Transition to Technological Adoption

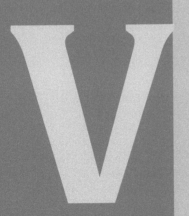

30 Operating Room Design and Efficiency

James Dowdell, Christopher M. Mikhail, and Andrew C. Hecht

Abstract:

New technologies in spine surgery are constantly being developed. These technologies are often aimed at improving operating room (OR) efficiency, ease of operation, and patient safety. The OR suite size and setup must be able to accommodate all personnel and equipment while improving sterile technique. Consistency in the anesthesia, nursing, and surgical teams and concomitant setup and breakdown of the OR significantly reduced OR time and expense. Finally, the introduction of robotics and navigation has reduced the misplacement of hardware but have yet to reduce operative times. The purpose of this study is to provide a narrative review of the current concepts in OR design, efficiency, and intraoperative robotics and navigation in spine surgery. Ultimately, it is prudent for the surgeons and medical institutions at large to be aware of the data and adapt their perioperative protocols as such.

Keywords: robotics, navigation, design, efficiency, spine, surgery

30.1 Introduction

As surgical innovation accelerates specifically in the field of spine surgery, new technologies are seemingly continuously introduced into the operative suite. Some of these technologies, specifically navigated platforms and robotics, promise to be revolutionary, but their integration into the operative workflow has proven challenging. OR design and machine setup within that framework is crucial to a smooth operative experience. Meticulous preoperative planning, including consideration for machine placement, can make the difference between an effortless or a frustrating surgical case. As the indications for navigation and robotic technologies in spine surgery continue to expand, their intraoperative use rises in hand. However, efficient use can be a barrier to more widespread adoption. This chapter aims to describe some of the challenges and provide design solutions to improve the operative experience with these technologies.

30.2 Operating Suite Design

30.2.1 Operating Room Size

As surgical equipment grows increasingly larger, there has been a commensurate demand for adequately scaled operative suites. Historically, the standard operating room (OR) suite was approximately 400 square feet. According to Facility Guidelines Institute (FGI) guidelines published in 2014, the size requirement for general OR suites remains 400 square feet, or 600 square feet for procedures which require more staff and/or equipment.[1] The size required for a hybrid OR, a surgical theater that is equipped with an advanced medical imaging device such as a fixed C-arm, CT scanner, or MRI, will be even higher with estimates of around 1,000 square feet.[1] The typical spine surgery case involves numerous staff and equipment requirements including space for the anesthesia team, surgical team, nursing staff, tables for implants, vendors, a neuromonitoring team, a large C-arm, and occasionally a microscope. The FGI guidelines provide recommendations which account for the need for adequate space for personnel and equipment with minimal potential for contamination.[1] Procedures that use navigation will require a secondary computer/image registration hub that houses the navigation software, while a surgical robot will be required for robotic-assisted cases. These products will have significant spatial requirements and the operating room must evolve to meet these demands.

30.2.2 Minimizing Contamination while Driving Technological Advancements

The modern operating suite should be set up to have ample space for all necessary equipment as contamination rates in the OR correlate with OR traffic. Implementation of new design features in the operative suite should not compromise sterility in the OR or operative efficiency. Recently, technologies have begun to be introduced and designed to minimize hand contact and potential intraoperative contamination. For example, OR 21 is a novel OR lighting system that utilizes a hands-free overhead light/laminar air flow combination system intended to ultimately replace currently used more typical lighting systems attached to a boom (▶ Fig. 30.1). Still under investigation, this system obviates the need for surgeon manipulation of intraoperative lighting, a potential source for contamination, and simultaneously can improve intraoperative air quality, another potential source of contamination.

Breach in sterility has been documented during intraoperative fluoroscopy as well as microscope use. Specifically, C-arm contamination has been reported to occur in as many as 56% of cases.[2] Although perhaps easier to drape during room setup rather than immediately prior to use, prolonged C-arm drape time, in the setting of increased foot traffic, can lead to contamination. In the case of early draping, it is generally recommended to avoid contact with the C-arm and treat it as contaminated.[2] Other more technologically advanced imaging modalities may be used with the benefit to decrease contamination and increase efficiency by obviating the need for multiple C-arm rotations and repeated imaging throughout the procedure. These modalities will be discussed in a separate chapter; they include Brainlab CT scanner, Ziehm C-arm, and the O-arm which do not require continuous use of the conventional fluoroscopy.[3]

Postoperative culture of the surgical microscope (and drape) has revealed that contamination may occur anywhere from 12 to 44% of the time.[4] However, this contamination rate has not led to a similar increase in the infection rate.[4] Most commonly, contamination occurs around the optic eyepieces and the handles. Adequate OR space can allow more ideal microscope positioning and potentially less need for intraoperative handling. If the operative microscope should be handled intraoperatively, it is recommended to change outer surgical gloves to minimize contamination of the surgical wound.[4]

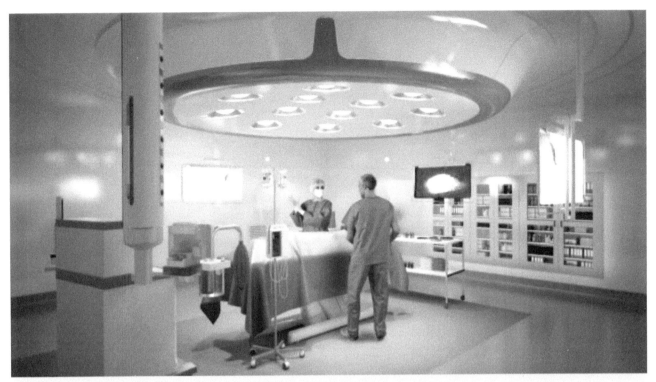

Fig. 30.1 Operating room 21—New lighting/laminar flow combination system to improve sterility.

30.2.3 Design of a Traditional Operating Suite

The operating suite should be designed to maximize efficiency, improving workflow for the assistive staff while simultaneously limiting traffic around the operative table. OR traffic has been implicated as a source of contamination.[2] Ideally, the operative suite should include the operating table in the center of the room, a space for anesthesia at the head of the table, an area for the OR back table that is at least 2 feet from any room traffic, and a dedicated area for the circulating nurse[1] (▶ Fig. 30.2). There should be access to the external corridor and a clean core from the OR, but these doors should not be able to be opened simultaneously so as not to allow turbulent air flow to cross the operative field.[5] An image display system (i.e., Picture Archiving and Communication System (PACS)) that projects images comfortably within the view of the operative table helps prevent surgeon traffic away from the operative table, limiting breaches in sterility. Similarly, with the introduction of robotics and navigation, a dedicated space should exist within the OR to store and use these devices without increasing the risk of contamination with their use.[3]

30.2.4 Design of a Hybrid Operating Room

The design of the hybrid OR for spine surgery should maintain all the necessary components of the traditional operating suite with the addition of advanced medical imaging device such as a fixed C-arm, CT scanner, or MRI. The estimate for space needed for a hybrid OR is about 1,000 square feet.[1,3] The most frequent imaging modality utilized in hybrid ORs for spine surgery has been a CT scanner. Hypothetically, with computer-assisted navigation (CAN), hybrid ORs can improve efficiency and minimize complications. CAN has already proven useful for minimizing radiation compared to conventional fluoroscopy.[3,6] A radiation-safe area should be implemented into the design of all hybrid ORs for the benefit of the surgeon and all OR staff.[3]

30.3 Efficiency in the Spine Operating Room

Operative suite design is one way to improve intraoperative efficiency; establishing an efficient workflow between operative staff team members is another. Each step of the operative day can be streamlined to be more efficient without sacrificing safety, but this increase in efficiency does not necessarily translate into increased case volume.[7] Although we generally think of patients progressing through the preoperative, intraoperative, and postoperative setting in a linear fashion[8] (▶ Fig. 30.3), parallel processing (e.g., simultaneously setting up anesthesia, placing leads for neuromonitoring, and setting up the back tables for the OR) can significantly improve timing and efficiency[8] (▶ Fig. 30.3). This requires the training of the preoperative nurses, anesthesia team, as well as the operative nursing team to know their specific roles during each portion of the case and how to multitask without negatively influencing patient outcomes.

30.3.1 Preoperative Efficiency

To discuss the efficiency of an OR, one must analyze the steps taken prior to OR roll back that lead to inefficiencies and waste in the perioperative setting. OR costs are high and each minute

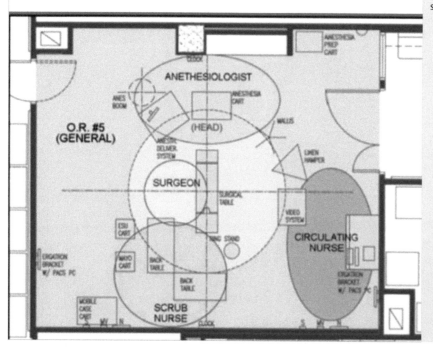

Fig. 30.2 Each operating room should have dedicated work zones to drive efficiency and safety.

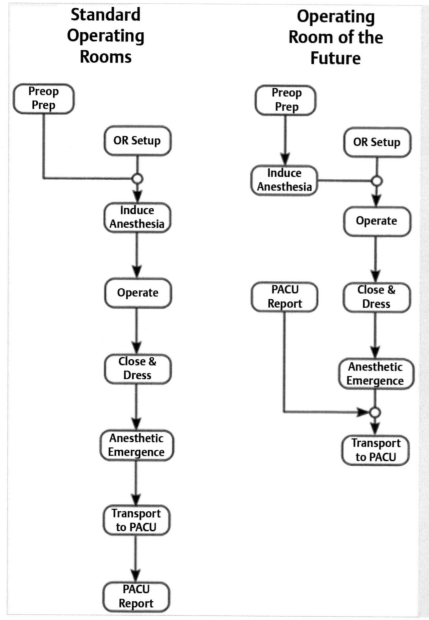

Fig. 30.3 Anesthesia work flow showing standard anesthesia protocol and parallel processing.

used for unnecessary tasks adds to the enormous cost burden and perioperative budget.[9,10] Several studies have evaluated the influence of preoperative checklist completion on OR day efficiency. Checklists may serve a dual purpose. Firstly, they ensure patient safety measures are taken prior to roll back. Secondly, they allow tracking of each teams' contribution to the preoperative evaluation,[11] including the roles of the surgical team, nursing team, anesthesiology team, and OR equipment team. Each team plays a unique and vital role in ensuring smooth operative flow. These checklists have been found to improve efficiency.

The flow of an OR day is often set by the first start. Being able to start the first case on time is critical in maximizing allotted block time. A recent study discussed the implementation of preoperative managers whose role was to ensure on-time first start times. They found that the addition of an OR facilitator reduced the amount of delayed first start cases by 50%.[9,10] Ensuring that preoperative checklists are completed in a timely fashion is critical for patient safety and OR workflow.[11]

OR turnover is also important for maintaining an appropriate workflow. It minimizes patient discomfort, maximizes surgeon block time, and ultimately enhances hospital revenue. Formally educating designated leaders (surgeons, anesthesiologists, and nursing staff) on the importance of turnover has done little to improve this issue. The six-sigma initiative in 2002 identified key factors in improving OR turnover times: surgeon at scrub sink during patient preparation, setup dismantled upon wound closure, clean up prior to patient out of room, case chart completed, and the surgeon consistently notified of room readiness. Improving these factors resulted in a 32% reduction in turnover time.[12] How applicable this study is to spine surgery can be debated, but recent literature focusing on efficiency in spine ORs has found that an initiative to consolidate trays and standardize instrumentation has a great benefit to both cost savings and decreased operative time.[13] This initiative was driven by communication between hospital OR staff, surgeon, and industry reps to focus only on needed equipment for any given surgery.[13] This allows a streamlined setup/clean-up, less chance for mistakes during surgery, and more efficient use of OR time. Our recommendation is that each surgeon streamlines the equipment needed for each case to derive maximum value and safety in the OR setting.

30.3.2 Intraoperative Efficiency

Comparison of Large and Small Community and University Hospitals OR Efficiency

Recent literature has suggested that private hospitals run more efficiently than university hospitals. Frequently, community hospitals have smaller surgical teams who have worked together before, while university hospitals may have larger surgical teams who work together less consistently.[14] A recent study showed that the total time from patient arrival at the hospital to anesthesia induction and the time from anesthesia induction to incision were shorter in the private rather than in the academic setting.[14] OR efficiency was reduced by a lack of consistency within the broader surgical teams. There was also a reduced amount of fluoroscopic time and exposure associated with radiology technicians with spinal surgery experience. More images, longer fluoroscopic time, and higher radiation

doses were administered in the university hospital system then in the private hospital setting. This was thought to be a result of higher staff turnover in the university setting with more frequent use of inexperienced, substitute, or night shift radiology technicians with less experience in the spine OR.

Understandably the university hospital setting results in multiple inefficiencies. The priority to teach trainees in their respective fields results in accepted increases in time of anesthesia induction, operative times, and room turnover. However, some training could reasonably be performed outside of the practical daily workflow that can improve these inefficiencies: for example, surgical residents attending workshops and courses to hone their surgical skills. Other members of the surgical team should also be provided educational resources to improve comfort and efficiency in the OR. Radiation technologists can utilize cadaver labs to practice obtaining appropriate imaging with less shots and fluoroscopic time.

Room Setup

An appropriately managed OR is essential for optimal OR efficiency. Room setup and turnover inefficiencies can negatively influence workflow in the OR. Appropriate setup includes having all necessary instruments and equipment for completion of a procedure by ensuring all appropriate trays are available for an operative day. It is imperative that this is overseen by the attending surgeon. Additionally, surgical representatives should be readily available, and be notified in advance of planned procedures. This can be done by the OR staff as well as the surgical team.[13]

To improve turnover time, patients should be allowed to enter the OR while sterile trays are still being opened and set up. This allows for concomitant setup for the surgical tech, while anesthesia begins their induction.

Patient Positioning

After anesthesia is administered, patient positioning should take place under the guidance of experienced surgical staff. Recent literature suggests that patient positioning can be a source of delay if not attended to by the surgical staff, secondary to the need for repositioning.[15] It is also important for a surgical team member to be present for positioning due to safety concerns, as improper positioning can lead to increased operative difficulties and complications such as nerve palsies, pressure sores, or even retinal ischemia. Neuromonitoring can be set up concurrently with anesthesia induction. The surgical site can be appropriately prepared and draped while the surgical team is starting to scrub for the procedure.

During the procedure, it is important to maintain a well-organized sterile setup. Experienced surgical technicians can anticipate instrument use and removal of unnecessary instruments, which can greatly improve surgical efficiency. In addition to improving surgical flow, this allows for concomitant setup and breakdown throughout the procedure. This allows containment of surgical sets, streamlined end of procedure counts, and room cleanup.[16] Allowing for overlap at each of these steps can dramatically reduce perioperative time from patient into the room, time to anesthesia, time from anesthesia to procedure start, and from surgical end time to time out of room.

Efficient Use of Navigation/Robotics

Intraoperative navigation and image-guided robotics can be utilized for simpler cases such as microdiskectomy and posterolateral lumbar fusion and more advanced cases such as three column spinal osteotomies, resection of intradural tumors, and deformity cases with distortion of normal anatomy.[3] Additionally, these platforms may mitigate much of the harmful radiation exposure in minimally invasive surgery to which the patient, surgeon, and ancillary OR staff are subjected.[3] Spine surgery relies upon meticulous motor skills to manipulate neural elements while exploiting small working corridors utilizing exposures that minimize collateral damage. This can predispose a surgeon to mental and physical fatigue that can potentially be mitigated with the use of navigation or robotic assistance. Recent innovation within computer-assisted 2D and 3D navigation as well as surgical robotics have the potential of improving outcomes. However, given the initial cost of these products, surgeons must demonstrate their superiority to traditional techniques currently being used. Nevertheless, these technologies are going to continue to evolve and become more efficient as they mature.

Multiple new navigation technologies have been studied in recent years that can improve operative room efficiency. For instance, newer navigation modalities can result in a lower number of misplaced pedicle screws and can theoretically improve both operative outcomes and decrease operative time, although this has not been shown consistently to this point. Han et al showed a significant increase in efficiency of navigation-guided screw placement over fluoroscopy with an average of 2.54 versus 4.56 minutes per screw, respectively ($p < 0.001$).[17] This must be weighed against the increases in time during other portions of the procedure including obtainment of images for guidance and robot/computer setup time. It is also important to understand that OR efficiency is closely intertwined with patient safety. Decreased operative time with open spinal procedures has been correlated to lower short-term complications. Thus, the effect of efficiency on healthcare cost burden is twofold. Firstly, a decrease in complication rate will result in lower cost to the healthcare system, as readmission and reoperation rates may decrease. Additionally, the ability to increase case volume and decrease operative time can lead to higher revenue.

Ideal Placement of Navigation/Robotic Systems within the OR

The ideal placement of navigation systems is dictated by surgeon comfort and experience. In our experience, the ideal placement of navigation systems depends on the case being performed. For a lumbar case, we typically place the noninvasive tracker with the tracking end more distal (▶ Fig. 30.4). We will then place a sterile drape over the tracker to allow for a spine with our mobile CT scanner (Ziehm C-arm), which comes in from the side opposite the surgeon (▶ Fig. 30.5, ▶ Fig. 30.6). It is important to hold respiration during the C-arm spin to prevent motion artifact which could impact navigation accuracy. We will then register the C-arm with the navigation camera so that the navigation camera is linked to the CT scan images. We place the navigation camera and monitor at the foot of the bed (▶ Fig. 30.7). For cervical and thoracic cases, we will place the navigation camera and monitor at the head of the bed.

Training Operative Staff

The nursing staff and scrub technologists are an integral part of operating efficiency. In the private hospital setting, the operative staff will frequently remain the same on a recurring basis and this will allow increasing efficiency. This continuity can occur in the teaching hospital setting as well, but it is rarer and can create the potential for delay secondary to operative staff not knowing setup, positioning, and equipment needs. It is recommended that a surgeon has a written set of instructions to give OR staff about OR setup, equipment/implants needed, and operative steps/instruments needed in detail to avoid questions and delays during the case.

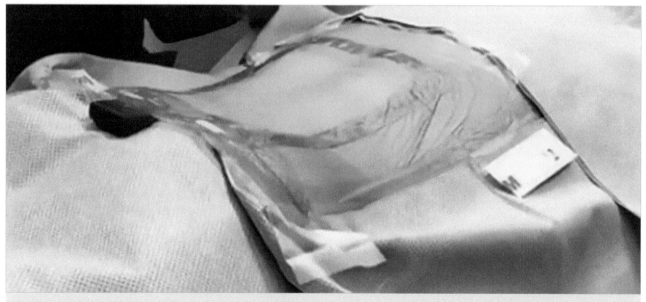

Fig. 30.4 Tracker is placed distal to where surgery will be performed.

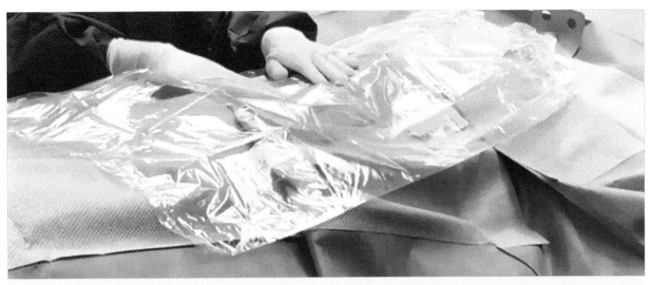

Fig. 30.5 Sterile drape over the surgical field/tracker.

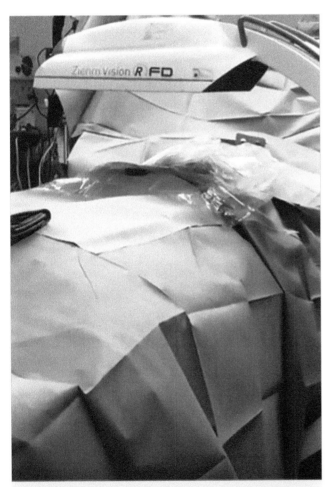

Fig. 30.6 Mobile CT scanner (Ziehm) approaching from the side opposite the surgeon.

Staff turnover can also have a great effect on efficiency as one inexperienced team member can contribute to significant surgical delays. While it would be difficult to change the culture of the teaching hospital completely, improvements could be made to training that would allow staff to feel more able to contribute early in their careers. There are a variety of software-based simulation units, one of which is called PeriopSim, which have been shown to help the training of surgical nurses and scrub technologists. This simulation training has been clinically shown to improve recognition of instruments, improve operative setup efficiency, and have staff readier to contribute in the early phase of their careers.

As technology advances, surgical team members must be active in learning to avoid excessive inefficiency. This concept applies to every member of the surgical team including X-ray technicians. Learning curves are expected; however, using new technology in a simulated fashion may decrease technical difficulties early on which can potentially improve operative times and decrease complication rates. It is therefore important to ensure that the implementation of these new systems is done so in an efficient manner and that all personnel who must operate these machines feel comfortable to do so. It is known that experienced X-ray technicians lead to less fluoroscopic time, less images taken, and overall lower radiation exposure.

30.4 Conclusion

The thought process of OR design should include technologies that exist today, but also include the potential for new technology to be implemented in the future. As new technologies develop it is imperative that they are implemented in the OR in a safe and streamlined fashion to avoid any potential for patient or surgical team member harm. As these new technologies mature and ORs evolve, it is going to be vital that each team

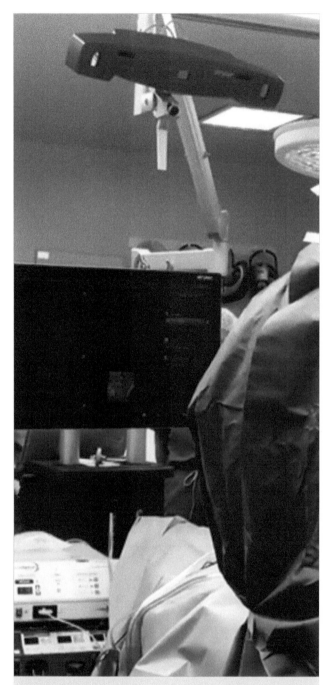

Fig. 30.7 Position of navigation camera and monitor.

involved in perioperative care be able to use these technologies efficiently. With advancements in perioperative care flow, simulated training, and streamlined surgeon-guided OR setups, there is likely to be a great improvement in OR efficiency.

References

[1] Shine TSJ, Leone BJ, Martin DL. "Specialized Operating Rooms." 2012 Operating Room Design Manual, ASA, 2012: 44–56. Available at: www.asahq.org/resources/resources-from-asa-committees/operating-room-design-manual. Accessed June 26, 2019

[2] Ahn DK, Park HS, Kim TW, et al. The degree of bacterial contamination while performing spine surgery. Asian Spine J. 2013; 7(1):8–13

[3] Overley SC, Cho SK, Mehta AI, Arnold PM. Navigation and robotics in spinal surgery: where are we now? Neurosurgery. 2017; 80 3S:S86–S99

[4] Basques BA, Golinvaux NS, Bohl DD, et al. Use of an operating microscope during spine surgery is associated with minor increases in operating room times and no increased risk of infection. Spine. 2014; 39(22):1910–1916

[5] Spagnolo AM, Ottria G, Amicizia D, Perdelli F, Cristina ML. Operating theatre quality and prevention of surgical site infections. J Prev Med Hyg. 2013; 54 (3):131–137

[6] Miller JA, Fabiano AJ. Comparison of operative time with conventional fluoroscopy versus spinal neuronavigation in instrumented spinal tumor surgery. World Neurosurg. 2017; 105:412–419

[7] Agnoletti V, Buccioli M, Padovani E, et al. Operating room data management: improving efficiency and safety in a surgical block. BMC Surg. 2013; 13:7

[8] Friedman DM, Sokal SM, Chang Y, Berger DL. Increasing operating room efficiency through parallel processing. Ann Surg. 2006; 243(1):10–14

[9] Dexter F, Epstein RH. Typical savings from each minute reduction in tardy first case of the day starts. Anesth Analg. 2009; 108(4):1262–1267

[10] Dhupar R, Evankovich J, Klune JR, Vargas LG, Hughes SJ. Delayed operating room availability significantly impacts the total hospital costs of an urgent surgical procedure. Surgery. 2011; 150(2):299–305

[11] Panni MK, Shah SJ, Chavarro C, Rawl M, Wojnarwsky PK, Panni JK. Improving operating room first start efficiency - value of both checklist and a pre-operative facilitator. Acta Anaesthesiol Scand. 2013; 57(9):1118–1123

[12] Adams R, Warner P, Hubbard B, Goulding T. Decreasing turnaround time between general surgery cases: a six sigma initiative. J Nurs Adm. 2004; 34 (3):140–148

[13] Abrams J, Dekutoski M, Chutkan N. Maximizing operating room efficiency in spine surgery: a process of tray consolidation, instrument standardization and cost savings. In: ISASS 17: General Session Outcomes and Value in Spine Surgery. 2017. Available at: https://www.isass.org/abstracts/isass17-oral-posters/isass17-477-Maximizing-Operating-Room-Efficiency-in-Spine-Surgery-A-Process-of-Tr.html. Accessed June 27, 2019

[14] Wasterlain AS, Tran AA, Tang C, et al. Can we improve workflows in the OR? A comparison of quality perceptions and preoperative efficiency across institutions in spine surgery. Bull Hosp Jt Dis (2013). 2015; 73(1):46–53

[15] Asiedu GB, Lowndes BR, Huddleston PM, Hallbeck S. "The Jackson Table is a pain in the…": a qualitative study of providers' perception toward a spinal surgery table. J Patient Saf. 2018; 14(1):21–26

[16] Foglia RP, Alder AC, Ruiz G. Improving perioperative performance: the use of operations management and the electronic health record. J Pediatr Surg. 2013; 48(1):95–98

[17] Han W, Gao ZL, Wang JC, et al. Pedicle screw placement in the thoracic spine: a comparison study of computer-assisted navigation and conventional techniques. Orthopedics. 2010; 33(8):8

31 Mounting the Learning Curve with New Technologies

John E. Ziewacz

Abstract:
Adopting a new technique or technology in surgery requires overcoming an initial learning curve, during which complication rates can increase and efficiency can decrease. Strategies to mitigate complication risk and increase efficiency while on the learning curve before mastery of a technique are paramount to ensure patient safety and the safe and effective adoption of new techniques. This chapter will address the learning curve for adoption of new techniques/technologies in surgery and examine barriers to adoption and strategies for navigating the learning curve safely and effectively.

Keywords: learning curve, barriers to adoption, robotics, navigation, hi-fidelity simulation

31.1 Introduction

The adoption of any new technology requires navigating an initial learning curve prior to attaining mastery of the new technique and its adoption into routine practice. The learning curve can be defined as the time (or in the case of surgery, number of cases) it takes to attain a reproducible and steady level of mastery of a new technique or technology. Surgically, this translates into reaching a state with the lowest possible complication rate and shortest case length attainable to achieve that rate. Surgical techniques/technologies vary in their relative ease or difficulty of mastery based on various factors including technical difficulty, resources necessary, need for specialized training, etc. The learning curve for a procedure is typically referred to as steep when a procedure is thought to be difficult to master or incorporate into regular practice. However, graphically, a steep learning curve is actually desirable as it indicates a smaller number of cases to attain the highest attainable competence (see ▶ Fig. 31.1, ▶ Fig. 31.2).

In surgery there is an inherent tension between adoption of new technologies that eventually make treatments safer and more effective and navigating the learning curve for those technologies as they are being adopted.[1,2] The difficulty with the surgical learning curve is that while on the slope of the curve a higher complication rate is typically identified, and this can translate into patient harm. Due to the ethical primacy of "primum non-nocere," or first do no harm, it is difficult to accept performing a new procedure that may take longer or carry a higher complication risk initially than the gold standard a surgeon is more familiar with. In fact, governing bodies have stated that there should be no learning curve in surgery when it comes to complications.[1,2] However, it is widely acknowledged that all new techniques/technologies have some learning curve associated. Given the desirability of adopting technological and procedural advancement, and given this adoption comes at an initial cost in inefficiency and increased complications, it is of paramount importance to understand the learning curve and to identify ways to steepen the curve for rapid and safe mastery of new technologies. This chapter will discuss barriers to adoption of new technology in spinal surgery, examine the learning curve for new technology in spinal surgery, and discuss potential means to steepen the learning curve for new techniques/technologies in spinal surgery.

31.2 Barriers to Adoption of New Technology

Prior to considering specific mechanisms to steepen the learning curve, it is worth considering the barriers to adoption of new technologies, since mounting the learning curve to begin with depends on the decision to adopt a new technology and since barriers to adoption can cause providers to fall off the learning curve entirely.

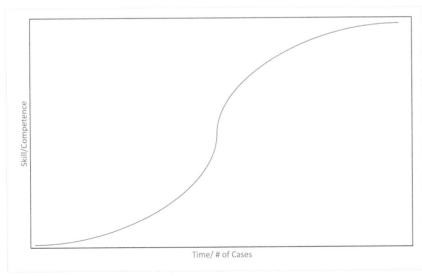

Fig. 31.1 Learning curve for a difficult technique/procedure.

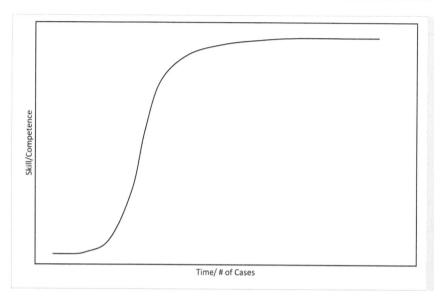

Fig. 31.2 Learning curve for an easier technique/procedure.

Barriers to adoption typically fall into two categories: (1) factors associated with the technology itself and (2) contextual factors surrounding the technology to be adopted.[3] Factors associated with the technology itself include a perceived difficulty of use, cost to the system, surgeon investment in time/energy learning the new technique/technology, and lack of perceived volume of cases or appeal to patients and providers.[3,4] In the case of robotics/navigation, direct costs to an institution can be in the six or seven figures and in the case of at least one of the manufacturers of robotic technology for spinal surgery, surgeons must travel to company headquarters to receive onsite formal training prior to being certified to perform robotic spinal operations. Contextual factors include the perceived benefit of a new technology versus existing technologies, patient desire/appeal, evidence for superiority established in the literature, marketing by companies, and adoption by surgeon or thought leaders/local competition.[3] While some of these barriers are difficult to alter or influence, such as the direct cost of the technology, others are more amenable to intervention—particularly study of a new technology.

When a new technology that is at face value appealing also has a compelling evidence-basis for its use in the literature, its adoption is more likely, as it is eventually seen as a standard of care and surgeons/institutions would lag behind peers if the technology is not adopted.[3] While technology in healthcare and spinal surgery in particular continues to progress rapidly, and its study is welcomed and necessary, its assessment continues to lag.[5] One of the reasons for this is described as Buxton's law.[6] This asserts that a new technology is too new to be studied until it is too established to be studied.[6] This means that there is a reticence to study a new technology, while early adopters are on the initial slope of the learning curve for fear that the promising technology, which may be of significant benefit once practitioners reach the asymptote of the learning curve (the point of maximal efficiency and minimal complication risk), will fare poorly against established procedures. However, once such a new technology has achieved widespread adoption, there is a further lack of desire to study it, given that practitioners believe they would now be delivering less than the new

standard to revert to the established procedure. As such, many new technologies have not undergone the rigorous study that would typically be required to establish them as superior to established procedures and as new standards of care.[3] The extent to which a new technology can be studied rigorously to establish equivalency and hopefully superiority compared to established techniques is an important factor in prompting surgeons to more quickly adopt the new technology to remain on the forefront of surgical technology development and not be left behind by advancements in the field. Ideally, a new technology would be studied both on the slope of the learning curve and at the asymptote, to both understand risks/complications while on the curve and define the learning curve, in addition to establishing equivalency/superiority compared to established techniques once the asymptote for adoption of the new technology has been reached.

In summary, new technologies face multiple barriers to adoption, both inherent to the procedure and cultural/contextual. Some barriers are more amenable to intervention than others. In short, providing a solid evidence basis for a new technology, making the technology as cost-effective as possible, minimizing time/energy expenditure by the practitioner adopting the technology, and fostering a supportive cultural environment for adoption of promising technologies help overcome these barriers.

31.3 Defining the Learning Curve for New Technologies in Spinal Surgery

Prior to determining ways to steepen the learning curve it is necessary to define the learning curve for a new technology/procedure. For emerging technologies, including robotics and navigation in spine surgery, the literature is nascent but instructive. First, initial studies must establish that a new technology can eventually be performed safely and effectively as compared to existing technology. While in the case of robotics, an initial study demonstrated improved accuracy with freehand techniques,[7] several subsequent studies of robotics and navigation in spinal surgery have confirmed that safe and effective placement of instrumentation is achievable, with eventual successful pedicle screw/instrumentation placement rates comparable or improved compared to freehand techniques.[8,9,10,11,12,13,14] Studies dealing specifically with the learning curve for robotics suggest the asymptote of the learning curve is achieved between 20 and 30 cases.[9,10,15] This is comparable to the published learning curve for other minimally invasive techniques in spinal surgery including microendoscopic diskectomy and minimally invasive transforaminal interbody fusion (TLIF), with the asymptote being reached for these procedures from 30 to 44 cases, respectively.[16,17,18] One study noted a rise in screw misplacement after the first five cases using the robot compared to the first five, with a peak at case 20, and subsequent decrease afterward.[15] It was thought that this was due to the loosening of supervision after the first five cases coupled with an increase in confidence, despite not having mastered the technique. Based on these results, the authors suggested supervision of cases for the first 25 robotic procedures.[15] Hu and Lieberman noted successful robot-assisted pedicle screw placement in 82% of their initial 30 patients, with a leveling off from 91 to 95% in their subsequent 120 patients.[9] Of note, the majority of the initial studies on robotic-assisted spinal surgery were performed by experienced attending/consultant surgeons. In a study of robotic-assisted surgery assessing trainees (residents and fellows), pedicle screws were safely and accurately placed, with decreasing time and radiation use per pedicle screw placement with increasing volume of cases.[14] However, no trainee performed more than seven cases, so an asymptote to the learning curve could not be assessed. Interestingly, there was no difference in time to screw placement across junior and senior residents, or those with a specialized interest in spinal surgery.[14] This result suggests the robot may decrease the skill necessary to accurately place pedicle screws, which has positive potential implications for widespread adoption. Of note, however, all trainees were under close supervision by an experienced attending surgeon.[14] The authors rightly point out, though, that ethically it would not be feasible to study the technique in trainees, particularly junior trainees, without adequate supervision.[14]

In summary, studies of navigation and robotics demonstrate these modalities are capable of assisting in pedicle screw placement that is at least as accurate and safe as conventional techniques, with a learning curve estimated at 20 to 30 cases, and evidence suggesting the learning curve may not be dependent on initial level of training.

31.4 Strategies to Accelerate the Learning Curve for Adopting a New Surgical Technology

Given the low tolerance for increased complications while navigating the learning curve in new surgical technologies, it is of paramount importance to determine methods for steepening the learning curve for cases when it comes to complications, so that the minimum number of cases to the acceptable asymptote on the learning curve can be achieved. With respect to navigation and robotics in spinal surgery, there is a paucity of studies specifically assessing this topic; however, there are valuable lessons from the available literature and from the literature addressing strategies for accelerating the learning curve for other surgical technologies.

The simplest way to accelerate the learning curve as it relates to complications is to actually broaden the learning curve initially as it relates to time. While efficiency and decreased case times are goals of adoption of a new technology and a part of the learning curve, initially minimizing the complication risk is the most important precept, so sacrificing time is an acceptable trade-off. Practically, this means scheduling extra time for robotic/navigation cases, avoiding scheduling cases when a flight or pressing scheduling matter is present, and avoiding scheduling cases on-call, whenever possible. Eventually, once the procedure is mastered, improving case times and efficiency can then be addressed.

Based on the acknowledged learning curve for robotic-assisted pedicle screw placement of approximately 20 to 30 cases, it has been recommended that these first cases be supervised/observed.[15] This level of supervision is ideal and may be practical in many academic settings. However, this may not be practical in many real-world private practice settings where obtaining supervision for 20 to 30 cases from an expert in the technology could be resource and cost-prohibitive. In this regard, a reasonable substitute may be to have another attending/partner scrub. Hasan et al, studying the learning curve for the Ross procedure for aortic root surgery, initiated a formal protocol wherein attending/consultant surgeons would assist each other after first performing the procedure with an expert, with no increase in complications.[2]

It is possible that the use of video may enhance or substitute for the ability of an expert to supervise the initial cases on the slope of the learning curve. Recent advances have led to the use of video in the preoperative, intraoperative, and postoperative settings. In the preoperative setting, surgeons can view multiple other surgeons' similar cases for tips on technique, complication avoidance, etc.[19] Intraoperative video with live streaming can allow for direct telementoring from remote surgeons, which may obviate to a degree the need for a physical presence for observation of the initial cases on the learning curve. Finally, postoperative use of video allows the opportunity for surgical "coaching"/mentoring from expert surgeons, hopefully accelerating the learning curve by constructive critique of actual cases performed by the training surgeon.[19] While formal evaluation of the effects of video on accelerating the learning curve for surgery are lacking, it is an exciting arena that has the potential to contribute greatly to the acceleration of the learning curve for navigation and robotics in spinal surgery, mitigating in part the difficulty practicing surgeons have in accessing experts to supervise/observe cases physically.

Hi-fidelity simulation represents another promising avenue for accelerating the learning curve for new technology in spinal surgery. While hi-fidelity simulation has become commonplace in general surgery and other specialties, it is less common for neurosurgery and spinal surgery.[20] However, there is mounting evidence in these fields that simulation can lead to improved performance in a range of procedures and that feedback from participants is positive overall.[21] Navigation and robotics are ideal technologies for simulation since the actual technology/ skills being used in the operating room can be employed in the simulations, on either cadavers or sawbones. Robotics in particular is engineered for reproducible successive iterations of a standardized process (i.e., pedicle screw placement), which would allow the practitioner ample opportunity to simulate real-world instrumentation placement multiple times in a standardized fashion using the actual technology in a simulated setting. While the effects of simulation in navigation and robotics in spinal surgery have not been studied in detail, owing to the characteristics of the technologies, a compelling logic exists that hi-fidelity simulation could accelerate the learning curve associated with their adoption.

It is likely that a structured approach to adoption of a new technology with stepwise processes and graded responsibility is best for accelerating the learning curve for new surgical technologies and minimizing complications. Accordingly, Hasan et al[2] followed a structured strategy to incorporating a new technique in aortic root surgery that included formal didactic training, simulating the technique in cadavers, undertaking the first operation with experts, and attendings/consultants assisting each other on the operation.[2] Their results demonstrated no increase in morbidity or mortality compared to the established literature.[2] This strategy could be followed when introducing navigation and robotics to spinal surgery. Formal didactics could be pursued at national meetings, academic centers, or through the manufacturers; hi-fidelity cadaver or sawbones simulation could be offered through specialized courses at meetings or through manufacturers; and observation and assistance from experts, either live or via video could be utilized for the initial 20–30 cases, which represent the approximate learning curve for the adoption of navigation and robotics. This structured approach requires study but provides a logical framework for accelerating the learning curve for adoption of new technologies in spinal surgery, and therefore limiting the complications associated with the adoption of new technologies in spinal surgery.

In summary, given the paramount importance of minimizing complications while navigating the learning curve of new technologies in spinal surgery, multiple steps can be taken to accelerate the learning curve for adoption of new technologies. These include allowing extra time for the initial procedures; following a structured process for adoption; and incorporating formal didactics, hi-fidelity simulations (cadaver or sawbones), and observation of initial cases, either physically or through video assistance (see ▶ Table 31.1).

Table 31.1 Strategies to accelerate the learning curve for adopting a new surgical technology

1. Formal didactic instruction/courses in the new technique/procedure
2. Structured cadaveric training
3. Hi-fidelity simulation
4. Close supervision/proctoring for the initial slope of the learning curve (~ 30 cases)
5. Video telementoring
6. Attending assistance while on the learning curve
7. Broaden the learning curve for time to steepen the learning curve for complications

31.5 Conclusion

New technologies in surgery face barriers to adoption and are inevitably associated with a learning curve prior to mastery. Minimizing the barriers to adoption better allows surgeons to initially mount the learning curve and to stay on the learning curve once a new technology has been initially adopted. Given the paramount importance of minimizing complications while on the slope of the learning curve, efforts at accelerating the learning curve and minimizing complications are necessary. Multiple strategies exist for accelerating the learning curve which should be employed and studied when adopting navigation and robotic technologies in spinal surgery.

References

[1] Edwards J, Mazzone A, Crouch G. Minimally invasive mitral surgery: dangerous to dabble. J Extra Corpor Technol. 2012; 44(1):51–54
[2] Hasan A, Pozzi M, Hamilton JR. New surgical procedures: can we minimise the learning curve? BMJ. 2000; 320(7228):171–173
[3] Wilson CB. Adoption of new surgical technology. BMJ. 2006; 332(7533):112–114
[4] Athanasiou T, Ashrafian H, Rowland SP, Casula R. Robotic cardiac surgery: advanced minimally invasive technology hindered by barriers to adoption. Future Cardiol. 2011; 7(4):511–522
[5] Herndon JH, Hwang R, Bozic KJ. Healthcare technology and technology assessment. Eur Spine J. 2007; 16(8):1293–1302
[6] Buxton MJ. Problems in the economic appraisal of new health technology: the evaluation of heart transplants in the UK. In: Drummond MF, ed. Economic Appraisal of Health Technology in the European Community. Oxford: Oxford Medical Publications; 1987:103–18
[7] Ringel F, Stüer C, Reinke A, et al. Accuracy of robot-assisted placement of lumbar and sacral pedicle screws: a prospective randomized comparison to conventional freehand screw implantation. Spine. 2012; 37(8):E496–E501
[8] Bai YS, Zhang Y, Chen ZQ, et al. Learning curve of computer-assisted navigation system in spine surgery. Chin Med J (Engl). 2010; 123(21):2989–2994
[9] Hu X, Lieberman IH. What is the learning curve for robotic-assisted pedicle screw placement in spine surgery? Clin Orthop Relat Res. 2014; 472(6):1839–1844
[10] Joseph JR, Smith BW, Liu X, Park P. Current applications of robotics in spine surgery: a systematic review of the literature. Neurosurg Focus. 2017; 42(5):E2
[11] Lee M-H, Lin MH-C, Weng H-H, et al. Feasibility of intra-operative computed tomography navigation system for pedicle screw insertion of the thoracolumbar spine. J Spinal Disord Tech. 2013; 26(5):E183–E187
[12] Macke JJ, Woo R, Varich L. Accuracy of robot-assisted pedicle screw placement for adolescent idiopathic scoliosis in the pediatric population. J Robot Surg. 2016; 10(2):145–150
[13] Onen MR, Simsek M, Naderi S. Robotic spine surgery: a preliminary report. Turk Neurosurg. 2014; 24(4):512–518
[14] Urakov TM, Chang KH-K, Burks SS, Wang MY. Initial academic experience and learning curve with robotic spine instrumentation. Neurosurg Focus. 2017; 42(5):E4
[15] Schatlo B, Martinez R, Alaid A, et al. Unskilled unawareness and the learning curve in robotic spine surgery. Acta Neurochir (Wien). 2015; 157(10):1819–1823, discussion 1823
[16] Lee JC, Jang H-D, Shin B-J. Learning curve and clinical outcomes of minimally invasive transforaminal lumbar interbody fusion: our experience in 86 consecutive cases. Spine. 2012; 37(18):1548–1557
[17] Lee KH, Yeo W, Soeharno H, Yue WM. Learning curve of a complex surgical technique: minimally invasive transforaminal lumbar interbody fusion (MIS TLIF). J Spinal Disord Tech. 2014; 27(7):E234–E240
[18] Nowitzke AM. Assessment of the learning curve for lumbar microendoscopic discectomy. Neurosurgery. 2005; 56(4):755–762, discussion 755–762
[19] Ibrahim AM, Varban OA, Dimick JB. Novel uses of video to accelerate the surgical learning curve. J Laparoendosc Adv Surg Tech A. 2016; 26(4):240–242
[20] Konakondla S, Fong R, Schirmer CM. Simulation training in neurosurgery: advances in education and practice. Adv Med Educ Pract. 2017; 8:465–473
[21] Kirkman MA, Ahmed M, Albert AF, Wilson MH, Nandi D, Sevdalis N. The use of simulation in neurosurgical education and training. A systematic review. J Neurosurg. 2014; 121(2):228–246

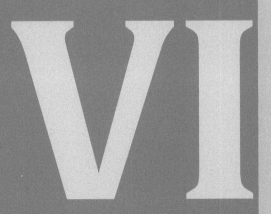

Part VI
Future Directions

32 Artificial Intelligence

Jaykar R. Panchmatia and Trishan Panch

Abstract

This chapter aims to define artificial intelligence (AI), machine learning, and deep learning; study the current usage of AI in healthcare; explore potential uses for AI in spinal surgery; and identify potential ethical challenges posed by AI. Spinal surgery is ideally suited to the early adoption of AI. Our specialty poses complex diagnostic and management challenges that can be overcome by the smart application of AI. The data required to train algorithms already exists in the form of outcome registries, as well as clinical and radiological electronic health records. However, in order for all patients to derive the full benefits of AI, it is imperative that spinal surgeons play a central role in the development, application, and oversight of this new technology.

Keywords: artificial intelligence, machine learning, deep learning, spinal surgery

32.1 Introduction

Artificial intelligence (AI) is a discipline at the intersection of computer science, medicine, and philosophy that aims to understand and replicate human intelligence using machines, typically computers. The most tangible manifestation of this field is *machine learning*: a field within computer science focused on the creation of computer programs that can learn associations from real-world examples—a task that has to date required human intelligence. Current examples of machine learning are all "narrow" AI: systems designed to perform a specific task such as analyze a photo, create a melody, or interpret written text. The ultimate challenge in AI is the creation of artificial general intelligence, also called "broad" AI: a machine that matches or exceeds the holistic nature of human intelligence.

32.2 Machine Learning: Making Associations from Real-Word Examples

The process of machine learning involves creating a computer program that itself makes associations based on examples from real-world data, and then uses these associations to predict future events. The task of developing associations is performed by an *algorithm* or process that creates a model to describe associations between elements of the data known as *features*. The rapid growth in both data and computational power has supported a commensurate increase in the performance and variety of machine learning algorithms. One type of algorithm that has recently gained prominence is the *Artificial Neural Network* or *Neural Net*. These algorithms were first proposed 70 years ago as a way of representing the information-processing capabilities of human neurons *in silico*. They have more recently enjoyed a renaissance through wins with tasks as diverse as image recognition and autonomous transportation—situations where vast quantities of structured, digitally available data is present. The increase in performance is due to more structured data, and with more data greater sophistication of the neural nets themselves: adding more layers and a control mechanism known as *back propagation*. These advances created *deep* neural networks (the depth referring to the number of layers of neurons) and a new science of *deep learning*.

32.3 Supervised versus Unsupervised Learning

Deep learning is unique in that the algorithm is designed to learn associations in the data without any supervision by a human as to which examples, or which elements of an example, are interesting. This form of learning is called *unsupervised* and is contrasted with *supervised learning* which requires an initial dataset labeled by a human expert that is used to train an algorithm such that it can produce useful outputs.

The difference between supervised and unsupervised learning can be better understood by extrapolating from Google's landmark 2012 study.[1] In the case of supervised learning, a machine is fed a series of pictures labeled "cat" and a series of pictures labelled "human"; this is the training dataset. If the machine is subsequently shown new pictures, it should be able to identify them as either "cat" or "human." The machine will get better at identifying cats and humans as it is shown more pictures. In the case of unsupervised learning, a machine can browse through millions of randomly selected images on the Internet and teach itself to categorize these pictures into different groups corresponding with "humans" and "cats," and also other groups such as "horses," "hamsters," et cetera, without the need for a human expert. As the machine scans bigger and bigger datasets, the risk of incorrectly classifying a picture is reduced and its confidence is said to increase. The quality and quantity of healthcare data is expanding with, for example, the roll out of electronic health records, and the online publication of research and outcomes. These increasingly large datasets will support both supervised and unsupervised machine learning.

32.4 Artificial Intelligence and Medicine

It can be argued that all tasks in medicine are in essence tasks of information processing, and that there are two high-level streams of information processing work: diagnosis and management. *Diagnosis* is the task of inference based on data (reported from patients as symptoms, elicited as signs, or received from investigations). *Management* is the task of implementing and monitoring a process to achieve a therapeutic endpoint. Surgery involves combinations of these tasks as the surgeon assesses the patient (akin to diagnostic inference), and takes the next action to deliver the surgical intervention (akin to management).

We propose that machine learning algorithms will provide support to clinicians in two key areas: *diagnosis support* and *decision support*. Current applications of machine learning involve automation of diagnosis. However, initiatives are under way to use machine learning to optimize clinical decision making/management and create personalized, adaptive management algorithms at scale.

32.5 Current Applications of Artificial Intelligence in Medicine

Examples of *diagnosis support* can be found in fields such as dermatology. Using deep neural networks and a training dataset of 129,450 clinical images, a supervised machine learning system achieved results equivalent to 21 board-certified dermatologists when classifying keratinocyte carcinomas, versus benign seborrheic keratoses, and malignant melanomas, versus benign nevi.[2] In orthopaedic subspecialties other than spinal surgery, deep neural networks have also been used to classify upper and lower extremity plain radiographs and identify the presence of fractures with an accuracy of over 90% and 83%, respectively.[3]

Evidence of *decision support* using AI exists in cardiology. A dataset including 40 patient factors such as gender, presence of cardiomyopathy, treatment delivered (angioplasty versus coronary artery bypass graft), and outcome was used to train a neural network. The network was subsequently applied to the data of two cohorts of patients. The first cohort was comprised of patients that survived for at least 5 years following treatment. The second cohort was comprised of patients that had died within five years of treatment. In those patients who died, neural networks were more likely to have proposed an alternative treatment plan to that which was actually carried out. Consequently, the authors suggested that, had a neural network been included as part of the team making the actual treatment plan, the 5-year survival of patients would likely have been better.[4]

32.6 Current Applications of Artificial Intelligence in Spinal Surgery

There is already early evidence of AI use in spinal surgery. For example, automated machine learning systems have been developed to facilitate the diagnosis of spinal pathologies. Machine learning systems are now able to diagnose and identify the vertebral level of compression fractures with a sensitivity of 95.7%, compared to a board-certified radiologist with 10 years' experience. Furthermore, grade of height loss (less than 25%, 26–40%, or greater than 40%) and fracture morphology (wedge, compression, or crush) were determined in the same study with an interobserver agreement of 68 and 95%, respectively.[5]

Machine learning can also be used to facilitate clinical decision making in spinal surgery by providing a patient-specific prediction of the rate of occurrence of postoperative complications. Kim et al first trained their artificial neural network model using 70% of a dataset of 22,629 patients, and then assessed their model using the remaining 30% of their dataset. The results of this study found that neural networks are more successful than a patient's American Society of Anesthesiologists grade at predicting complications such as venous thromboembolism, cardiac events, wound complications, and mortality.[6]

32.7 Future Applications of Artificial Intelligence in Spinal Surgery

The current use of AI in spinal surgery is in its nascency, even when compared to the usage of navigation and robotics. A combination of an aging population, increased patient expectations, and growth in affluence globally means that demand for spinal surgery is increasing. AI has the potential to aid service efficiency so that we can meet this increasing demand. The analysis of data will also help untangle some of the controversies that exist within spinal surgery, allowing the surgeon to offer the optimal operation using the optimal approach suited for each individual patient. Additionally, AI has the potential to build a *personalized* regimen of pre- and postoperative care for a given individual patient. This regimen would be based on the experience of previous similar patients undergoing the same procedure; adapting said regimen based on the given patient's progress; and even dynamically recruiting resources of the surgical system (such as physical therapists) where the given patient is most likely to benefit. In this way, the future with machine learning and digital delivery of care around surgical interventions offers the promise of a care experience that is not only *personalized* to each patient (drawing on the collective experience of past patients), and *adaptive* to an individual patient's progress, but is also *automated* and thereby scalable in a way that even the highest quality approaches cannot achieve today. Finally, surgical outcomes and improvement in patient function may be automatically incorporated into spinal registries, thereby ensuring that data used by AI remain *contemporaneous*.

To formally analyze this potential future impact of AI in spinal surgery, it is necessary to first identify a value chain of processes in spinal surgery. We propose a value chain from the patient's point of view that involves eight distinct and interrelated sets of processes (▶ Table 32.1). Each of these processes involves a set of information processing tasks, and many of these tasks are opportunities for the application of AI in general and machine learning in particular.

However, in order for our patients to derive the full benefits of AI, and for ethical and logistical challenges to be addressed, spinal surgeons and physicians more broadly need to be involved in the design and adoption of AI technology.

Table 32.1 Timeline for spinal surgery

Stage	Current management	AI enabled management
Self-management	Patient self-identification of symptoms Self-management, such as use of over-the-counter medication Use of lay referral networks and self-referral to primary care, or alternative therapies such as massage therapy	AI prognosis based on collective experience of previous similar patients Monitoring of self-management with patient-held digital health tools Appropriate referral into primary care in accordance with agreed national guidelines such as the American College of Physicians guidelines[7] Ability of spinal pathway service managers to predict demand and dynamically staff services, based on real-time monitoring of demand
Primary care	Triage Instructions for patient self-management and appropriate use of nonoperative management Referral for investigation (such as MRI) requiring secondary care analysis Planning follow-up	Patient flagged for assessment due to failure of progress with self-management Evidence-based use of nonoperative management AI monitoring of patient-held digital health tool to monitor treatment response after visit Proactive screening for secondary complications (such as failure to progress or neurological deterioration) with automated referral to primary care physician for reassessment MRI ordered in primary care and analyzed automatically using AI in community Based on positive findings, referral for spinal surgery assessment made by primary care physician decision support tool Patient referred with view to surgery based on AI decision support tool (reduction in inappropriate referrals)
Specialist spinal care	Initial outpatient consultation Investigations Outpatient consultation to discuss proposed treatment plan Case discussion at multidisciplinary team meeting	Referral screened and investigations requested using AI diagnostic tool. Salient data also collected at this stage, for example, comorbidities, smoking history, and current functional status Discussion at multidisciplinary team meeting. Interrogate AI to determine best procedure and best approach based on collective experience of previous cases, for example, decompression vs. fusion, anterior approach vs. posterior approach, and surgical levels requiring fusion Patient-specific consent prepared with analysis presented based on national outcomes databases of likely prognosis
Preoperation	Preoperative assessment by nursing team and anesthesia Schedulers coordinate operative team and implants	Monitoring of patient progress with preoperative care delivered using patient-held digital health tool Dynamic scheduling of preoperative assessments. Operative date based on patient progress and surgical team's operative schedule Appropriate implants automatically requested
Intraoperation	Intraoperative neuromonitoring with neurophysiologist present Physiological status manually monitored by anesthesia	Computer vision to monitor visual field of surgeon for extent of decompression, neuromonitoring changes, or physiological complications. Automated alerting of surgical and anesthesia team
Postoperation	Regular neurological and physiological monitoring with nursing team alerting physicians if any concerning features present	AI monitoring of patient in postoperative period tailored to patient and intraoperative parameters and calibrated according to progress
Outpatient follow-up	Patient discharged with generic clinic dates with both surgeons and physical therapists	Patient discharged with digital health follow-up plan AI vigilant system to monitor progress of patient with plan as per self-management and preoperative period Automated referral into primary physician-based care or specialist spinal services, on proactive monitoring of pain control, patient-reported outcome measures, and screening for complications
Long-term management	Patient expected to follow advice provided by physicians and physical therapists	Patient-held digital health tool for long-term health promotion to include longer term monitoring of patient-reported outcome measures related to spinal surgery. Data automatically uploaded to spinal registry AI enabled automated referral into primary care when recurrence or complications detected

Abbreviation: AI, artificial intelligence.

32.8 The Ethical Challenges Posed by the Use of Artificial Intelligence in Medicine

Supervised and unsupervised machine learning both rely on large, high-quality datasets. Ethically, the populations from which datasets are drawn should also be able to benefit from the technical advancements derived from their data. The existing norms of drug and implant trials–restricting the use of data from populations that will not derive any immediate or obvious benefit—do not extend well to the era of AI where enormous data sets are required to drive algorithm development, and where the contribution of any individual patient's data is not easily attributable. New norms will need to be formulated: broadly, health data will need to be viewed as a public good, rather than private capital, and governments and healthcare providers will need to view investments in high-quality data sets in the same way that they view other investments in core health infrastructure.

A further ethical challenge is ensuring that guidance provided by AI is truly objective. The design of machine learning algorithms needs to be robust so as to limit the impact of poor data, and to identify algorithms that may be biased due to subjectivity in the data or potential conflicts from sponsors of an algorithm. It might be theoretically plausible to implement management controls, akin to a Chinese wall, to separate the implementation of AI from those that derive monetary benefit from its application (such as pharmaceutical companies and medical device manufacturers). However, it will be much more difficult to control for biases in data, especially those that are due to the corrosive influence of unconscious factors, such as race or income, on the data upon which algorithms are built.

Where AI is being used to aid *diagnosis*, it is easy to regard it as a tool used by physicians to make a clinical decision, similar to imaging and lab tests. However, what is the position of a physician's advice if it differs from the *decision* offered by a machine learning algorithm? Alternatively, what is the status of a patient vis-a-vis funding their treatment if they opt for a solution that differs from that proposed by a machine learning algorithm supported by their healthcare provider? We suggest that, until the inner workings of machine learning algorithms are fully understood and the processes that underpin their inferences interrogable by physicians, machine learning will only act as a *decision support tool*. Similarly, guidelines with respect to responsibility in the event that AI fails also need to be established: does responsibility lie with the physician, manufacturer, owner of the algorithm, or the provider of the dataset on which the decision was based?

Finally, the exceptional nature of medicine also needs to be acknowledged. The trust that patients place in physicians is unique and consequently, before AI can be used to guide a patient's care with minimal physician oversight, it will need to be accepted by the wider population of patients and physicians. In this instance, an AI algorithm may need to be assessed using a challenge akin to Alan Turing's Imitation Game.[8] That is, an algorithm needs to be able to trick independent physician and patient interrogators into believing that its treatment plan was devised by a human physician (▶ Fig. 32.1). By meeting such a challenge, said algorithm may gain wider public acceptance. The involvement of spinal surgeons is integral to addressing these ethical considerations and also designing AI solutions to meet the clinical challenges that are faced by our patients.

32.9 Conclusion

Spinal surgery is ideally suited to the adoption of AI. It is a complex specialty posing diagnostic and therapeutic challenges due to the variety of pathologies treated and solutions available. Furthermore, diagnosis is reliant on radiological imaging, and endpoints are well defined with established outcome parameters (including patient-reported outcome measures, radiographic outcomes, and complication rates). In order to realize the benefits of AI, physicians, computer scientists, and ethicists will need to collaborate to apply AI effectively in spinal surgery.

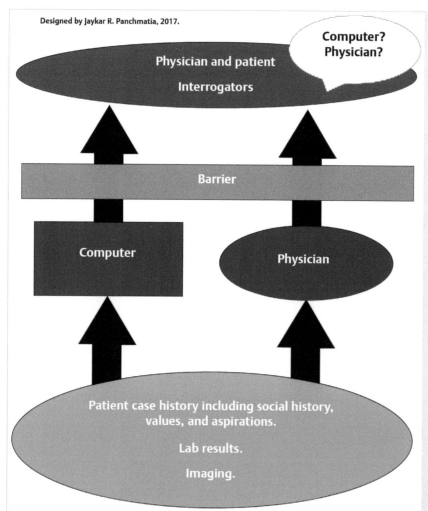

Fig. 32.1 Test to confirm equivalence of advice offered by physician and artificial intelligence.

References

[1] Le QV, Ranzato MA, Monga R, et al. Building high-level features using large scale unsupervised learning. Proceedings of the 29th International Conference of Machine Learning. 2012

[2] Esteva A, Kuprel B, Novoa RA, et al. Dermatologist-level classification of skin cancer with deep neural networks. Nature. 2017; 542(7639):115–118

[3] Olczak J, Fahlberg N, Maki A, et al. Artificial intelligence for analyzing orthopedic trauma radiographs. Acta Orthop. 2017; 88(6):581–586

[4] Buzaev IV, Plechev VV, Nikolaeva IE, Galimova RM. Artificial intelligence: Neural network model as the multidisciplinary team member in clinical decision support to avoid medical mistakes. Chronic Dis Transl Med. 2016; 2(3): 166–172

[5] Burns JE, Yao J, Summers RM. Vertebral body compression fractures and bone density: automated classification on CT images. Radiology. 2017; 284(3): 788–797

[6] Kim JS, Merrill RK, Arvind V, et al. Examining the ability of artificial neural networks machine learning models to accurately predict complications following posterior lumbar spine fusion. Spine. 2018; 43(12): 853–860

[7] Qaseem A, Wilt TJ, McLean RM, Forciea MA, Clinical Guidelines Committee of the American College of Physicians. Noninvasive treatments for acute, subacute, and chronic low back pain: a clinical practice guideline from the American College of Physicians. Ann Intern Med. 2017; 166(7):514–530

[8] Turing AM. Computing machinery and intelligence. Mind. 1950; 236:433–460

33 What We Can Learn from Other Industries

Nikola Kocovic and I. David Kaye

Abstract

The current landscape of technological innovation is a remarkable one. We are living in a time where various technologies are altering the way we experience everyday life, including entertainment, travel, and other aspects. This wave of innovation is one that has included medicine and is quite actively contributing to healthcare the patients receive today. Specifically, with the advent of robotic operative systems and minimally invasive operative systems and their use in spine surgery, technological innovation has played an evolving role in this discipline and will undoubtedly play a part in its future. This chapter will review how looking to advancement in other industries may benefit the specialty of spine surgery, and how certain emerging technologies such as virtual reality, augmented reality, haptic feedback, and autonomous robotics may especially contribute to spine surgery, its techniques, and ultimately patient care.

Keywords: spine surgery, virtual reality, augmented reality, haptic feedback, autonomous robotics, computer vision, minimally invasive surgery, robotic spine surgery

33.1 Introduction

Virtual reality is a computerized technology that generates realistic images, sounds, and sensations meant to simulate the user's presence in a virtual or imaginary environment, one that can be explored by and interacted with by that very user.[1] The effect can be created via a headset with a small screen that displays images in front of the user's eyes, a series of multiple large screens, or other specially designed areas that can simulate the user's presence in the virtual environment. Luckily, this technology has been expanded from its initial use as entertainment, and has found a place in several different disciplines with unbelievable implications. Currently, its technology allows for a vast application of its simulations, ranging from gorgeous, realistic, video game playing experiences to the training of chefs, airplane pilots, military personnel, and astronauts; to better understanding bias and other social constructs[2,3]; and to the treatment of anxiety disorders,[4] managing pain and anxiety in children,[5] and even the rehabilitation of stroke patients.[6,7] Its applications are far-reaching, and its ability to contribute to spine surgery is rooted in its ability to generate rich simulated experiences. As it stands, spine surgery is a specialty that requires first and foremost much training, along with great geometrical precision[8] and control once that training is completed, considering the delicate nature of working around the spinal cord and its associated structures.

33.1.1 Virtual Reality as a Training Module

As mentioned earlier, virtual reality has the ability to simulate an elegant and intricate environment. With this in mind, it is reasonably straightforward to understand how a technology such as this may properly simulate an operative experience and its many nuances. Coincidentally, virtual reality (hereafter referred to as VR) simulators are already relatively well established as training modalities for surgery, and more specifically spine surgery[9] (▶ Fig. 33.1). Research has shown, for now, that simulators are promising training modalities with a host of benefits. First, VR simulators provide trainees with a rich variety of training opportunities,[9] and that simulator training has led to improved speed and accuracy of various surgical skills.[10] These simulator-trained skills have resulted in improved

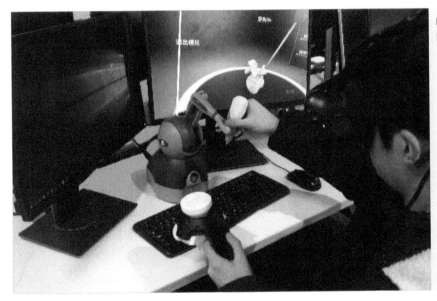

Fig. 33.1 Virtual reality training simulation for pedicle screw placement.

patient care and decreased patient discomfort.[11] In addition, VR simulations pose no risk to patients, and require fewer resources, as simulator training is inherently independent of patients and cadavers.[9] Furthermore, the increase in ease of access allows for an increase in the frequency of training. Finally, objective assessments of trainees and surgeons can be performed, as exact measurements can be performed by the simulation, allowing for recording of the accuracy of instrumentation.[12] This information can be used to evaluate the ability of surgeons, and further can even be used to investigate the effects of pharmacologic advancement of sleep-deprived physicians in the operating room.[13,14]

Many centers now employ the use of VR simulators as means of training and assessing individual's surgical skills.[9] However, for now, it seems as if its utility as a training module remains somewhat unclear for a couple of distinct reasons. First and perhaps most important, there is a lack of evidence regarding the study of patient outcomes.[9] Further adaptation of simulators will require improved study designs, longer term study periods, examination of nontechnical skills, and multidisciplinary team training.[9] As VR continues to improve, and as its applications continue to expand, it could potentially better simulate the operations performed by spine surgeons and further help train surgeons, residents, and students toward better patient outcomes. It is a technology that should be, and for now, has been, embraced by spine surgery as technology continues to produce unbelievable possibilities.

33.2 Augmented Reality

Augmented reality, not to be confused with, yet closely related to, VR, consists of a live direct or indirect view of a physical environment that is modified by other sensory inputs such as sound, video, and haptic feedback, among other modalities. Again, similarly with the roots and origins of VR, augmented reality finds its origins in the entertainment industry. Other industries are now finding applications for this type of experience enhancement, including the medical field, because of its ability to gather and share information rapidly.[14] Advanced augmented reality (hereafter referred to as AR) systems are able to overlay information regarding environments and its components in real time and in an interactive manner. Imagine someone wears glasses while driving that are able to relay real-time traffic information, or glasses that are able to project an updated flight itinerary while sprinting through a crowded airport. Now imagine this application in the operating room: existing images such as X-rays, ultrasounds, CT scans, and MRIs are blended together with surgical reference points and the patient lying on the operating table. Operating staff could potentially wear lenses that project patient's current vital signs, patient's relevant past medical history, and other information that may become relevant that would otherwise require breaking scrub.

33.2.1 Practical Applications in the Operating Room

What makes AR so exciting is that it already has some existing applications within the operating room. For example, AR is used as a means of projecting optimal port placement on abdomens prepared for laparoscopic surgery,[15] as a means to identify the position of lymph nodes during cancer surgeries,[16] and has found applications as specialized near infrared devices that can help detect tissue vascularity.[17] Furthermore, neurosurgical procedures have adopted some AR techniques during the management of extracranial–intracranial bypass surgery and intracranial arteriovenous malformation surgery.[18,19]

There are currently many devices that are capable of offering a variety of augmented and virtual realities, all of which contain different gadgets and technologies and different approaches to providing similar experiences. Imagine a device such as HoloLens finds its way into the operating room as eyewear; this head-mounted unit is a pair of smart glasses that contain an inertial measurement unit consisting of an accelerometer, gyroscope, and magnetometer, along with a camera, four environment understanding sensors, microphone, and an ambient light sensor that are used to record surroundings and integrate them into an image of altered reality[20] (▶ Fig. 33.2). This technology

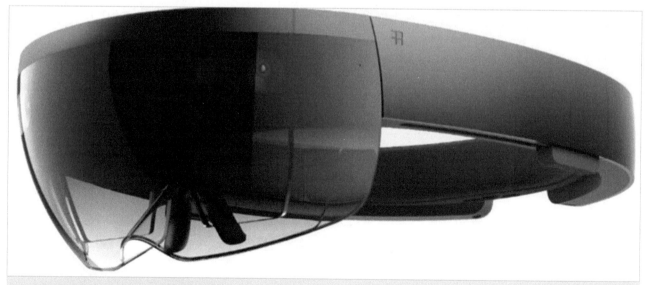

Fig. 33.2 Example of Microsoft HoloLens.

in fact already has applications within the medical field, as both Case Western Reserve University and the Cleveland Clinic are using them in a digital human anatomy course.[20,21] Picture that this device, or other similar devices, is programmed with software targeting patient information mentioned previously. That spine surgery seems to benefit greatly from this technology is through image-based augmentation. Imagine a spine surgeon is able to view preoperative diagnostic images intraoperatively, helping guide surgical planning in terms of incision, instrumentation, and optimal approach,[14] all while being connected to a totality of patient information in safe way (▶ Fig. 33.3).

33.3 Virtual Reality and Augmented Reality as a Vehicle for Garnering Interest and Fostering Education

Apart from the applications of VR and AR previously mentioned, these simulation modalities also have a remarkable capacity of increasing the accessibility of information for those learning the art of spine surgery. Imagine the common scene where a medical student finds him/herself in a crowded operating room, struggling to see what the surgeon and residents are seeing within the operative field, attempting impossible and uncomfortable maneuvers to catch a glance of what is happening. Now imagine a scenario in which that same student is wearing a VR or AR headset, tucked away in the corner, out of the way, while being able to see a variety of multidimensional perspectives on the operation. And now imagine a scenario in which these perspectives are broadcasted worldwide. This technology could allow efficient sharing of information and techniques involved in spine surgery.[14] It also has implications for training residents. Junior residents would be able to virtually participate in complex cases, cases they are not yet qualified for in the operating room, helping them learn more quickly.[14]

Fortunately, firms such as Medical Realities are working to make this latter image a reality.[22] Individuals will be able to engage and learn in virtual operative settings by purchasing their software. In April 2016, Dr. Shafi Ahmed, a cofounder of Medical Realities, became the first physician to broadcast an operation via VR.[23] Now imagine a spine surgeon partakes in this concept, and students around the world are not only exposed to but able to interact with a virtual pedicle screw placement, a virtual posterior cervical laminectomy, or a virtual vertebroplasty. Other industries are also starting to take advantage of broadcasting information via VR. The Minnesota Vikings of the National Football League (NFL) just recently announced that they are partnering with VR firm Oculus and are launching an application that will allow for fans to view 360-degree footage within the stadium via VR simulation.[24]

33.4 Haptic Feedback Technology

Haptic feedback is a technology that re-creates the human sensation of touch via the application of force, vibration, or motion to the user of the device providing haptic feedback. A fine example of early haptic feedback is the familiar feeling of the violent shaking of the steering wheel when veering off the

paved road while playing our favorite arcade racing game. This technology has been used in arcade games and other video game derivatives for many years as a means of enhancing user experience. Starting with simple joysticks, steering wheels, and video game controllers, haptic feedback has evolved to the point where it can simulate using, handling, and moving a variety of objects[25] in more modern handheld devices, such as the Nintendo Switch. As with both VR and AR, the applications of haptic feedback quickly expanded to where it is now, being included in cellphones, personal computers, flight simulators, and various other forms of robotics. It is further advancing, and companies such as Disney[26] and Microsoft[27] are investigating the use of air vortex rings as a means of allowing users to interact with 3D projections while receiving tactile feedback. Haptic feedback allows for a more intuitive and natural use of robotics, and it is this very reason that it can benefit spine surgery so greatly.

33.4.1 Improving Existing Robotic Operative Systems

A current problem with robotic spine surgery, and robotic surgery in general, is the complete lack of transmission of sensory information from the operative field to the operating surgeon on the console. Haptic feedback provides the operating surgeon with the ability to better sense and regulate the amount of force that is applied to the various tissues being operated on, which in turn reduces the risk of unnecessary tissue damage.[28] Unfortunately, in general, it seems that the technology is still somewhat unconsolidated and unsure,[28] and there is a need for new developments in regard to haptic feedback.

Nonetheless, the future may very well lead to further advancements in this technology, as many robotic labs are working on improving this and many studies have been done evaluating the available technologies.[29,30,31,32,33,34,35,36,37,38] There are some robots that claim to have advanced this technology, but they require further evaluation. A specific example lies within the HeroSurg robot (▶ Fig. 33.4). The robot was designed in collaboration between Deakin's Institute for Intelligent System's Research and Innovation, Harvard University, and Deakin's School of Medicine with the idea that robotic operative systems do not have to be limited by a lack of tactile sensation. HeroSurg employs a complex haptic feedback system that purportedly allows for better differentiation of tissue composition, especially those affected by infection, inflammation, and cancerous processes.[39] Only time will tell how successful this robot's technology will be. However, it is useful to look at other disciplines in robotics, to see their approach to delivering the human sensation to robotic devices.

33.4.2 Enabling Better Healthcare

Apart from the direct benefit of enhancing robotic capabilities, haptic feedback technology may perhaps provide an indirect benefit of helping train future surgeons. As previously discussed, the implementation of VR in the training of medical professionals has offered some tangible benefits to spine surgery.[8] Thus, one would think that there is an advantage in making VR simulations as accurate as possible to further enhance the training experience. Coincidentally, this can be done with

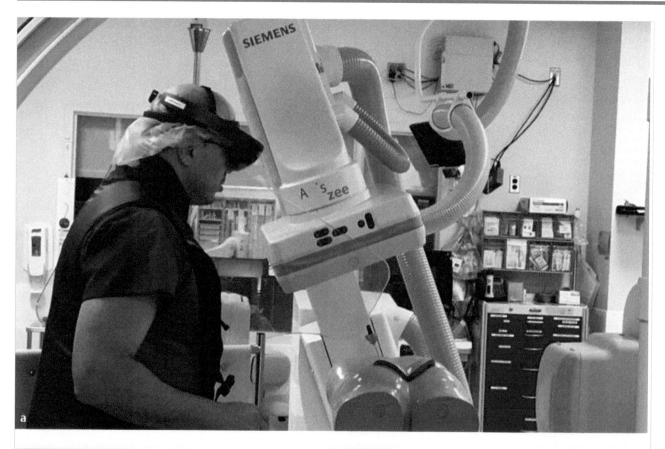

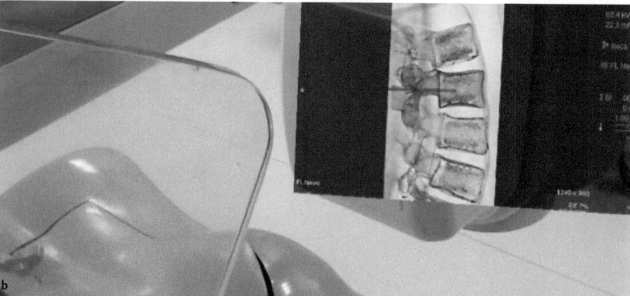

Fig. 33.3 (a) Simulation with surgeon wearing HoloLens head mount while directly viewing field for planned kyphoplasty and (b) actual surgeon view through the head mount which demonstrates simultaneous view of operative field on left and the superimposed deep surgical anatomy with the Jamshidi needle advancing into the vertebral body on right.

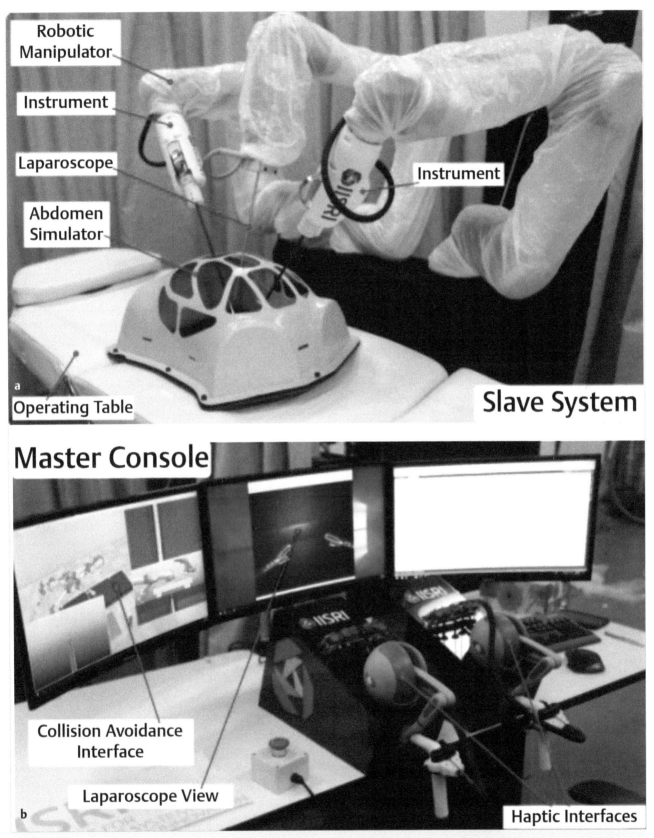

Fig. 33.4 HeroSurg robot allows remote control of robotic arms (**a**) and provides high fidelity haptic feedback through the master control (**b**).

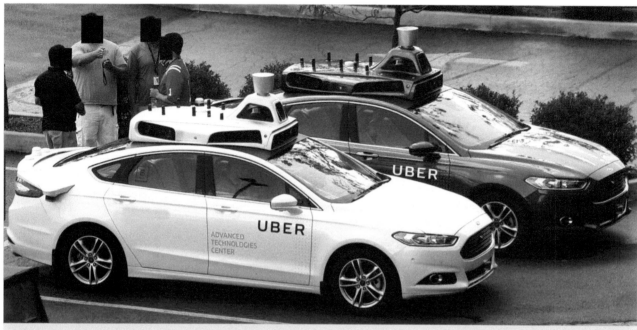

Fig. 33.5 Set of Uber autonomous vehicles seen on road in San Francisco.

haptic feedback technology, as it can produce more realistic simulations of operative procedures.

33.4.3 How Realistic Is Telesurgery?

Haptic technology also makes remote surgery (telesurgery) an idea that can be entertained within the medical field, albeit a faraway one. Via furthering the advancement of robotics and haptic feedback, a spine surgeon could potentially "feel" the incision he or she is making on a patient while sitting at a telesurgical platform separated by a distance of hundreds or even thousands of miles, along with every other maneuver necessary for a successful operation. While this type of venture obviously has many financial, legal, ethical, and technological challenges before it,[40] at the root of this idea is the ability to somehow improve upon the robotic technology currently employed in the operating room.

33.5 Autonomous Robotics

Looking into the future requires a certain degree of speculation, and possibly, the most entertaining of questions regarding robotics is the possibility for eventual artificial intelligence and completely autonomous robots. With companies such as Google,[41] Amazon,[42] and Tesla[43] employing various forms of autonomous robotic technology, it becomes evident that self-sufficient robots have a place in the industrial setting. However, the more relevant question for spine surgery and the rest of medicine is if autonomous robots have a place in the operating room. As mentioned earlier, spine surgery is a specialty that benefits from geometrical precision,[7] and robots have helped aid in this endeavor. However, as it currently stands, the three major robotic systems cannot operate without heavy human intervention, whether it be in a telesurgical system where the robot is directly controlled by a surgeon,[44] or in supervisory or shared control systems, where immense planning is necessary on the surgeon's part. Understanding this question requires better understanding of the technologies that may contribute to its solution.

33.5.1 What Can Be Learned from Computer Vision

Computer vision, as a scientific field, deals with the issue of allowing computers to extract and understand information from images.[45] In other words, computer vision aims to build autonomous systems that can perform some of the tasks that the human visual system can perform.[45] The implications of this type of technology are limitless, as it could potentially be the bridge to allowing artificial software systems to interpret data adaptively, effectively, and in a time-efficient way. Imagine a robotic operative system that has processed millions of images in various imaging modalities, and is able to distinguish between human anatomy and its associated pathologies, and ultimately is able to adapt to different operative scenarios, independent of human intervention. Even though this type of inference and adaptation is most likely far from realization, computer vision does have some current practical applications.

33.5.2 Computer Vision and Autonomous Vehicles

To understand computer vision and its implications for medicine and spine surgery in the future, our attention can be turned to the automobile industry. Autonomous driving is complex, and with companies such as Uber recently announcing that they may have a large fleet of autonomous vehicles,[46] self-driving cars have been a hot topic of conversation. Autonomous vehicles employ a variety of technologies, including Simultaneous Location and Mapping (SLAM) algorithms,[47] which allow for information bridging between multiple sensors and maps into updated location estimates,[47] and have started to utilize deep neural networks as a means of processing massive amounts of imaging inputs, and allowing for recognition of objects such as cars and lane annotations during highway driving.[48] These deep neural networks have made some recent strides and seem promising in regard to large-scale image and video recognition,[49,50,51] and have current practical implications, at least in terms of autonomous driving on highways.[48] In other words, these programs are able to "learn" and distinguish objects from each other in a relatively sophisticated way. Of course, a highway is in many ways simpler than an operative field, but perhaps these deep neural networks will eventually be advanced enough to distinguish pathology from healthy in the clinical sense.

References

[1] Li L, Yu F, Shi D, et al. Application of Virtual Reality technology in clinical medicine. Am J Transl Res. 2017; 9(9):3867–3880

[2] Groom V, Bailenson JN, Nass C. The influence of racial bias in immersive virtual environments. Soc Influence. 2009; 4(3):231–248

[3] Kilteni K, Bergstrom I, Slater M. Drumming in immersive virtual reality: the body shapes the way we play. IEEE Trans Vis Comput Graph. 2013; 19(4):597–605

[4] Maples-Keller JL, Bunnell BE, Kim S-J, Rothbaum BO. The use of Virtual Reality technology in the treatment of anxiety and other psychiatric disorders. Harv Rev Psychiatry. 2017; 25(3):103–113

[5] Arane K, Behboudi A, Goldman RD. Virtual reality for pain and anxiety management in children. Can Fam Physician. 2017; 63(12):932–934

[6] Vanbellingen T, Filius SJ, Nyffeler T, van Wegen EEH. Usability of videogame-based dexterity training in the early rehabilitation phase of stroke patients: a pilot study. Front Neurol. 2017; 8:654

[7] Colomer C, Llorens R, Noé E, Alcañiz M. Effect of a mixed reality-based intervention on arm, hand, and finger function on chronic stroke. J Neuroeng Rehabil. 2016; 13(1):45

[8] Taylor RH. Medical robotics and computer-integrated surgery. In: Handbook of Industrial Robotics. Springer; 2007:1213–1227

[9] Pfandler M, Lazarovici M, Stefan P, Wucherer P, Weigl M. Virtual reality-based simulators for spine surgery: a systematic review. Spine J. 2017; 17(9):1352–1363

[10] McGaghie WC, Issenberg SB, Cohen ER, Barsuk JH, Wayne DB. Does simulation-based medical education with deliberate practice yield better results than traditional clinical education? A meta-analytic comparative review of the evidence. Acad Med. 2011; 86(6):706–711

[11] de Visser H, Watson MO, Salvado O, Passenger JD. Progress in virtual reality simulators for surgical training and certification. Med J Aust. 2011; 194(4):S38–S40

[12] Gallagher AG, O'Sullivan GC. Fundamentals of Surgical Simulation. London: Springer; 2012

[13] Sugden C, Housden CR, Aggarwal R, Sahakian BJ, Darzi A. Effect of pharmacological enhancement on the cognitive and clinical psychomotor performance of sleep-deprived doctors: a randomized controlled trial. Ann Surg. 2012; 255(2):222–227

[14] Khor WS, Baker B, Amin K, Chan A, Patel K, Wong J. Augmented and virtual reality in surgery-the digital surgical environment: applications, limitations and legal pitfalls. Ann Transl Med. 2016; 4(23):454–454

[15] Volonté F, Pugin F, Bucher P, Sugimoto M, Ratib O, Morel P. Augmented reality and image overlay navigation with OsiriX in laparoscopic and robotic surgery: not only a matter of fashion. J Hepatobiliary Pancreat Sci. 2011; 18(4):506–509

[16] Tagaya N, Yamazaki R, Nakagawa A, et al. Intraoperative identification of sentinel lymph nodes by near-infrared fluorescence imaging in patients with breast cancer. Am J Surg. 2008; 195(6):850–853

[17] Diana M, Dallemagne B, Chung H, et al. Probe-based confocal laser endomicroscopy and fluorescence-based enhanced reality for real-time assessment of intestinal microcirculation in a porcine model of sigmoid ischemia. Surg Endosc. 2014; 28(11):3224–3233

[18] Cabrilo I, Bijlenga P, Schaller K. Augmented reality in the surgery of cerebral aneurysms: a technical report. Neurosurgery. 2014; 10 Suppl 2:252–260, discussion 260–261

[19] Cabrilo I, Schaller K, Bijlenga P. Augmented reality-assisted bypass surgery: embracing minimal invasiveness. World Neurosurg. 2015; 83(4):596–602

[20] Microsoft HoloLens: Partner Spotlight with Case Western Reserve University. GameZone. Available at: http://www.gamezone.com/videos/microsoft-hololens-partner-spotlight-with-case-western-reserve-university-4nf. Accessed December 27, 2017

[21] Couric K. Cleveland Clinic uses hologram technology to bring medical students inside the human body. Yahoo! News. Available at: https://www.yahoo.com/katiecouric/cleveland-clinic-uses-hologram-technology-bring-medical-students-inside-human-body-181136417.html. Accessed December 27, 2017

[22] Platform. Medical Realities. Available at: https://www.medicalrealities.com/. Accessed December 16, 2017

[23] Volpicelli G. What's next for virtual reality surgery? WIRED. Available at: https://www.wired.co.uk/article/wired-health-virtual-reality-surgery-shafi-ahmed. Accessed December 27, 2017

[24] Bradley L. Minnesota Vikings first in NFL to Launch Virtual Reality App for Oculus. SportTechie. Available at: https://www.sporttechie.com/minnesota-vikings-first-nfl-launch-virtual-reality-app-oculus/. Accessed December 27, 2017

[25] Nintendo's HD Rumble will be the best unused Switch feature of 2017. Engadget. Available at: https://www.engadget.com/2017/01/13/nintendos-hd-rumble-will-be-the-best-unused-switch-feature-of-2/. Accessed June 17, 2019

[26] Sodhi R, Poupyrev I, Glisson M, Israr A. AIREAL: Interactive tactile experiences in free air. ACM Trans Graph. 2013; 32(4):1–134

[27] Gupta S, Morris D, Patel SN, Tan D. AirWave: Non-contact Haptic Feedback Using Air Vortex Rings. Proceedings of the 2013 ACM International Joint Conference on Pervasive and Ubiquitous Computing. UbiComp '13. New York, NY: ACM; 2013:419–428

[28] Amirabdollahian F, Livatino S, Vahedi B, et al. Prevalence of haptic feedback in robot-mediated surgery: a systematic review of literature. J Robot Surg. 201 8; 12(1):1:1–25

[29] Tezuka M, Kitamura N, Miki N. Micro-needle electro-tactile display. Conf Proc IEEE Eng Med Biol Soc. 2015; 2015:5781–5784

[30] Sengül A, van Elk M, Rognini G, Aspell JE, Bleuler H, Blanke O. Extending the body to virtual tools using a robotic surgical interface: evidence from the crossmodal congruency task. PLoS One. 2012; 7(12):e49473

[31] Seifabadi R, Iordachita I, Fichtinger G. Design of a teleoperated needle steering system for MRI-guided prostate interventions. Proc IEEE RAS EMBS Int Conf Biomed Robot Biomechatron 2012:793–798

[32] Sun Z, Ang RY, Lim EW, Wang Z, Ho KY, Phee SJ. Enhancement of a master-slave robotic system for natural orifice transluminal endoscopic surgery. Ann Acad Med Singapore. 2011; 40(5):223–230

[33] Sutherland GR, Maddahi Y, Gan LS, Lama S, Zareinia K. Robotics in the neurosurgical treatment of glioma. Surg Neurol Int. 2015; 6 Suppl 1:S1–S8

[34] Reilink R, Kappers AM, Stramigioli S, Misra S. Evaluation of robotically controlled advanced endoscopic instruments. Int J Med Robot. 2013; 9(2):240–246

[35] Reilink R, Stramigioli S, Kappers AM, Misra S. Evaluation of flexible endoscope steering using haptic guidance. Int J Med Robot. 2011; 7(2):178–186

[36] Khan F, Pearle A, Lightcap C, Boland PJ, Healey JH. Haptic robot-assisted surgery improves accuracy of wide resection of bone tumors: a pilot study. Clin Orthop Relat Res. 2013; 471(3):851–859

[37] King CH, Culjat MO, Franco ML, Bisley JW, Dutson E, Grundfest WS. Optimization of a pneumatic balloon tactile display for robot-assisted surgery based on human perception. IEEE Trans Biomed Eng. 2008; 55(11):2593–2600

[38] King CH, Higa AT, Culjat MO, et al. A pneumatic haptic feedback actuator array for robotic surgery or simulation. Stud Health Technol Inform. 2007; 125:217–222

[39] University D. Deakin builds robotic surgical system with sense of touch. Deakin. Available at: http://www.deakin.edu.au/about-deakin/media-releases/articles/deakin-builds-robotic-surgical-system-with-sense-of-touch. Accessed December 27, 2017

[40] Hung AJ, Chen J, Shah A, Gill IS. Telementoring and telesurgery for minimally invasive procedures. J Urol. 201 8; 199(2):355–36-9

[41] Simonite T. Google's CEO is excited about seeing AI take over some work of his AI experts. MIT Technology Review. Available at: https://www.technolo-

gyreview.com/s/607894/why-googles-ceo-is-excited-about-automating-arti-ficial-intelligence/. Accessed December 27, 2017

[42] Nick Heath | January 26, 2016, 7:02 AM PST. Amazon, robots and the near-future rise of the automated warehouse. TechRepublic. Available at: https://www.techrepublic.com/article/amazon-robots-and-the-near-future-rise-of-the-automated-warehouse/. Accessed December 27, 2017

[43] Elon Musk unveils Tesla factory video to showcase full automation. Futurism. Available at: https://futurism.com/elon-musk-unveils-tesla-factory-video-to-showcase-full-automation/. Accessed December 27, 2017

[44] Ryan H, Tsuda S.. History of and Current Systems in Robotic Surgery. Essentials of Robotic Surgery. 2014:1–12

[45] . CERN Document Server, 1996, cds.cern.ch/record/400313/files/p21.pdf. Accessed August 10, 2019. 2f400313%2ffiles%2fp21.pdf&p=DevEx,5067.1. Accessed December 28, 2017

[46] Burke K. Uber re-focuses on self-driving initiative. Automotive News. Available at: http://www.autonews.com/article/20171126/OEM06/171129826/uber-volvo-autonomous-technology. Accessed December 27, 2017

[47] Durrant-Whyte H, Bailey T. Simultaneous localization and mapping: part I. Simultaneous localization and mapping: Part I - IEEE Journals & Magazine. Available at: http://ieeexplore.ieee.org/document/1638022/. Accessed December 28, 2017

[48] Huval B, Wang T, Tandon S, et al. An Empirical Evaluation of Deep Learning on Highway Driving. April 15 ADAD

[49] Simonyan K, Zisserman A. Very Deep Convolutional Networks for Large-Scale Image Recognition. April 2015

[50] Simonyan K, Ziserman A. Two-stream convolutional networks for action recognition in videos. CoRR abs/1406.2199, 2014. Published in Proc. NIPS; 2014

[51] Sermanet P, Eigen D, Zhang X, Mathieu M, Fergus R, LeCun Y. OverFeat: Integrated Recognition, Loacalization and Detection using Convolutional Networks. In Proc. ICLR; 2014

34 Future Growth in Navigated and Robotic Spinal Surgery

Darian R. Esfahani, Prateek Kumar, Kimberly Hu, Zachary Tan, Brandon L. Neisewander, and Ankit I. Mehta

Abstract

As technology advances at a rapid pace, contemporary surgery is becoming more efficacious, precise, and safe, with new options offering promise for some of the most challenging diseases. In this chapter, the authors review several emerging technologies in navigated and robotic spinal surgery, discuss legal questions, and outline future challenges for an evolving field. Augmented reality, including modern heads-up displays such as Google Glass and Microsoft HoloLens, is first reviewed, along with recent systems able to superimpose 3D anatomy with the surgeon's hand and instrumentation. Advances in imaging, including diffusion tensor imaging, are then explored, and potential utilities in tumor resection are discussed. Progress in nanotechnology is covered next, including nanoknife and nanoscaffolds, as well as nanorobots designed to selectively target tumor cells and administer a chemotherapy payload. Legal questions are then investigated, including Food and Drug Administration (FDA) approval and legal liability for robots. The chapter concludes with a discussion of ongoing challenges in robotic spine surgery, including cost-effectiveness, miniaturization, artificial intelligence, and ethical considerations of the robot as a surgeon.

Keywords: augmented reality, diffusion tensor imaging, ethics, heads-up display, legal, nanorobotics, nanotechnology, neuronavigation, robotics, technology

34.1 Introduction

Augmented reality (AR) is the projection of computer-generated images onto the user's view of the real world. Although only in its infancy, AR has been subject to growing interest in surgical training as well as certain procedures to improve precision and minimize trauma.[1] Several AR systems are being tested for spinal applications, including commercial heads-up displays (HUD) such as Google Glass and Microsoft HoloLens, as well as AR surgical navigation devices.

34.1.1 HUD AR—Google Glass and Microsoft HoloLens

Over the last several decades, the ergonomics of AR systems have evolved into wearable technology with increasing ease of use. Contemporary HUD devices are mounted over the eyes and allow the surgeon to view imaging overlays of CT or MR data without needing to look off the surgical field.[2] Google Glass (Google, Mountain View, CA) consists of a miniature computer, screen, and projector mounted onto a pair of glasses that allows the user to view projected images on the top right of their right eye (▶ Fig. 34.1). Google Glass has found utility in displaying intraoperative monitoring data for dorsal rhizotomy procedures,[3] as well as live, updating data from neuronavigation devices to monitor pedicle screw placement.[2]

The Microsoft HoloLens (Microsoft, Seattle, WA) consists of a visor that can project three-dimensional (3D) images in space and has paired speakers to create virtual surround sound cues. The HoloLens utilizes gaze commands, such as head tracking, as well as gestures and voice inputs to allow the user to interact with projected images. The HoloLens has been used, for example, in a proof of concept study to project holograms of spinal deformity patients, allowing for surgical planning in a 3D space and later postoperative review.[4]

34.1.2 Augmented Reality Surgical Navigation

A recently developed augmented reality surgical navigation system (Philips Healthcare, Best, the Netherlands) has been subject to recent study as an aid to pedicle screw placement. The system consists of multiple high-resolution video cameras mounted on a C-arm used to track markers placed on the skin around the surgical site. After creation of a 3D image with rotation of the C-arm, a 3D volume on the screen is seen, a screw insertion path is planned, and the C-arm automatically rotated to the axis of the planned screw. On the display screen, the screw path is then overlaid in real time over the patient's underlying anatomy to guide screw trajectory and depth[5] (▶ Fig. 34.2). Initial results on a cadaveric model revealed superiority of the AR system in achieving optimal screw placement and avoiding breaches versus the freehand technique.[5]

34.2 Diffusion Tensor Imaging

Diffusion tensor imaging (DTI) is a magnetic resonance imaging technique used to render 3D images of white matter tracts in the CNS.[6] The presence of a mass within a white matter tract causes deviations of the tract's normal path through the brain or spinal column, allowing the surgeon to visualize the location of the tumor in 3D space based on altered tract pathways[7] (▶ Fig. 34.3). Visualization of white matter tracts helps the surgeon plan approaches to avoid injuring pathways which can create neurologic deficits.

While potentially useful as a surgical adjunct, DTI has been criticized as unreliable in its current state due to the noise involved in constructing 3D images.[9,10] Diffusion-weighted imaging on its own is low resolution, and when coupled with fiber orientation and complex tracking algorithms can produce results that are challenging to replicate.[10] For intradural masses, opening of the dura and release of cerebrospinal fluid (CSF) can also cause movement of the spinal cord, making images unreliable. These shortcomings have led some authors to argue that DTI is not refined enough to be used in routine clinical practice until acquisition and rendering techniques are improved.[9]

Improvements in DTI under investigation include more robust models of data acquisition such as spatiotemporally encoded (SPEN) magnetic resonance imaging, which has been shown to provide more reliable data compared to DTI-rendered

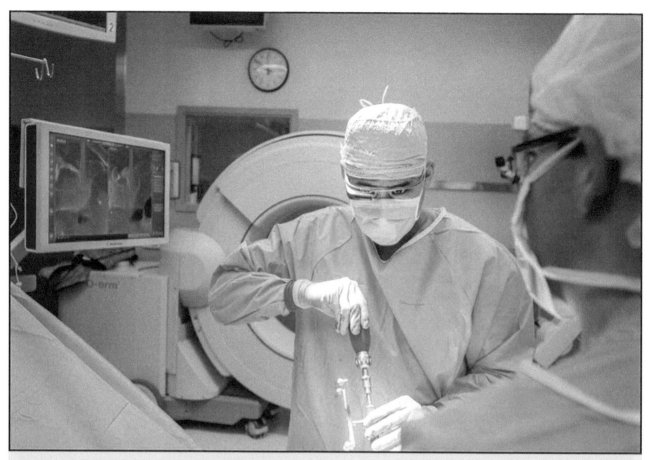

Fig. 34.1 Surgeon using Google Glass to monitor neuronavigation images during pedicle screw placement. (Reproduced with permission from Yoon et al.[2])

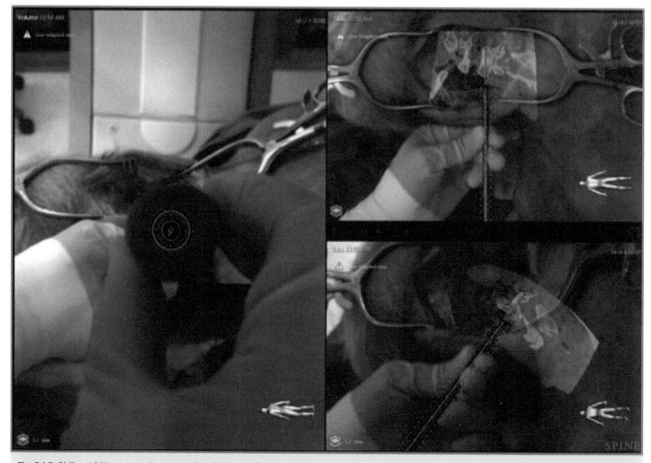

Fig. 34.2 Philips ARSN system. Augmented reality view of virtual path of screw alignment and trajectory. (Reproduced with permission from Elmi-Terander et al.[5])

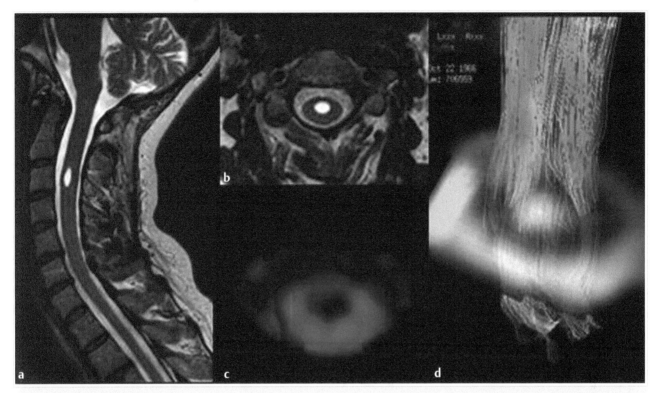

Fig. 34.3 Sagittal (**a**) and axial (**b**) weighted T2 images showing an intramedullary mass. Anisotropic (**c**) and diffuse tensor imaging (DTI) (**d**) maps illustrate tract displacement around the mass. (Reproduced with permission from Lerner at al.[8])

images.[11] SPEN improves image reliability by decreasing noise present in diffusion motion, resulting in more robust data acquisition in tissues that display chemical heterogeneity.[11] Other potential improvements include the addition of feedback mechanisms, such as ultrasound monitoring, which can account for spinal cord movement on dural opening and allow images to be updated with new positions.

34.3 Nanorobotics

Renowned physicist Richard Feynman, credited with introducing the concept of nanotechnology in 1959, suggested that machines might one day reduce in size to the extent that one could, in effect, "swallow the doctor."[12] Once the subject of science fiction, nanotechnology has evolved from a futuristic concept into a mainstream research initiative with potential applications in all fields of science including medicine and surgery. Governments around the world are increasingly investing in nanotechnology,[13,14] while medical specialties are eagerly examining applications for the detection and treatment of disease.[13,15,16,17]

Nanomaterials and devices are structured on the order of 10^{-9} to 10^{-7} meters (1–100 nanometers),[18] with a nanometer roughly the size of a molecule.[17] Due to their small size, nanoparticles and nanotools can decrease the risk of injury during surgery and make accessible anatomically challenging regions of the body.[19]

Nanorobotics is the branch of technology dealing with the design, construction, operation, and application of robots that have components at or near the scale of a nanometer. To date,

various nanomedicine applications have been investigated clinically and are being incorporated into nanorobotics for targeted drug delivery, imaging, diagnostics, tissue engineering, surgery, and intraoperative navigation. Polymeric nanoparticles, liposomes, and dendrimers can deliver drugs, growth factors, and genetic material across selective membranes including the blood–brain barrier.[15,20] For diagnosis, nanoparticles can be magnetized or conjugated to specific cell markers, and light-emitting quantum dots or metallic nanoparticles can be used as contrast agents or to detect specific biomolecules.[20] Nanoelectromechanical systems (NEMS) and microelectromechanical systems (MEMS), machines composed of miniaturized electrical and mechanical apparatuses such as actuators, beams, sensors, pumps, resonators, and motors, have been explored as tools to monitor physiological variables such as CSF pulsatility, intracranial pressure, weight load, and strain.[19] Finally, tools such as femtosecond laser systems, nanoneedles, and nanotweezers enable molecular ablation, dissection, penetration, and transfer at the subcellular level, and have been subject to growing interest.[18,20]

34.3.1 Nanotechnology in Surgery

Nanotechnology is beginning to be used for spine surgery, including treatment for spinal cord injury, peripheral nerve repair, and neuronal regeneration. Platforms for individual axon repair have involved tools such as the 40-nm-diameter nanoknife and dielectrophoresis, which uses electrical fields to manipulate polarizable objects in space.[20,21] Fusion between ends of transected axons can be induced via electrofusion, polyethylene glycol, or lasers, among other methods.[21] In addition, nanoscaffolds consisting of carbon nanotubes, nanowires, or polymer nanofibers can provide a structural framework to promote axon regeneration or to augment bone tissue regeneration and enhance osseointegration of implants.[17,22]

Biogenesis using nanomaterials can also be used in spinal fusions. One biomimetic approach involves nanocrystal-induced formation of organoapatite on surgically implantable structures such as foils and meshes.[16,20,22] Scaffolds formed by self-assembly of molecular nanofibers interspaced with mineralized hydroxyapatite crystals morphologically resemble collagen fibrils.[23,24] These scaffolds, when seeded with stem cells, have been demonstrated to generate cartilage and bone tissue in vivo, and therefore have found potential utility in improving bone growth after fusion, repairing annular defects, or regenerating the nucleus pulposus.[23,24]

34.3.2 Nanorobotics in Surgery

An aspiration of nanotechnology is to create autonomous or semiautonomous nanorobots that can circulate throughout the body and selectively perform therapeutic interventions, such as treatment of metastases.[15] Proposed nanorobot designs have included flagella for propulsion with receptors designed to release a chemotherapy payload upon contact with surface features on tumor cells.[21,25]

Nanorobotics may find utility in surgical navigation as well. Research has suggested that incorporation of nanorobots into tumor resection may improve intraoperative mapping and resection of tumor margins.[21] Rather than using injections the day prior to surgery, nanorobots could be administered intravascularly or intrathecally during procedures; after localizing to tumor tissue, robots could send electromagnetic or other localizing signals to the surgeon for mapping.[14,21]

Growth in robotic spinal surgery inevitably will involve nanotechnology. Recent developments have already given rise to interventions expected to expand surgical capabilities, allowing for less invasive and more accurate techniques for diagnosis and treatment.[14,19,20] Further growth requires an interdisciplinary approach between fields including microelectronics, molecular biology, and tissue engineering. Although the image of billions of nanorobots streaming through blood vessels toward their targets is many decades away, current nanotechnology applications are poised to become integrated into modern spinal surgery.[20]

34.4 Legal Questions

34.4.1 The Food and Drug Administration

The Food and Drug Administration (FDA) is tasked with regulating all medical devices, including robotically assisted surgical devices (RASDs), which are considered class II devices that pose moderate risk.[26] To be approved, RASDs must be demonstrated to be equivalent to a previously approved device and have the same intended use.[26] The da Vinci surgical system (Intuitive Surgical Inc., Sunnyvale, CA) was the first RASD approved by the FDA in 2000. In 2011, Renaissance (MAZOR Surgical Technologies [HQ] Ltd., Orlando, FL) was approved by the FDA for

spine surgery, while recently the first robotic system with Haptic Feedback, Senhance (TransEnterix Surgical Inc., Morrisville, NC), was approved by the FDA in October 2017.[27] Traditionally, FDA approval has been difficult for RASD manufacturers to obtain; as technology advances and safety profiles improve, however, the process of FDA approval is anticipated to accelerate.[28]

34.4.2 Legal Liability for Robotic Surgery

Product malfunction and medical malpractice remain controversial in robotic surgery. Since RASDs are approved by the FDA, manufacturers are technically subject to product liability and can be tried for failure to warn, defective design, or faulty manufacturing.[29] Unlike other products, however, many RASDs are held to an amended standard for failure to warn. Due to evidence that patients typically do not read detailed medical information and potential disruption of the doctor–patient relationship caused by individualized warnings from manufacturers, contemporary law utilizes the Learned Intermediary (LI) doctrine.[29] The LI doctrine states that since the physician is in the best position to weigh the benefits and risks of a surgical procedure, the ultimate responsibility for problems with a medical device lies with the physician, not the manufacturer or patient, so long as the manufacturer provides adequate education and warnings to the surgeon.[29] In most states, courts have upheld LI as a protection against pharmaceutical and device companies, but the doctrine continues to be debated. Furthermore, as procedures move into the realm of cyberspace, where a surgeon can operate from a remote site with the aid of a robot and Internet connection, liability for a telecommunications provider, in the event of an outage midsurgery, has remained an unanswered question.[29]

34.5 Future Challenges in Robotic Spine Surgery

34.5.1 Cost-Effectiveness

Many factors contribute to the costs of robotic surgery including capital acquisition, limited-use tools, maintenance and repair, training, and operating room renovation and setup.[30] The da Vinci robot, for example, costs around $2 million, with annual maintenance ranging from $100,000 to $200,000 or 10% of the initial cost of the robotic system.[30,31] Although hospitals typically charge more for robotic surgeries, a financial analysis conducted at one medical center found that 349 robotic surgery cases would need to be conducted annually to reach a breakeven point, far beyond the hospital's capability.[31] Cost savings may be obtained, however, from better outcomes. In spine surgery, improved accuracy in pedicle screw placement, decreased recovery times, lower repetitive use injury in surgeons, and faster return to usual activities are potential sources of savings.[30,32]

34.5.2 Education

Training for surgical robotic systems typically consists of online modules and a training course provided by the manufacturer, as mandated by the FDA, and a period of supervision implemented by the hospital's credentialing committee.[33] The lengthy learning curve associated with robotically assisted spine procedures is well documented,[32] with residents typically receiving limited training in robotic surgery. Surgical simulators such as ImmersiveTouch (ImmersiveTouch, Chicago, IL) have shown promise in improving trainee skills in procedures such as percutaneous spinal fixation and pedicle screw placement,[34] with recent models allowing for the unique characteristics of patients to be programmed in, allowing the surgeon to "rehearse" the procedure.[30]

34.5.3 Technology Limitations

The application of robotics in surgery was initiated by the National Aeronautics and Space Administration (NASA) in the 1970s with the goal of providing surgical care to astronauts using robots remotely controlled by physicians.[35] Although this goal has not yet been achieved, advances in telesurgery are under way with the first transatlantic pig surgery completed almost two decades ago.[36] Several major technological limitations of robotic surgery platforms persist, however, and limit the type of procedures and clinical settings in which robots can be used. The most obvious limitation of products is the size of the platform.[28,30] As new generations of devices are developed, however, systems such as SpineAssist and Renaissance (MAZOR Surgical Technologies) have become small enough to attach to the patient.[37]

Despite advances in technology, surgical robotic systems continue to serve as an extension of the surgeon controlling them, and are vulnerable to technical limitations as well as errors in judgment.[28,30] Advances in artificial intelligence (AI), however, have been proposed to allow for increasing autonomy of robotic systems. Early steps, for example, include automation of suturing by allowing the physician to draw a line that a robotic system could automatically suture along.[30] Although fully automated surgical robots are many years away, advances in AI have also included training robotic surgery systems using heuristic knowledge which can be applied to future cases.[28,30] A team in Spain, for example, developed a robotic scrub technician that can recognize 82 spoken instructions, locate 27 surgical instruments, select the appropriate instrument from a tray, and determine if instruments are missing.[38]

34.5.4 The Robot as a Surgeon

With AI and automated robots positioned to advance in the coming century, will the human surgeon become obsolete? In a well-publicized analysis of 702 occupations by Frey and Osborne, physicians and surgeons were identified as among the least susceptible professions to be computerized, with an estimated risk of 0.4%.[39] Compared to other professions, such as accountants, at 94%, the "bottleneck" to computerization for surgeons was significant levels of perception, manipulation, and social intelligence needed, qualities not easily replicated by robots. The final aspect, social intelligence, is perhaps the most important. Despite the appeal of AI and computerized, surgical precision, could a robot pick up social cues, like a long pause in conversation, suggesting problems at home? Could it weigh the role of mental health and social challenges on chronic disease?

Could a robot, one-on-one, build trust with a patient?[40] These questions tap into the unique humanity of the surgeon, which, despite the rapid growth of new technology, is not easily replaced.

34.6 Conclusion

Advancing technology in navigated and robotic spinal surgery has allowed for surgery that is more effective, accurate, and safe than ever before. New progress in augmented reality, fiber tract imaging, nanotechnology, and nanorobotics offer promise to make the most challenging diseases treatable, and familiar, easier, and less dangerous. At the same time, legal questions persist, including the liability of robots, manufacturers, and telecommunication providers in surgeries conducted remotely. Finally, despite many advances, challenges persist in the adoption of robotic technology, ranging from cost-effectiveness to ethical considerations of the robot as a surgeon. Taken together, in a discipline already at the forefront of its field, robotics is poised to invigorate spinal surgery more than ever before.

References

[1] Madhavan K, Kolcun JPG, Chieng LO, Wang MY. Augmented-reality integrated robotics in neurosurgery: are we there yet? Neurosurg Focus. 2017; 42(5):E3

[2] Yoon JW, Chen RE, Han PK, Si P, Freeman WD, Pirris SM. Technical feasibility and safety of an intraoperative head-up display device during spine instrumentation. Int J Med Robot. 2017; 13(3)

[3] Golab MR, Breedon PJ, Vloeberghs M. A wearable headset for monitoring electromyography responses within spinal surgery. Eur Spine J. 2016; 25(10): 3214–3219

[4] Choudhry OJ, Mundluru SN, Morley C, Ahmed F, Buckland AJ, Frempong-Boadu AK. P56 - Augmented reality for evaluation of spinal deformity and spinal pathologies. Spine J. 2017; 17(10) Suppl:S200–S201

[5] Elmi-Terander A, Skulason H, Söderman M, et al. Surgical navigation technology based on augmented reality and integrated 3D intraoperative imaging: a spine cadaveric feasibility and accuracy study. Spine. 2016; 41(21):E1303–E1311

[6] Le Bihan D, Mangin JF, Poupon C, et al. Diffusion tensor imaging: concepts and applications. J Magn Reson Imaging. 2001; 13(4):534–546

[7] Ducreux D, Lepeintre JF, Fillard P, Loureiro C, Tadié M, Lasjaunias P. MR diffusion tensor imaging and fiber tracking in 5 spinal cord astrocytomas. AJNR Am J Neuroradiol. 2006; 27(1):214–216

[8] Lerner A, Mogensen MA, Kim PE, Shiroishi MS, Hwang DH, Law M. Clinical applications of diffusion tensor imaging. World Neurosurg. 2014; 82(1–2): 96–109

[9] Duffau H. Diffusion tensor imaging is a research and educational tool, but not yet a clinical tool. World Neurosurg. 2014; 82(1–2):e43–e45

[10] Nimsky C. Fiber tracking–we should move beyond diffusion tensor imaging. World Neurosurg. 2014; 82(1–2):35–36

[11] Solomon E, Liberman G, Nissan N, Frydman L. Robust diffusion tensor imaging by spatiotemporal encoding: principles and in vivo demonstrations. Magn Reson Med. 2017; 77(3):1124–1133

[12] Feynman RP. There's plenty of room at the bottom. Eng Sci. 1960; 23(5):22–36

[13] Morigi V, Tocchio A, Bellavite Pellegrini C, Sakamoto JH, Arnone M, Tasciotti E. Nanotechnology in medicine: from inception to market domination. J Drug Deliv. 2012; 2012:389485

[14] Cavalcanti A, Freitas RA, Jr. Nanorobotics control design: a collective behavior approach for medicine. IEEE Trans Nanobioscience. 2005; 4(2):133–140

[15] Gharpure KM, Wu SY, Li C, Lopez-Berestein G, Sood AK. Nanotechnology: future of oncotherapy. Clin Cancer Res. 2015; 21(14):3121–3130

[16] Sullivan MP, McHale KJ, Parvizi J, Mehta S. Nanotechnology: current concepts in orthopaedic surgery and future directions. Bone Joint J. 2014; 96-B(5): 569–573

[17] Silva GA. Introduction to nanotechnology and its applications to medicine. Surg Neurol. 2004; 61(3):216–220

[18] Elder JB, Liu CY, Apuzzo MLJ. Neurosurgery in the realm of 10(-9), part 1: stardust and nanotechnology in neuroscience. Neurosurgery. 2008; 62(1):1–20

[19] Mattei TA, Rehman AA. "Extremely minimally invasive": recent advances in nanotechnology research and future applications in neurosurgery. Neurosurg Rev. 2015; 38(1):27–37, discussion 37

[20] Leary SP, Liu CY, Apuzzo ML. Toward the emergence of nanoneurosurgery: part III–nanomedicine: targeted nanotherapy, nanosurgery, and progress toward the realization of nanoneurosurgery. Neurosurgery. 2006; 58(6): 1009–1026, discussion 1009–1026

[21] Saadeh Y, Vyas D. Nanorobotic applications in medicine: current proposals and designs. Am J Robot Surg. 2014; 1(1):4–11

[22] Walmsley GG, McArdle A, Tevlin R, et al. Nanotechnology in bone tissue engineering. Nanomedicine (Lond). 2015; 11(5):1253–1263

[23] Hartgerink JD, Beniash E, Stupp SI. Self-assembly and mineralization of peptide-amphiphile nanofibers. Science. 2001; 294(5547):1684–1688

[24] Li W-J, Tuli R, Huang X, Laquerriere P, Tuan RS. Multilineage differentiation of human mesenchymal stem cells in a three-dimensional nanofibrous scaffold. Biomaterials. 2005; 26(25):5158–5166

[25] Lenaghan SC, Wang Y, Xi N, et al. Grand challenges in bioengineered nanorobotics for cancer therapy. IEEE Trans Biomed Eng. 2013; 60(3):667–673

[26] Discussion Paper FDA. Robotically-Assisted Surgical Devices. Paper presented at the FDA Public Workshop; 2015; Silver Spring, MD

[27] FDA clears new robotically-assisted surgical device for adult patients [press release]. October 13, 2017

[28] Camarillo DB, Krummel TM, Salisbury JK, Jr. Robotic technology in surgery: past, present, and future. Am J Surg. 2004; 188(4A) Suppl:2S–15S

[29] McLean T. The complexity of litigation associated with robotic surgery and cybersurgery. Int J Med Robot. 2007; 3:23–29

[30] Herron DM, Marohn M, SAGES-MIRA Robotic Surgery Consensus Group. A consensus document on robotic surgery. Surg Endosc. 2008; 22(2):313–325, discussion 311–312

[31] Tedesco G, Faggiano FC, Leo E, Derrico P, Ritrovato M. A comparative cost analysis of robotic-assisted surgery versus laparoscopic surgery and open surgery: the necessity of investing knowledgeably. Surg Endosc. 2016; 30 (11):5044–5051

[32] Schatlo B, Martinez R, Alaid A, et al. Unskilled unawareness and the learning curve in robotic spine surgery. Acta Neurochir (Wien). 2015; 157(10):1819–1823, discussion 1823

[33] Bric J, Connolly M, Kastenmeier A, Goldblatt M, Gould JC. Proficiency training on a virtual reality robotic surgical skills curriculum. Surg Endosc. 2014; 28 (12):3343–3348

[34] Luciano CJ, Banerjee PP, Bellotte B, et al. Learning retention of thoracic pedicle screw placement using a high-resolution augmented reality simulator with haptic feedback. Neurosurgery. 2011; 69(1) Suppl Operative:ons14–ons19, discussion ons19

[35] Marescaux J, Diana M. Robotics and remote surgery: next step. In: Kim K, ed. Robotics General Surgery. New York, NY: Springer; 2014:479–484

[36] Marescaux J, Leroy J, Gagner M, et al. Transatlantic robot-assisted telesurgery. Nature. 2001; 413(6854):379–380

[37] Tian W, Han X, Liu B, et al. A robot-assisted surgical system using a force-image control method for pedicle screw insertion. PLoS One. 2014; 9(1): e86346

[38] Perez-Vidal C, Carpintero E, Garcia-Aracil N, et al. Steps in the development of a robotic scrub nurse. Robot Auton Syst. 2012; 60(6):901–911

[39] Frey CB, Osborne MA. The future of employment: how susceptible are jobs to computerisation? Technol Forecast Soc Change. 2017; 114 Suppl C:254–280

[40] Senior T. Being replaced by a robot. Br J Gen Pract. 2016; 66(649):436–436

Index

Note: Page numbers set **bold** or *italic* indicate headings or figures, respectively.